MEDICAL SCHOOL SCHOLARSHIPS, GRANTS & AWARDS

INSIDER ADVICE ON HOW TO WIN SCHOLARSHIPS

SAMIR P. DESAI, M.D.
ANAND D. TRIVEDI, M.D.
HIRSH D. TRIVEDI, M.D.
RAM JAGANNATHAN, M.D.
SAMISH A. PATEL, M.D.
AVA J. GHALILI, MBBS

FROM THE AUTHOR OF THE SUCCESSFUL MATCH

PUBLISHED BY

MD2B

HOUSTON, TEXAS

www.MD2B.net

Medical School Scholarships, Grants & Awards: Insider Advice on How to Win Scholarships is published by MD2B, PO Box 300988, Houston, TX 77230-0988.

www.MD2B.net

NOTICE: The authors and publisher disclaim any personal liability, either directly or indirectly, for advice or information presented within. The authors and publishers have used care and diligence in the preparation of this book. Every effort has been made to ensure the accuracy and completeness of information contained within this book. The recommendations made within this book have come from the author's personal experiences and interactions with medical students over many years. There is considerable variability in the selection of scholarship and award recipients from one program to another. Therefore, the recommendations are not universally applicable. No responsibility is assumed for errors, inaccuracies, omissions, or any false or misleading implication that may arise due to the text.

Printed in the United States of America

ISBN # 9781937978044

Dedication

To all of the individuals who have taught us important lessons and helped us throughout our careers: our mentors, our teachers, our students, and our patients.

ABOUT THE AUTHORS

Samir P. Desai, M.D.

Dr. Samir Desai serves on the faculty of the Baylor College of Medicine in the Department of Medicine where he is actively involved in medical student and resident education. He is a member of the Clerkship Directors in Internal Medicine, and the recipient of multiple teaching awards. He is an author and editor, having written sixteen books that together have sold over 200,000 copies worldwide.

His book *Success in Medical School: Insider Advice for the Preclinical Years* provides preclinical students with detailed knowledge and guidance to excel and position themselves for match success later in medical school. In 2009, he co-authored *The Successful Match: 200 Rules to Succeed in the Residency Match*, a well-regarded and highly acclaimed book that has helped thousands of residency applicants match successfully. He is also the co-author of *Success on the Wards: 250 Rules for Clerkship Success*. This book has helped thousands of medical students make the difficult transition from the preclinical to clinical years of medical school. *Success on the Wards* is a required or recommended resource at many U.S. medical schools, providing proven strategies for success in patient care, write-ups, rounds, and other vital areas.

As a faculty member, he serves on the medical school admissions and residency selection committees. His commitment to helping premedical and medical students reach their professional goals led him to develop the website TheSuccessfulMatch.com. The website's mission is to provide medical school, residency, and fellowship applicants with a better understanding of the selection process.

After completing his residency training in Internal Medicine at Northwestern University in Chicago, Dr. Desai had the opportunity to serve as chief medical resident. He received his M.D. degree from Wayne State University School of Medicine in Detroit, Michigan, graduating first in his class.

Anand D. Trivedi, M.D.

Dr. Anand Trivedi is currently an internal medicine resident at the University of Illinois at Urbana-Champaign (UIUC). He is a resident member of the American College of Physicians and serves on the resident curriculum committee at UIUC. Having completed his medical degree at Sri Ramachandra Medical College in Chennai, India, he has had the pleasure of working with diverse groups of patients, physicians and medical students. He now enjoys regularly working with and educating medical students as they rotate with him on the medical wards. As an international medical graduate who has faced the challenges of securing a competitive residency position, Dr. Trivedi understands what it takes to achieve success. He hopes that this book will be a valuable resource for medical students as they strive to become competitive applicants themselves. In his free time Dr. Trivedi enjoys spending time with his family and traveling.

Hirsh D. Trivedi, M.D.

Dr. Hirsh Trivedi is an internal medicine resident at St. Elizabeth's Medical Center, a Tufts University Medical School affiliate program, in Boston, Massachusetts. He is an active member of the resident committee at St. Elizabeth's Medical Center, and he is also involved in the Medical Interview and Doctor Patient Relationship program where he teaches interviewing and clinical examination techniques to Tufts University medical students. Through his participation in teaching during clinical rounds, he has established himself as an excellent resident teacher. Having recently gone through the residency application process, he understands the challenges that medical students face in securing a competitive residency position. He plans to continue working with medical students in order to help them maximize their chances in securing these positions. After the completion of his Internal Medicine residency, he plans to pursue a career in Gastroenterology and Hepatology.

Ram Jagannathan, M.D.

After completing his medical education at Sri Ramachandra University in Chennai, India and an internship at Providence Hospital in Southfield, Michigan, Dr. Jagannathan resides in Chicago, Illinois where he is a Resident Physician in Anesthesiology at Rush University Medical Center. Having recently been through the residency application process, Dr. Jagannathan is passionate about teaching, guiding, and learning from medical students he works with. Dr. Jagannathan's academic interests include airway management, regional anesthesia, and perioperative transesophageal echocardiography. Following residency, Dr. Jagannathan aspires to contribute to the growth of these fields while continuing to be a part of student education. In his spare time, Dr. Jagannathan enjoys spending time with his family and traveling to further learn from others' customs and cultures.

Samish A. Patel, M.D.

Dr. Samish Patel is currently an internal medicine resident at North Shore Long Island Jewish Medical Center. He was born and raised in Southern California. After his undergraduate training at University of California, San Diego, he went on to complete his medical degree at Ross University School of Medicine. Having done rotations throughout the country, he has had the opportunity to work with many medical educators in a variety of health care systems. He now enjoys regularly working with and educating medical students as they rotate with him in Long Island. He helped author this book with the hope that it will provide medical students with unique opportunities that will help them reach the forefront of medicine and develop relationships with leading physicians. After completing his residency in internal medicine he plans to pursue a career in either hospital medicine or adult primary care.

Ava J. Ghalili, MBBS

Dr. Ava Ghalili is an emergency department registrar (senior resident) at Royal Prince Alfred Hospital in Sydney, Australia and a medical school graduate of the University of Notre Dame, Western Australia. She has had international exposure in her field through various community and county hospitals in the USA. She is actively involved in teaching students and presenting at conferences/symposiums on topics of acute medicine. Throughout her training and career she has been involved in research relevant to women's health and evidence-based medicine outcomes in Emergency Departments. Much of her extracurricular time has been spent overseas in the developing world, working for various organizations addressing public health concerns and ethical humanitarian standards. She hopes to continue with these endeavors and to complete in the near future a fellowship in pediatric emergency medicine.

CONTENTS

How to Use This Book

1) The first part of this book describes the scholarship application and process with a focus on strategy. The second part of this book is an extensive listing and description of scholarships and awards with profiles of award winners.

2) Scholarships and awards are listed in the following categories: Research, Gender, Ethnicity, Minority, Global Health, Writing, Leadership, Osteopathic, Specialty, and Geography by State. Each category has been given its own chapter. See Table of Contents for more information.

3) Awards that are not easily categorized into one of these groups are listed in Chapter 18 (Miscellaneous Scholarships, Awards, & Grants).

4) In each chapter, scholarships and awards are listed in alphabetical order.

5) Some scholarships are listed in multiple chapters. For example, scholarships awarded by the Osteopathic Foundation of Central Washington are listed in Chapter 17 (Osteopathic Awards & Scholarships). These scholarships are only open to medical students in certain states. Therefore, you will see that we have also listed these scholarships in Chapter 40 (Scholarships in Alaska), Chapter 50 (Scholarships in Idaho), Chapter 64 (Scholarships in Montana), Chapter 75 (Scholarships in Oregon), and Chapter 85 (Scholarships in Washington). We chose this approach to ensure that students do not miss out on important opportunities. When awards are repeated in different chapters, you will be referred to a particular chapter for the award description.

6) We do list and describe scholarships by State. In these chapters, however, you will not see scholarships and awards that are only open to students at a single medical school. Donors at every medical school have provided funds to establish scholarship programs. These school-specific scholarships are not presented in this book because they will be readily accessible to you through your school's Office of Financial Aid.

Chapter 1

Introduction

According to the Association of American Medical Colleges (AAMC), the median four-year cost to attend medical school for the class of 2014 was over $218,000 and $286,000 for public and private schools, respectively.[1] The following table shows how the median cost of attendance has changed over time.

Change in 4-Year Median Cost to Attend Medical School (AAMC Data)[1-2]		
Year	Public	Private
2000	$100,215	$161,760
2008	$159,396	$225,215
2014	$218,898	$286,806

Although the average annual cost to attend medical school has risen at a rate that has outpaced inflation, this has not prevented a record number of students from applying to medical school. In 2013, there were over 48,000 applicants to U.S. medical schools, breaking the mark set in 1996.

Medical schools have been graduating more students than ever, the result of a nationwide effort to meet the needs of an anticipated physician manpower shortage. As these students fulfill their professional dreams of becoming physicians, they leave medical school with considerable debt. AAMC research indicates that the median education debt for the class of 2013 was $175,000.[1]

Fortunately, there are hundreds of scholarships available to medical students to help offset the cost of medical school education. Although there are few "full-ride" scholarships, there are many awards that can significantly lessen the burden. "Every $1,000 in scholarship support reduces a student's potential indebtedness by more than $8,400," writes the Wake Forest School of Medicine.[3]

Although financial relief is a major reason to pursue scholarships, the benefits of receiving such awards and honors extend well beyond money. Does winning a medical student award or scholarship make a difference in the residency match? It certainly does with multiple research studies demonstrating that awards provide a competitive edge.

Election to the Alpha Omega Alpha Honor Medical Society (AOA) is perhaps the most well studied award as it relates to residency admission. Eligibility is limited to only allopathic medical students, and members are selected based on academic achievement, leadership, professionalism, and commitment to service by school chapters. According to the AOA Constitution, no more than 1/6 of the graduating class can be elected into the school's chapter. In 2012, the National Resident Matching Program, the organization that administers the Match, surveyed 1,960 residency programs representing 21 specialties about the importance of various residency selection criteria.[4] Overall, membership in AOA was cited by 51% as a factor in selecting applicants to interview. Membership in AOA was also an important factor in the ranking of applicants. Overall, it received a mean rating of 3.4 on a scale of 1 (not at all important) to 5 (very important). Data for the individual specialties is presented in the table below.

Percentage Of Residency Programs Citing AOA As A Factor In Selecting Applicants To Interview By Specialty[4]	
Specialty	**% of Programs**
Anesthesiology	69%
Dermatology	57%
Emergency Medicine	57%
Family Medicine	24%
General Surgery	60%
Internal Medicine	51%
Neurosurgery	76%
Obstetrics & Gynecology	47%
Orthopaedic Surgery	68%
Otolaryngology	76%
Pathology	40%
Pediatrics	55%
Physical Medicine & Rehabilitation	26%
Plastic Surgery	75%
Psychiatry	38%
Radiation Oncology	61%
Radiology	66%

Although osteopathic students are not eligible for AOA induction, both allopathic and osteopathic students may be elected into the Gold Humanism Honor Society (GHHS). Started in 2002 by the Arnold P. Gold Foundation, GHHS honors medical students for "demonstrated excellence in clinical care, leadership, compassion and dedication to service."[5] In a study conducted to determine if GHHS membership influences residency selection, the authors wrote that "membership in GHHS may set candidates apart from their peers and allow PDs to distinguish objectively the candidates who demonstrate compassionate medical care."[6] In the 2012 NRMP Program Director Survey, 23% reported using Gold Society Membership as a factor in selecting applicants to interview.[4]

AOA and GHHS are not the only awards or honors viewed favorably by residency programs. In a survey of over 1,200 residency program directors in 21 specialties, Dr. Marianne Green, Associate Dean of Medical Education at the Northwestern University Feinberg School of Medicine, determined the relative importance of various residency selection criteria.[7] Dr. Green found that medical school awards (non-AOA) were tenth in importance among a group of 14 residency selection criteria. Although not as important as USMLE Step 1 scores, clerkship grades, and letters of recommendation, awards were ranked higher than such factors as preclinical grades, research while in medical school, and published medical school research.

Benefits of winning medical school awards and scholarships include the following:

- Awards can provide a significant boost to the strength of your residency application, and distinguish you from your peers. Awards and scholarships can easily be placed in the residency application, MSPE (Dean's Letter), letters of recommendation, and CV. We have found that interviewers often ask about awards during residency interviews.

Did you know...

In 2013, Justin Berk, a medical student at Texas Tech University School of Medicine, received the American Medical Association Foundation Leadership Award. "For Justin, it's obviously a huge accolade and something that will follow him for the rest of his medical career," said Dr. Tedd Mitchell, President of Texas Tech Health Sciences Center, in an interview with *The Daily Toreador*. "As he's applying for residency programs, it will stand out."[8]

Did you know...

Alexander Gallan, a medical student at the Boston University School of Medicine, was the recipient of the 2012 American Society of Clinical Pathology Academic Excellence Award. "The award was a common topic during my residency interviews. I believe it helped my residency application immeasurably by providing justification for all the hard work I have done."[9]

- Competitive specialties and residency programs value students who have been recognized with awards. There is belief among educators that you will make similar contributions as a trainee.

Did you know...

When Casey DeDeugd, a medical student at the University of Central Florida, won the Medical Student Achievement Award from the Ruth Jackson Orthopaedic Society, she enhanced her visibility in the field. "Your accomplishments thus far are very impressive!" wrote Dr. Gloria Gogola, Chair of the Society's Scientific Committee. "We look forward...to welcoming you to our field of orthopaedic surgery."[10]

Did you know...

In 2008, Brian Caldwell, a medical student at the University of Arkansas for Medical Sciences, was the winner of the Dr. Constantin Cope Medical Student Research Award from the Society of Interventional Radiology. "Brian carried the whole project with very little help and really did a nice job," said Dr. William Culp, Professor of Radiology and Surgery. "I am so pleased that he won the national SIR award, because his participation in the conference introduced him to national leaders in interventional radiology and will help jumpstart his career."[11]

- You gain visibility in your school, and bring recognition to the institution.

Did you know...

When Ramy El-Diwany, an M.D./Ph.D. student at Johns Hopkins University, won the 2014 Excellence in Public Health Award from the U.S. Public Health Service (USPHS) Physician Professional Advisory Committee, his institution was also lauded. "This award is a testament to the education provided by the Johns Hopkins University School of Medicine and to the high caliber of its students," wrote USPHS Lt. Cmdr. Kimberly Smith. "We hope that this award will encourage other Johns Hopkins faculty and students to continue their strong work in public health."[12]

Did you know...

After Rahul Vanjani received the AMA Foundation Leadership Award, Dr. Scott Schroth, Senior Associate Dean of Academic Affairs at George Washington University, took pride in his student's accomplishment. "Rahul's commitment to the community and leadership of service efforts are unparalleled. He exemplifies the sort of creativity and dedication that we look for in medical students at GW, and we are extraordinarily proud of him as a winner of the AMA Foundation's 2011 Leadership Award."[13]

- Recipients have found that awards have made them more attractive for other awards and scholarships. Awards follow you throughout your career, and can make you more competitive for future opportunities, programs, and employment.

- You further your professional reputation and enhance your credibility in the areas that form the basis for the award.

- Winning an award or scholarship can give you the confidence to pursue other goals.

- Applying for an award requires the support of advocates who become reference letter writers. Strengthening these relationships over time allows faculty members to write strong letters of recommendation for residency.

Did you know...

In applying for awards, you often have to submit reference letters. Over time, your letter writers become even stronger advocates with a vested interest in furthering your career. After David Leverenz won the Southwestern Medical Foundation Ho Din Award, his mentor had this to say. "Dr. Leverenz has done exceptionally well in medical school, performed research, worked, volunteered, and completed multiple mission trips," said Dr. David Balis, his faculty mentor at UT Southwestern Medical Center. "But what strikes me most about David is his caring, sincere, compassionate personality." Dr. Leverenz is now a resident at Vanderbilt University.[14]

Did you know...

Winning a scholarship may also affect the way in which you view your specialty choice. "This scholarship has allowed me the freedom to broaden my thoughts about what field I want to pursue," said Mike Bosworth, a medical student at Tulane University. "My focus is more on how I can help patients versus what I can make."[15]

It is clear that there are compelling reasons to pursue medical school scholarships, awards, and grants. In this book, we'll show you how to maximize your chances of winning these awards. Although our book includes an extensive list of scholarships and awards, we've also placed considerable emphasis on strategy. Some examples of what you'll find in our book include:

- Although we encourage you to apply for the most competitive scholarships and awards, we also show you how to identify awards that are easier to win. There is considerably less competition for these awards, and we'll show you how you can significantly enhance your chances of winning.

- Since letters of recommendation are a critical component of most scholarship applications, how can you work closely with your letter writers to have the best possible letters written?

- The personal essay is an opportunity for you to stand out from the rest of the applicant field. What's the best approach to take with the essay? What makes an essay particularly compelling to the scholarship committee? How can you avoid common errors?

- Scholarship programs may ask you to submit a CV or enter information from your CV directly into the application. Content and appearance are important factors in the way your CV will be assessed, and we'll show you how to create one with maximum impact.

Our recommendations are based on data from a full spectrum of sources. Whenever possible, we present evidence obtained from scientific study and published in the academic medical literature. We also take an insider's look at the entire process based on our experiences. For years, we've helped applicants match successfully into competitive specialties and residency programs. We've worked with medical students at all levels, and we always try to identify scholarship and award programs that will bolster their credentials. In the process of helping students win scholarships and awards, we've gained insight into the factors that lead to success. There's much that can be learned from your predecessors, and we've included the profiles of past scholarship winners. Reading about their stories will help guide your strategy and application. Although it's been a joy for us to help medical students win scholarships and awards, we know that the process is difficult. Although success is never guaranteed, our advice and perspectives provide the specific, concrete recommendations that will maximize your chances of being an award recipient.

A Medical Student Scholarship Winner Speaks...

"The scholarship will greatly ease the trouble and distraction of growing debt so that I can focus on my studies, my family and my community. It is a generous gift, and I am reminded that it is an investment in my future. I know that it is my role in the future to give back to my community as a physician."[16]

References

[1] AAMC. Available at: https://www.aamc.org/download/152968/data/debtfactcard.pdf. Accessed April 2, 2014.

[2] AAMC Physician Education Debt and the Cost to Attend Medical School: 2012 Update. Available at: https://www.aamc.org/download/328322/data/statedebtreport.pdf. Accessed April 4, 2014.

[3] Wake Forest School of Medicine. Available at: http://www.wakehealth.edu/School/Alumni-Affairs/Scholarship-Endowment.htm. Accessed June 12, 2014.

[4] 2012 NRMP Program Director Survey. Available at: http://www.nrmp.org/wp-content/uploads/2013/08/programresultsbyspecialty2012.pdf. Accessed June 20, 2014.

[5] Arnold P. Gold Foundation. Available at: http://humanism-in-medicine.org/. Accessed June 22, 2014.

[6] Rosenthal S, Howard B, Schlussel Y, Lazarus C, Wong J, Moutier C, Savoia M, Trooskin S, Wagoner N. Does medical student membership in the gold humanism honor society influence selection for residency? *J Surg Educ* 2009; 66 (6): 308-13.

[7] Green M, Jones P, Thomas JX Jr. Selection criteria for residency: results of a national program directors survey. *Acad Med* 2009; 84(3): 362-367.

[8] The Daily Toreador. Available at: http://www.dailytoreador.com/news/article_4512fb50-758f-11e2-a99f-0019bb30f31a.html. Accessed June 3, 2014.

[9] American Society of Clinical Pathology. Available at: http://www.ascp.org/Newsroom/ASCP-Academic-Excellence-Award-Crucial-to-Medical-Students-Career-Path.html. Accessed June 24, 2014.

[10] University of Central Florida College of Medicine. Available at: http://today.ucf.edu/ucf-medical-student-wins-national-orthopaedic-award/. Accessed June 2, 2014.

[11] University of Arkansas for Medical Sciences. Available at: http://www.uams.edu/update/absolutenm/templates/news2003v2.asp?articleid=7594&zoneid=15. Accessed June 2, 2014.

[12] Johns Hopkins Medicine. Available at: http://www.hopkinsmedicine.org/news/media/releases/johns_hopkins_mdphd_student_wins_us_public_health_award. Accessed June 23, 2014.

[13] George Washington University School of Medicine. Available at: http://smhs.gwu.edu/news/gw-medical-student-wins-prestigious-ama-leadership-award. Accessed June 23, 2014.

[14] UT Southwestern Medical School. Available at: http://www.utsouthwestern.edu/newsroom/center-times/year-2013/may/award-ho-din.html. Accessed June 3, 2014.

[15] Tulane University School of Medicine. Available at: http://tulane.edu/news/newwave/120511_adopt_a_student.cfm?RenderForPrint=1. Accessed June 3, 2014.

[16] Virginia Commonwealth University School of Medicine. Available at: http://wp.vcu.edu/somdiscoveries/page/14/. Accessed June 24, 2014.

Chapter 2

Scholarship Myths

Myths abound in applying for medical school scholarships, and these assumptions may prevent qualified applicants from pursuing opportunities or lead to errors in the application process. Below we dispel some common myths.

Myth # 1   **I don't qualify for financial need. There is no need to even apply.**

There are three types of scholarships – need-based, merit-based, and a combination thereof. At some medical schools, 85 - 90% of students receive some type of financial assistance. The Financial Aid Office at the Duke University School of Medicine administered $36 million in loans and scholarships to 87% of the student body during the academic year 2011-2012.[1] Merit-based scholarships are open to every student, irrespective of financial need.

Did you know...

Medical schools award some merit scholarships based on information provided by students during the admissions process. Other merit scholarships require separate applications.

Myth # 2   **Only academic superstars win merit-based scholarships.**

Although class rank and GPA are factors with some merit-based scholarships, many awards are based on community service, leadership, or research. There are also awards for teaching, writing, mentoring, and advocacy. Grades are not used in the selection process for many of these scholarships.

When GPA or class rank is a factor, scholarship programs may simply look to see that you meet a threshold value. If your academic credentials exceed this value, you may be on equal par with applicants having higher grades.

Even when academic achievement is an important factor, it's often one criterion among a group which the selection committee will consider. We have seen applicants who are particularly strong in a nonacademic area win awards over academically superior students lacking notable accomplishments or contributions. In other words, the transcript isn't everything.

Did you know…

"Privately endowed scholarships at the medical school are a combination of need-based and merit-based awards," writes the Virginia Commonwealth University School of Medicine. "When each fund was established, donors outlined the criteria used to select the student recipients. Some scholarships support students considering a certain specialty or from a particular geographic region. Others reward those who have distinguished themselves through community service or academic merit."[2]

Did you know…

Overcoming key barriers is an important part of success for scholarship winners. Major barriers include fear of failure, not believing you are smart or talented enough, or assuming that only academic superstars win these awards. We have seen that it is often not the academic superstar who snags these awards but the student who is willing to work harder, smarter, and more strategically.

Myth # 3   **Medical school awards are primarily given to minority students.**

There are certainly many scholarships available for minority medical students. However, such awards are a small percentage of the total number of awards available throughout the country. In chapter 13, we discuss medical scholarships and awards for minority medical students. Regardless of your background or ethnicity, our book will show you how you can increase your chances of being an award recipient.

Myth # 4   **You have to win these awards before medical school. I'm too late.**

Although many awards are available to incoming medical students, some awards are restricted to students in the second, third, or fourth years of medical school. No matter where you are in the medical education process, there are awards available for you.

> **Tip # 1**
>
> Become knowledgeable about scholarship opportunities and requirements as soon as possible. This will allow you to develop a strategy for success and then utilize the time available to improve your chances of winning. We have seen many deserving candidates lose out because of late planning. With the benefit of time, you can make the most of your volunteer and extracurricular activities. You will see that many scholarship programs heavily value involvement outside of the classroom.

Myth # 5   **The same approach that served me well to get into medical school will help me win scholarships.**

The scholarship application bears similarities to the medical school application. Strategic planning is required to be successful for both but the scholarship application process mandates its own specific strategy. Award recipients are successful because they identify the purpose and goals of the scholarship program, understand the type of candidate that is considered "ideal" to the program, and tailor their application to emphasize their fit with the scholarship program's mission. We'll show you how to do just that.

> **Did you know…**
>
> For scholarship recipients, it's more than luck that nets these awards. Our conversations with winners have revealed that a tremendous amount of effort developing and implementing strategy was crucial to their success.

Myth # 6   **I should devote all my efforts to a few awards to increase my odds of success.**

Your chances of winning an award increase with the number of scholarships programs you apply to. You may believe that this approach would spread you too thin but you can streamline the process by recycling material from one application to another. The most effort and time is expended preparing the first several applications. After that, applicants often find the process easier and less time consuming. If you're able to follow this advice, you'll be able to apply for more awards without sacrificing the quality of your application. The more scholarships and awards you apply for, the more you're likely to win.

Tip # 2

The availability of hundreds of scholarships makes it difficult for the busy medical student to apply to all programs. That said, after you complete several scholarship applications, you will find that the time needed to complete subsequent applications will decrease. You will see that scholarship applications often ask for the same information. Therefore, you can recycle material from one application to another, making adjustments as needed.

Myth # 7   Bigger is always better

If you're the recipient of five $1,000 awards or the winner of a $5,000 scholarship, you've accomplished the same goal. Smaller awards do add up, and are often renewable. In addition, smaller scholarships tend to be less competitive.

Did you know...

Applying for scholarships or awards of minimal or even no value may be worthwhile. If you win these prizes, they can strengthen your application for awards of higher monetary value.

Myth # 8   I don't have enough extracurricular activities to be seriously considered.

With extracurricular activities, quality often trumps quantity. With the demands placed on time, it's understandable that most medical students will not have a long list of extracurricular activities. Considerably more important is the depth of your involvement in these activities. What have you done in your extracurricular activities? How has your involvement set you apart from other applicants?

Myth # 9   I should avoid applying to scholarship programs that require too much time or effort.

It's true that some scholarship programs are easier to apply to than others. Some will require only a CV while others ask applicants to submit multiple letters of recommendation and personal essays. As you can imagine, programs that are easier to apply to receive the most scholarship applications.

Tip # 3

Remember this rule of thumb: the less effort that is required, the more competition you will face.

Tip # 3

The Saint Louis University School of Medicine encourages students to build a scholarship portfolio to make the process of applying for scholarships faster and easier. "Include things like personal statements, Curriculum Vitae, transcripts (undergraduate, graduate, and medical school), copies of diplomas, and copies of honors, awards, or certificates received."[3]

Myth # 10   One spelling error is unlikely to affect my chances of winning the scholarship.

Since scholarship programs receive so many applications, it's common for programs to screen applications and discard those that fail to meet basic requirements. A surprising number of applications have the following errors:

- Missed deadlines
- Spelling errors
- Incorrect information
- Omitted information
- Failure to include required application materials
- Failure to follow directions (e.g., submitting a 525-word essay when the essay specifically requests a response of < 500 words)

The details matter in the scholarship application process, and your ability to be detail-oriented will help you avoid the mistakes that so many applicants make.

References

[1]Duke University School of Medicine. Available at:
http://medschool.duke.edu/education/financial-aid-office. Accessed June 25, 2014.
[2]Virginia Commonwealth University School of Medicine. Available at:
http://www.medschool.vcu.edu/giving/funding/scholarships.html. Accessed July 4, 2014.
[3]Saint Louis University School of Medicine. Available at:
https://www.slu.edu/Documents/medicine/sfs/Scholarships%20Search%20tips1 314.pdf. Accessed June 28, 2014.

Chapter 3

Basics of the Scholarship Search

To win a scholarship, award, or grant, you must first identify and research the available programs. What's the biggest reason students fail to win? By far, it's a lack of awareness that the scholarship exists. In this chapter, we'll provide you with tools that will leave you well informed of scholarship opportunities.

Search High and Low

Although there are hundreds of scholarship opportunities, some are obviously more known than others. Understandably, well-known awards are harder to win because of increased competition. Fewer students will spend the extra time and effort to identify the less publicized awards. With these awards, there is considerably less competition, and therefore you have an increased chance of winning.

Tip # 4

Although some awards receive thousands of applications, others only get a handful. The most popular scholarship programs are those with the highest monetary value. Everyone would love to win the $10,000 scholarship but the less popular $2,500 award may be easier to win. Smaller awards may be renewable every year. At the end of four years, you may have won an equivalent amount of money.

Harness the Power of the Internet

Twenty plus years ago, the search for scholarships started with large printed scholarship directories. Although these are still available, the Internet has supplanted directories as the starting point for today's medical student. The advantage of the Internet is that information is readily available and can be updated much faster.

Although technology has made the scholarship search process easier, it's important to understand its limitations. Not all scholarship information is available nor is all information found accurate. An excellent list of medical school scholarships is available at the University of Pennsylvania website but the school cautions students to understand its limitations. "The Office of Admissions and Financial Aid has compiled a directory in an effort to help you locate outside scholarships," writes the University of Pennsylvania Perelman School of Medicine. "This information has been compiled from financial aid directories and announcements sent to the Med School. Please note that this listing is by no means complete."[1]

Tip # 5

The Internet is an excellent place to start your scholarship search but not all scholarships will be found on the Web. Local scholarship programs often lack a Web presence. Also, what's easily found on the Internet will be more competitive. Our advice is to start online and then move offline.

Tip # 6

Use Internet search engines to identify scholarships. Your ability to find opportunities will depend upon the keywords you use. Some recommended keywords include "medical school" and the following: financial aid, scholarships, grants, awards, fellowships, money, and minority scholarships. An effective technique is to place quotation marks around the terms to generate the most specific results. Specific results are also generated by using the advanced search function.

Tip # 7

Many scholarship programs are featured in newspapers and magazines. Cengage Learning operates HighBeam Research, an information service that provides access to thousands of published sources. The resource offers access to over 6,500 publications, and has more than 80 million articles. Visit http://highbeam.com for more information. We have found this to be a valuable resource in the scholarship search.

An increasing number of scholarship programs are engaging students through social media. Use Facebook to "like" and Twitter to follow so that you can receive alerts about the scholarship. To learn more about the sponsoring organization, visit YouTube. The knowledge you gain will be useful in developing essays and preparing for scholarship interviews.

Tip # 8

Set a Google Alert for key words related to medical school scholarships so that you're notified when a new article is written.

Visit the Library

With so much information available on the Internet, it's easy to overlook the library. Your city, county, college, and medical library system will be staffed with knowledgeable librarians eager to help you with your scholarship search. Some libraries have placed scholarship resources in a reference area. Ask where books, catalogs, and directories are kept. Find out what information is available in electronic databases subscribed to by the library.

Tip # 9

Since a variety of associations offer scholarships and awards, wouldn't it be great if there was a directory of associations? Fortunately, there is. Ask the librarian if you can look through the reference *Encyclopedia of Associations*.

Utilize Scholarship Databases

There are a number of Internet scholarship databases available to medical students. In fact, you may be familiar with some if you've used databases to find money for college. A database is essentially a directory of scholarships that allows you to search for opportunities in an organized manner.

Databases take the leg work out of the scholarship search process by consolidating information in one location. That's particularly appealing to the busy and overstretched medical student.

Each database will claim that its information is the most comprehensive. Don't be swayed by these claims. Take time to learn about the available databases so that you can determine which one to use in the limited time that you have. Of key importance is to know how to analyze and investigate the available databases.

Databases should be part of your scholarship search process but don't view these resources as comprehensive. Although national scholarships tend to be included in these directories, our experience has shown that local, regional, and state awards are often missed.

Scholarship Databases for Medical Students	
EducationPlanner.org	ScholarSite.com
Fastweb.com	ScholarshipExperts.com
FinAid.com	Scholarships101.com
Sallie Mae	SchoolSoup.com
Scholarships.com	Studentawards.com
ScholarshipMonkey.com	StudentScholarshipSearch.com

Investigating and Analyzing Scholarship Databases

- Determine if the database contains the information you need for each scholarship opportunity. You need more than just the name and amount of the award. Does the database include sponsoring organization, address, phone numbers, contact names, website addresses, eligibility requirements, criteria for judging or selection, application materials, and deadlines?

- What type of search function is provided? Databases may utilize a browsing or matching system to search for scholarships.

- With the browsing system, you will be able to investigate scholarships by category.

- In the matching system, you will complete information fields, allowing the database to create a profile of you based on your background and credentials. This profile will be used to identify awards and scholarships that fit with your profile.

- There are advantages and disadvantages to both systems. With both systems, you assume that the developers have been exhaustive in identifying and including scholarship programs. In the matching system, you also assume that the developers have found a way to match you with every award you would be eligible for. Unfortunately, awards will be missed, and you can never be certain how many are missed.

- In the browsing system, you can search through every scholarship in a particular category. The disadvantage with this approach is that it takes considerably more time, energy, and effort to do so. That can present a problem for the busy medical student.

Go Above and Beyond in your Research

Students who take the time to extensively research the award will often fare better. Not long ago, I worked with a motivated scholarship applicant who was looking for an edge in the scholarship application process. He was interested in a highly competitive national award that several students from his school had won in the past. I encouraged him to locate these previous winners and contact them. He really took my words to heart, and he was able to gain valuable insight and perspective through discussions with them. After determining the factors that led them to be successful, he was able to tailor his scholarship application strategy accordingly to meet the needs of the scholarship program committee. The end result was a winning application, and one very happy medical student.

Look to the Future

You will be tempted to devote all your energy and effort on scholarships you are eligible for now. That's understandable but the savvy scholarship applicant will make note of future scholarship opportunities. Why? By becoming familiar with the criteria for selection, you will understand your competitiveness for the award. If you find that you are not yet the ideal candidate, you have the luxury of time to become one. Are you lacking in extracurricular activities, service, or leadership? Take steps to strengthen your candidacy as you see fit. Then when you are eligible for the award later in medical school, you will have turned your weaknesses into strengths. Your chances of winning the award have increased.

Tip # 10

You will find that some scholarship programs only consider applicants who are members of a certain group. Consider joining these groups. As an example, consider the American Medical Women's Association (AMWA) Service Recognition Award. Criteria for selection includes a minimum of 50 cumulative hours of service with AMWA, participation in a project aligned with AMWA's mission, and recommendation from a supervising AMWA leader. If you come to learn of this opportunity as a freshman medical student, you could join the organization. Your contributions to the organization over time could make you eligible for the award later.

Tip # 11

Pay particular attention to the words used to describe what the program is seeking in candidates. What are the values important to the scholarship committee?

Tip # 12

Some scholarship programs post information about previous winners. Detailed profiles may be available, and you may able to identify what these winners have in common.

Tip # 13

As you become familiar with available scholarships, you will see that programs are often very interested in extracurricular activities. Take stock of your activities by considering the depth and breadth of your involvement. Being involved in multiple activities demonstrates interest and well-roundedness. Making significant contributions in one or more activities is a sign of depth. Aim for both to attract the attention of scholarship committees.

Know Thyself

Do you volunteer in an organization? Is your father a member of a professional organization? Are your parents employed by the government? By answering these types of questions, you may find that you are eligible for awards and scholarships you had never considered or imagined. The table on the next page is a starting point to uncover these frequently overlooked sources of support.

Behold the Power of Organization

Too many medical students approach the scholarship process in haphazard fashion. Your time as a medical student is limited, and a disorganized scholarship approach can easily take you away from your studies. With an organized approach, you remain efficient and spend no more time than is needed.

We recommend that you set up an organizational system that you will use throughout medical school. Every time you come across a scholarship opportunity, create a separate file for it. Print out the application, and store it in your file. Organize these scholarship opportunities by deadlines. We have found that the biggest medical school scholarship winners have such systems in place.

Tip # 14

The savvy scholarship applicant will read the scholarship description carefully to understand the reasons why the sponsoring organization is doling out money. By understanding the reasons, you will be better able to paint the picture of the ideal candidate. This will allow you to tailor the application accordingly. If you have the luxury of time before the application is due, you can make considerable efforts to strengthen your candidacy.

Question	Significance
Where were you born? Parents? Grandparents?	You may be eligible for certain scholarships based on your country of birth.
What is your ethnicity/race?	Ethnic groups award scholarships.
What is your gender?	A number of awards are available to female medical students.
Are you a member of an underrepresented minority group?	African American, Native American, Alaska Native, Native Hawaiian, Hispanic, and mainland Puerto Rican applicants are eligible for certain awards.
What is your religion? Parents? Grandparents?	Churches, temples, synagogues, and mosques provide awards.
Do you have any family members who are serving or have served?	The military offers scholarships to children of service members.
Where do you work? Parents? Grandparents?	Current and previous employers are a source of support.
Are you a member of a professional organization? Parents? Grandparents?	Professional organizations often have scholarship programs open to members or relatives of members.
What is your sexual orientation or gender identity?	Some scholarships are only open to gay, lesbian, or transgender applicants.
What high school did you attend?	High school booster and alumni groups may award scholarships.
Who is your local state representative or congressman?	Politicians may sponsor scholarship programs.
Are your parents or grandparents members of a union?	Scholarships have been awarded by unions.
Are your parents or grandparents employed by the government?	Awards are available at the federal, state, and local level.
Do any members of your family volunteer?	Volunteer organization may have funds set aside for scholarships.

Tip # 15

If you are unable to access a scholarship application online, send an email to the contact person. In some cases, you may have to call. Make note of any correspondence in your file, including the date of communication. This will allow you to follow up later if you don't receive the application materials.

References

[1]University of Pennsylvania Perelman School of Medicine. Available at: http://www.med.upenn.edu/financialaid/externalscholarships.shtml. Accessed July 2, 2014.

Chapter 4

Your Medical School
and the Scholarship Process

After you receive an offer of admission to medical school, one of your initial inquiries should be with your school's Financial Aid Office. This office will be staffed with knowledgeable people who are well informed about need-based and merit-based scholarships and awards. It is routine for many scholarship programs to contact schools to inform them of their opportunities. Schools are particularly familiar with awards specific to the local community, region, or state.

Tip # 16

Start your scholarship search as soon as you are admitted to medical school. Many awards are available to incoming students but only if you meet deadlines.

Many schools have devoted a section of their website to scholarships. It's best not to rely fully on the website because schools vary on how often they update this information. Scholarship programs will contact schools throughout the academic year so visit the Financial Aid Office regularly. During your initial visit, ask staff if there is a cabinet or binder listing scholarship opportunities, a bulletin board where new information is posted, or a database that you can access. "A listing of outside scholarships is published in the Financial Aid Resource Guide which is available in the Financial Aid Office," writes the Case Western Reserve University School of Medicine.[1]

Schools often have internal scholarships set aside for incoming students. At the Pritzker School of Medicine of the University of Chicago, approximately $10 million dollars in scholarship money is available for M.D. students. "This fellowship and scholarship money has been given as gifts to the University by grateful alumni, families of alumni, grateful patients of the University Hospitals, former faculty, and a host of friends of the University and University Hospitals."[2]

Some internal scholarship awards will be given to incoming students at the discretion of the admissions committee or dean. For example, at Duke University, the Dean's Tuition Scholarship is awarded to students whose background will add to the diversity of the class. It does not require an application.[3] Campus-based awards at Wright State University Boonshoft School of Medicine are "made from information gathered from the AMCAS application and/or from the FAFSA."[4]

Tip # 17

With some internal awards, you may only be eligible if you express interest or apply. Begin by visiting your school's website for financial aid information. Some schools list available scholarship opportunities. Don't hesitate to contact the financial aid office for further information.

Tip # 18

Schools may have a list of former students who have won scholarships. Take note of the awards won by these students so that you can investigate these opportunities.

Less well appreciated by medical students is the availability of scholarships oriented toward specific specialties. These may be internal awards granted by a medical school department. At the New York University School of Medicine, the Eve R. Flechner Memorial Award is given to a female student for excellence in the Internal Medicine Clerkship. The Ferrari Award for Academic Excellence in Pediatrics is presented to the medical student who achieves the highest grade in the pediatric clerkship at West Virginia University School of Medicine. The Dr. Atwood P. Latham Memorial Prize in Anatomy is awarded to the first-year medical student deemed most proficient in anatomy at the University of Louisville.

Tip # 19

Specialty departments can also enlighten you about national scholarship opportunities. I have seen medical students discover awards not known to their school's Financial Aid Office through departmental inquiries. Some of these awards may require the department to nominate a student. For example, in order to be eligible for National Outstanding Medical Student Award bestowed by the American College of Emergency Physicians, the chair of emergency medicine, emergency medicine program director or the medical student clerkship director is asked to choose one emergency medicine bound medical student who fulfills the award criteria.

> **Tip # 20**
>
> A quick review of medical school websites will show you that some schools have larger lists of scholarship opportunities than others. We encourage you to go beyond your own school's website.

If you are an incoming or returning medical student seeking need-based aid, you will have to complete the Free Application for Federal Student Aid (FAFSA). Many schools also ask students to complete a school-specific financial aid application.

The importance of submitting the financial aid application before the deadline seems obvious but many students fail to do so. What happens if you're late? Institutional funding is limited, and you may not receive support if funds are exhausted. "Students who do not complete a FAFSA...will not be considered for scholarships," writes the UMKC School of Medicine.[5] "Late applicants may be excluded from consideration for institutional funding since these funds are limited," writes the Tufts University School of Medicine.[6] Unfortunately, there are students every year who qualify for institutional funds but do not receive support because of late applications. Of note, late applications have no effect on federal student aid eligibility but applying late may result in delays with the processing of your application and the availability of your funds.

> **Did you know...**
>
> Parental information is not required if you are applying for federal loans. If you are seeking institutional funds, you will have to submit parental financial information. "Although students may wish to declare independence from their parents...most U.S. medical schools, requires parental income statements from all applicants," writes the Geisel School of Medicine at Dartmouth University.[7] Failure to provide parental information may disqualify you from being considered for institutional funds. "Lack of parental information may disqualify you from receiving some scholarships and low-interest loans," writes Howard University Health Sciences.[8]

> **Tip # 21**
>
> According to the U.S. Department of Education, many applicants fail to complete the FAFSA because "it's too hard" or "takes too long to complete." Research indicates that it takes most applicants 23 minutes to complete.[9]

Common Errors Made By Applicants Seeking Need-Based Medical Scholarships/Awards

The following are common mistakes made on financial aid applications:

- Not applying for need-based awards because of failure to quality for awards as an undergraduate
- Failure to complete these forms in their entirety
- Not making note of all filing deadlines
- Submitting forms after the deadline
- Not recognizing that these forms need to be completed annually
- Misunderstanding terms on the form
- Not checking with the financial aid office to ensure that your application is complete
- Failure to write down your institution's correct federal code
- Submitting FAFSA or other forms for the wrong academic year
- Providing conflicting data
- Leaving spaces blank. Best to write "not applicable."
- Omitting zip codes from addresses
- Failure to provide telephone numbers
- Not providing references if requested
- Not signing and dating applications
- Forgetting to have your parents sign tax forms

Did you know…

Do I have to notify the financial aid office if I win an external scholarship? If you are receiving need-based funds, you should be familiar with federal laws. These laws indicate that funds received from all sources cannot exceed the cost of medical school attendance. This means that if you receive an external award, you will have to notify the financial aid office. If you have an over award, the office may have to reduce your institutional or federal funding. This is generally to your advantage because it reduces your indebtedness. If your loan amount is reduced, you will have less interest that accrues over the lifetime of your loan.

Did you know…

"It is up to the student to take the initiative and work with the Financial Aid Administrator in identifying and pursuing the sources of funds that are available," writes the Case Western Reserve University School of Medicine.[1]

Did you know…

"We've found that successful scholarship recipients:

- Apply for all relevant opportunities.
- Adhere strictly to guidelines for each application.
- Provide supporting documents before deadlines.

To enhance your chances of getting a scholarship, we recommend that you:

- Adhere to deadlines and pay attention to applications with multiple deadlines for different portions of the application.
- Make sure you have quick access to secure transcripts from your previous schools."

- University of Michigan Medical School[10]

Did you know…

Some scholarship programs will only consider medical students who have been nominated by their medical school. If you come across such an award, you will have to express your interest to the medical school. Make inquiries with your school to determine who makes nomination decisions. Then explain why you are a particularly good candidate for the scholarship. Give compelling reasons but be tactful without disparaging other candidates. On the following page is a template that can be used in communicating with your school's administration about awards that require you to be nominated.

Sample Letter of Request for Consideration of Nomination

Your Name
Address

Date

Name
Title
Address

Dear _____:

I recently learned about the [scholarship program] sponsored by [organization]. This is an award that is given for [describe scholarship].

In order to be considered for the scholarship, students must first be nominated by their medical school. As a medical student who has been actively involved in [describe leadership, community service, extracurricular activity along with contributions], I believe that I am eligible for this award.

I have enclosed my [CV, additional information] to help you decide whether my nomination for the scholarship program is appropriate.

The deadline for the nomination is [date]. If you require any further information, please contact me at [phone number] or [email address]. Thank you very much for your consideration.

Sincerely,

Signature/Name

References

[1]Case Western Reserve University School of Medicine. Available at:
http://casemed.case.edu/financial_aid/scholarships/outside.cfm. Accessed July
2, 2014.
[2]Pritzker School of Medicine at the University of Chicago. Available at:
https://pritzker.uchicago.edu/admissions/financialaid/sources.shtml. Accessed
June 3, 2014.
[3]Duke University School of Medicine. Available at:
http://medschool.duke.edu/education/financial-aid-
office/httpmedschooldukeedu/scholarships. Accessed June 22, 2014.
[4]Boonshoft School of Medicine at Wright State University. Available at:
http://www.med.wright.edu/admiss/financialaid. Accessed June 2, 2014.
[5]UMKC School of Medicine. Available at: http://med.umkc.edu/bamd/finance/.
Accessed June 2, 2014.
[6]Tufts University School of Medicine. Available at: http://www.tufts.edu/tufts-
test/med/staging/about/offices/finaid/faqs/mdfaq.html. Accessed June 12, 2014.
[7]Geisel School of Medicine at Dartmouth University. Available at:
https://geiselmed.dartmouth.edu/admin/fin_aid/policy.shtml. Accessed June 14,
2014.
[8]Howard University Health Sciences. Available at:
http://healthsciences.howard.edu/education/schools-and-
academics/medicine/admissions/financial-aid%20Aplication. Accessed June 2,
2014.
[9]U.S Department of Education Blog. Available at:
http://www.ed.gov/blog/2014/01/7-common-fafsa-mistakes/. Accessed July 22,
2014.
[10]University of Michigan Medical School. Available at:
http://medicine.umich.edu/medschool/education/md-program/financial-
aid/how-apply/scholarships-grants/other-scholarship-sources. Accessed June
22, 2014.

Chapter 5

Canvass Your Local Community

Local scholarship opportunities tend to be less known, and therefore fewer applicants compete for these awards. Community groups often have foundations that collect donations to support various initiatives, including scholarships. Investigate groups and organizations in your community by performing a search with your city, county, or region and the word "scholarships." Below we have included a list of community organizations to contact.

Community Groups and Organizations Offering Medical School Scholarships	
American Legion	Lions Club
American Red Cross	Masons
Boy Scouts of America	National Association for the
Girl Scouts of America	Advancement of Colored People
Chamber of Commerce	National Honor Society
Circle K	Odd Fellows and Rebekah
Daughters of the American	Lodges
Revolution	Optimist International
Daughters of the Confederacy	Parent-Teacher Association
Delegate and Senatorial	Rotary Club
Scholarships	Ruritan
Disabled American Veterans	Sons of the American
Elks Club	Revolution
Jaycees	Soroptimist International
Junior League	Urban League
4-H Club	Veterans of Foreign Wars
Key Club	YMCA
Kiwanis International	YWCA
Knights of Columbus	

Local businesses are another source of scholarship support. Department stores, banks, credit unions, newspapers, radio stations, television stations, and power companies are some businesses that have been known to support students. Banks often hold or administer scholarship funds for a variety of organizations. An underutilized but effective technique is to contact banks to learn about opportunities. Not everyone at the bank will have this information so you will have to determine who is in the know.

Did you know…

Hospitals may offer scholarships to medical students. The Washington Hospital Healthcare Foundation offers two scholarships to college students pursuing medical degrees. To be eligible, the student "must be a resident or former resident of the Washington Township Health Care District or have significant ties to the District."[1]

If you are working while attending college or medical school, make inquiries with your employer as to the availability of scholarship opportunities. If your immediate supervisor is not aware of scholarships, reach out to the personnel office, human resources department, or national headquarters. Your parents should also look for scholarship opportunities with their employers.

Religious organizations should not be ignored. Although organizations generally provide support only to members, some awards are made available to nonmembers. Begin your search for these awards by using scholarship directories and databases but be sure to also contact organizations directly. Some medical students have been able to secure funds through direct contact.

Members of underrepresented minority groups are eligible for numerous scholarships and awards. There are dedicated directories and databases for minority scholarships.

If you are a war veteran or relative of a war veteran, you may be eligible for a variety of scholarships. Awards are also available for disabled veterans.

Applicants with disabilities are eligible to receive scholarships from many sources. The American Association on Health and Disability awards the Frederick J. Krause Scholarship to an undergraduate or graduate student with a disability who is enrolled in coursework related to field of health and disability. Specific disease foundations may also be a source of support. The Lupus Inspiration Foundation for Excellence provides merit-based assistance to college and graduate school students with Systemic Lupus Erythematosus. Some medical students have received awards from organizations and foundations because of a family member with disability or disease.

Tip # 22

If you or your parents are members of a fraternity or sorority, you may be eligible for awards. Visit the national website or write to the national headquarters for more information. The Omega Psi Phi Fraternity bestows the W. Montague Cobb Award to support a brother who is enrolled full-time in an accredited school of medicine and has demonstrated service to the fraternity during the year of application.

Tip # 23

Where are you from? Where have you lived? Where did you go to high school? The answers to these questions may make you eligible for certain awards and scholarships. Certain regions or areas of the country produce relatively few physicians. Awards may be available if you are from a certain region, and there may be few applicants.

Although the internet can be a useful way to start your local scholarship search, we have seen that many local awards and scholarships are not featured on the Web. It's worthwhile to contact local groups directly. Approach the local chapter or branch in your city, country, region, or state. If you are having difficulty finding contact information, call the national headquarters for this information. Below is dialogue you can use as a template:

My name is _____ and I'm a medical student here in [City]. I was wondering if your organization has scholarships or awards that are available for students in the area.

If scholarships are available, ask for additional information and an application. Some scholarship programs may only send materials after they receive a written request. On the following page is a template that you can use to make the written request.

Tip # 24

An excellent resource to search for local organizations offering scholarships is the Yellow Pages. You will find contact information for governmental agencies, civic organizations, service clubs, and businesses.

SAMPLE REQUEST FOR SCHOLARSHIP APPLICATION

Your Name
Address

Date

Name of Organization
Scholarship Program Name
Address

To whom it may concern:

I recently learned about the scholarship program sponsored by your organization. I would like to receive an application. Please also include any available information about guidelines, criteria, and deadlines. This information can be sent to:

Name
Address

If you require any further information, please contact me at [phone number] or [email address]. Thank you very much.

Sincerely,

Signature/Name

References

[1]Washington Hospital Healthcare System. Available at: http://www.whhs.com/community/scholarship-opportunities/. Accessed July 22, 2014.

Chapter 6

Scholarship Application

Programs will receive hundreds of applications for a few awards. To whittle down this large group into a more manageable number, scholarships programs will assign an administrative staff member to quickly look over all applications. During this screening process, the application will be examined to determine if it should be sent to the scholarship committee for further consideration.

Did you know…

Too many applicants complete scholarship applications as if they are filling out just another form. Scholarship recipients recognize that considerable thought, skill, and effort are required to develop a winning application.

Did you know…

In the initial screening process, scholarship programs will look to see if your application is neat, complete, and professional. "This stage is also where MOST applications end up in that big 'NO' pile, never to be seen again," writes Laura DiFiore, a noted scholarship expert. "In many cases, up to 90% of applications are 'killed' right here."[1] To survive this stage, submit neatly typed applications that are complete, free of spelling errors, and accurate. Make sure all required supporting materials are included.

Unless the application form is online, begin by making multiple copies of the scholarship application. This will allow you to initially fill in the fields in pencil, and then edit your responses over time until you are satisfied.

Although your initial work may be in pencil, scholarship applications should be typed on a computer or typewriter. You may have received great praise for your handwriting but the best penmanship pales in comparison to the professional look of a typed document.

As you complete the application fields, you may realize that space is limited. If that's the case, add additional information on attached sheets as needed. Do this only if the application form permits you to do so. With some forms, it will not be clear if the addition of extra sheets is allowed. In these cases, don't hesitate to contact the scholarship program.

On many forms, you will be asked to list extracurricular activities, leadership roles, community service involvement, and awards. Unless you have nothing at all to list, do not leave any of these fields blank. If possible, use the entire space available. If you don't have enough material for a particular field, a useful and recommended approach is to add detail to what you have listed. For example, in listing your involvement as a medical student peer tutor, you can provide a description of the contributions you have made as a tutor.

In the process of polishing the application, you will go through a series of drafts. Be sure to save these drafts as separate files. We recommend using the date of the draft as part of the name. You may decide later that an earlier draft was better, and you will easily be able to retrieve it. Saving your work will allow you to readily recycle information for future scholarship applications.

Many scholarship applicants simply list their extracurricular activities, leadership roles, and community service involvement. We believe that it is far better to use powerful words to show the reader what you have done. Action verbs such as organized, coordinated, founded, and led are particularly effective. Chapter 7 includes a list of these powerful verbs.

Take care in the order in which you present your activities or involvement. Lead with what is most important. How do you decide? Consider the scholarship or award, and ask yourself which activity would make the most favorable impression on the scholarship committee? Is the activity particularly relevant to the scholarship? If you've made strong contributions in an activity or held prominent leadership positions, do not bury these notable accomplishments in the middle or end of the description field. The way in which you order the list will vary from one scholarship program to another.

Scholarship applications may ask you to provide a list of awards and honors. As with activities, present the list in descending order of importance. Of course, this is a judgment call but, in general, state or national awards carry more weight than local or regional awards. Think also about awards received that are related to the scholarship. Such awards need to be placed higher on the list. In listing honors and awards, include language to enlighten the scholarship committee about the significance of the award. Remember that awards familiar to you may not be easily understood by others. If this is the case, add explanations for these awards.

Tip # 25

Assuming you have enough time before the deadline, you can send your scholarship by regular U.S. mail. Of course, if the application is due in the next day or two, send it by USPS Express Mail, UPS, or FedEx. Be sure to follow up with the program to ensure its receipt. If the deadline is rapidly approaching, send the application with certified mail with a return receipt requested card. Spending a few extra dollars now will provide you with the peace of mind that it has arrived at the destination.

Components of the Scholarship Application

Scholarships programs generally ask for some combination of the following:

Scholarship application
Photo
CV or resume
Letters of recommendation
Extracurricular activities
Transcript (college, medical school)
Standardized exam scores
Financial aid form
Letter of good standing (or proof of enrollment) from medical school
Dean's letter
Personal statement/essays
Proposal/budget for research grants and awards

Tip # 26

As you prepare the scholarship application, never lose track of what the organization considers the ideal scholarship applicant. This will allow you to tailor your application to meet the needs of the program.

Did you know...

Scholarship programs can be very strict with respect to guidelines and rules. "Applications that contain more than the specified number of pages, or letters will be rejected out of fairness to candidates who adhere to the guidelines," writes Triangle Community Foundation, which sponsors the Gertrude B. Elion Mentored Medical Student Research Award. "In addition, applications that are not properly organized or that do not include all of the requested materials will be rejected."[2]

References

[1]University of Florida College of Medicine. Available at: http://finaid.med.ufl.edu/scholarships/understanding-the-judging-process/. Accessed July 1, 2014.
[2]Triangle Community Foundation. Available at: http://www.trianglecf.org/grants_support/view_scholarships/gertrude_b._elion_mentored_medical_student_research_award/. Accessed July 2, 2014.

Chapter 7

Curriculum Vitae

Curriculum vitae is a Latin expression, meaning the "course of one's life." Known as CV for short, this document provides an overview of a candidate's academic and professional background. The CV is an important component of many scholarship applications. Creating a good CV requires time, effort, and a thorough examination of your training and achievements. The overall appearance of your CV needs to be impeccable. The proofreading must be perfect. Each individual line should be positioned for maximum impact. Every pertinent aspect of your achievements must be included. Your CV will continue to be an important document throughout medical school. It is not a static document, but rather one that needs to be updated regularly as you progress through your career.

Utilize only the correct CV format and structure.

All CVs begin with your name and contact information. Since these items will be at the top of your CV, they can contribute to a positive first impression, and so should be visually appealing. Many applicants use the same font size for the name and contact information. However, your name should be a bit bigger and even bolder than the rest of the contact information. Don't add the words "curriculum vitae" to the top of the page, as many students tend to do. The reader recognizes a CV. Why waste valuable space stating the obvious?

Following your name and contact information should be an "education" section. From here, you will have considerable latitude in the order in which you present the remaining categories. It is preferable, however, to lead with your strengths.

If you have been particularly productive publishing as a student, have the "research experience" and "publications" sections follow "education" rather than placing it second to last. Weigh the impact of each section before deciding where to place it. Below are the standard sections of the CV.

Standard Sections of the CV	
Name	Research experience
Contact information	Publications
Education	Presentations
Postgraduate training	Committees/service
Employment experience	Licensure and certification
Honors/awards	Extracurricular activities
Professional memberships	Volunteer activities
Teaching experience	Personal interests

Always place items in chronological order.

Incorrect ordering is among the most common CV mistakes. In all sections of the CV, information should be presented in reverse chronological order. Using this order, one would list items such as jobs and awards with the most recent item first.

Every section and line of your CV must impress.

If you have a section with just one item, plan on eliminating it, unless it's an impressive accomplishment. A category with a single item looks decidedly unimpressive. It also wastes valuable lines of CV space. A single item can always be woven into another category. For example, a single honor earned during medical school can be listed in the "education" section.

Each line of your CV must pack the maximum impact. Study your CV line by line. In many cases, a description or explanation of an item will maximize its impact.

Tip # 27

As you read through your CV, question whether the reader would understand the significance of what you have written. If not, it may be assumed to have little value.

Tip # 28

Avoid unfamiliar acronyms or abbreviations. An abbreviation that is readily apparent to you may have no meaning to a scholarship committee. If an organization is not readily recognizable, a brief explanation of the group and its purpose should be included in the CV.

Tip # 29

The typical member of the scholarship committee is forced to quickly review a CV. Part of refining your CV, then, should be the two-minute glance over. Have you captured the reviewer's attention and conveyed your accomplishments?

Did you know...

"Students are encouraged to compile their CV in the first year of medical school...will allow them to quickly apply for scholarships and research grants throughout medical school," writes the Ohio State University College of Medicine.[1]

The language style you use makes a difference. Use only action verbs.

Use words that capture the reviewer's attention. The use of action verbs acts to strengthen your CV. Placed at the beginning of sentences, these verbs make more powerful statements.

In writing about your work, extracurricular, volunteer, and research experiences, use action verbs to emphasize your accomplishments. Many applicants simply describe their duties and responsibilities. It is far more powerful to stress what you accomplished.

Utilize the following extensive list of action verbs in order to highlight your accomplishments:

Action Verbs	
A	Abridged, accelerated, accomplished, accounted for, achieved, adapted, adjusted, administered, advanced, advised, allocated, analyzed, answered, approved, arranged, assembled, assimilated, assisted, attained, augmented
B	Balanced, broadened, built
C	Calculated, calibrated, cared for, categorized, catalogued, chaired, charted, clarified, classified, coached, collaborated, collected, compared, compiled, completed, composed, conceived, condensed, conducted, consolidated, constructed, consulted, contributed, coordinated, counseled, created, critiqued
D	Debated, defined, delegated, delineated, delivered, demonstrated, derived, designed, detected, determined, developed, devised, diagnosed, directed, discovered, displayed, distributed, documented, drafted
E	Edited, earned, educated, elicited, enabled, encouraged, enhanced, ensured, established, estimated, evaluated, examined, exceeded, exhibited, expanded, expedited, explained, explored
F	Facilitated, followed, formulated, found, founded, furthered
G	Gathered, generated, guided
H	Handled, headed, helped
I	Identified, illustrated, implemented, improved, increased, initiated, innovated, inspected, installed, instituted, instructed, interacted, interpreted, interviewed, invented, investigated
J	Judged, justified
L	Launched, lectured, led, logged
M	Made, maintained, managed, mastered, measured, met, modified, monitored, motivated
O	Observed, obtained, offered, operated, organized, oversaw
P	Participated, performed, pinpointed, pioneered, planned, prepared, presented, presided, prioritized, processed, produced, programmed, proposed, proved, provided
Q	Quantified
R	Raised, realized, received, recommended, recorded, redesigned, reported, researched, revamped, received, revised
S	Scheduled, screened, searched, secured, selected, served, set up, simplified, solved, spearheaded, started, streamlined, strengthened, studied, submitted, succeeded, summarized, supervised, supplied, supported, surpassed, surveyed, synthesized
T	Tabulated, tallied, taught, tested, traced, tracked, trained, translated, transmitted, tutored
U	Uncovered, undertook, updated, upgraded, used
V	Validated, verified, volunteered
W	Widened, won, worked, wrote

As you review this list, note the following:

- Some action verbs are more powerful than others. Use the most powerful verb you can without exaggerating your accomplishments.
- Do not downplay, diminish, or deflate your contributions by using verbs such as "assisted" or "helped."
- Avoid the much too commonly used phrases "Responsibilities for…" or "Duties included…"
- Avoid repeating the same verb if possible.
- For those activities or experiences with which you are currently involved, use the present tense. Use the past tense for completed work or past experiences.

Tip # 30

Provide tangible evidence whenever possible to support your claims. This means including numbers and facts to emphasize your accomplishments. Numbers can often drive home key points in ways that words can't.

Utilize multiple reviewers.

It doesn't matter how many times you review and revise your own CV. You should have several individuals review your CV prior to submission. We recommend having your CV reviewed by two faculty members, if at all possible. Don't submit your CV for review to faculty, though, until you feel that it is perfect.

You should ask someone with excellent writing and editing skills to review your CV. This type of careful review may lead to the discovery of spelling or grammatical errors, mistakes that can be very damaging to your candidacy.

Finally, consider the benefits of having a family or member or close friend critique your CV. Those who know you well on a personal level may point out accomplishments that you'd forgotten.

After collecting reviewer comments, consider them carefully. Compare reviewer comments with another. While you don't need to agree with all comments, if several of your reviewers make the same recommendations, take these comments seriously. If there is disagreement, solicit more opinions to help you make a more informed decision.

Avoid even a single spelling, typographical, or grammatical error.

Spelling, typographical, and grammatical errors are among the worst mistakes you can make on the CV. Even one misspelled word can make you look careless. Otherwise well-qualified applicants have been removed from consideration because of these errors. Ensure your CV is free of errors:

- If you created your CV using word processing, use the spell checker. However, the spell checker won't help if you misuse a word (e.g., substituting "there" for "their").

- Take the time needed to proofread your CV. Read it aloud, and sound out each word, syllable by syllable. Errors not apparent during a silent read may be picked up by this method.

- Read the CV backwards one word at a time, a technique used by many professional proofreaders. This allows you to focus on each individual word.

- Set the CV aside for a day before looking at it again. This allows you to look at your work with fresh eyes.

First impressions matter

The overall appearance of your CV is important as well. Scholarship programs must whittle down a large group of applications, and therefore every piece of the application becomes magnified in importance. Before reviewing your CV, the reader will form an impression of you based on its overall appearance. These recommendations should be used to create a CV with a professional appearance.

Margins

Allow for generous margins at the top, bottom, and sides of your CV. A margin of at least 1 inch is often recommended. Shrinking the margins to anything less than an inch will make the CV difficult to read.

Font

Use a font that is easy to read. Times New Roman or Arial are appropriate choices. After selecting a particular font, stick with it. The use of multiple fonts can appear unprofessional.

Font size is also an important consideration. Avoid a font size less than 10-point or one greater than 12-point. It is acceptable to use two font sizes, a larger one for headings and a smaller one for the content under each heading. The use of more than two font sizes is discouraged.

Spacing

Be consistent with spacing. Maintain enough white (open) space, especially between sections. If you use one line space between the end of one section and the beginning of another, maintain this with all sections. Rather than striking the space bar twice after each sentence, strike it only once to save space. If your CV exceeds one page in length, avoid splitting a section when going from page 1 to 2.

Design elements

It is acceptable to use the bold function to highlight your name and section headings (e.g., education). You can also consider bolding certain awards and leadership positions as a way to highlight these achievements. However, excessive use of the bolding technique can overwhelm the reader. If you bold an element such as "education," then you should bold similar elements as well (e.g., honors/awards). Keep headings consistent in style and size.

Limit the use of italics to the names of journals and foreign phrases such as *magna cum laude*. Underlining should also be used sparingly. The excessive use of underlining tends to focus the eyes on the underlined portion of the CV only. Occasional use of caps may be acceptable, but some consider it to be rude, akin to shouting.

Paper quality

Print your CV on one side only of high quality 8.5' X 11" bond paper (e.g., 24 to 28 lb). Do not use unusual or multicolored paper that may appear unprofessional. Select a white, off-white, natural, or cream colored paper.

Characteristics of an outstanding CV	Characteristics of a poor CV
Visually appealing, professional look	Weathered look (e.g., bent corners, stains)
Brief and concise	Long sentences/paragraphs
Easy to read	Lack of organization
Uniform margins with none < 1 inch	Too little white space ("crowded look")
No misspelled words or typos	Typos or misspelled words
Use of action verbs	Handwritten corrections
Moderate use of bolding, underling, and italics	Poor paper or printing quality

Start your CV now.

Your CV plays a key role in the scholarship application process. When should you start working on your CV?

Start now. The process of developing your CV will allow you to assess your strengths and weaknesses. You will be able to identify areas in your CV that can be maximized.

When you approach a faculty member for a letter of recommendation, you will provide a packet of information to assist them. Your CV is a standard component of that packet. The CV you provide must be in its final, perfected form, even at this stage. You need to make an impact with these individuals, who are advocating for your candidacy and have the power to sway scholarship committees.

Take adequate time to reflect on your experiences and accomplishments.

The process of identifying your unique characteristics, experiences, and accomplishments is not an easy one. It is critical that you take adequate time to reflect on your experiences and accomplishments. Start with brainstorming. Begin the process by writing down absolutely everything; this is not the time to edit your thoughts. Start by taking each section of the CV, and make a list of everything that you've done that related to that category.

In the pages that follow, we describe each section in detail. As you complete each section, write down everything you can possibly think of. After several initial brainstorming sessions, you should seek out other sources to help you come up with more ideas. Look at other books, websites, other examples of CVs, and speak to friends, family members, and colleagues. All of these sources may provide you with ideas. Later, you can edit this information.

You may find that you don't have anything to list in a particular category. Don't be alarmed – you're in good company. If you don't have anything to list under a section, then omit the section. However, if you are reading this book well in advance of the scholarship deadline, you do have time to improve your situation. Seek out opportunities, responsibilities, or experiences that would enhance your application.

Don't obsess over your first draft.

Once you have reviewed and written down your experiences and accomplishments, you can use this information to create the first draft of your CV. The ultimate goal is to present the information in such a way that it captures the interest and attention of the reader. However, your first draft doesn't need to be perfect.

Instead of agonizing over small details related to phrasing or formatting, take the information you have generated, transfer it to your word processing software, and arrange it in an organized manner. Once you've completed your first draft, you can then start agonizing over revisions. In the pages that follow, we present some important points about each section of the CV.

Contact Information

The CV begins with your contact information. It should include your name, address, telephone number, and e-mail address.

Avoid these mistakes...

- Avoid nicknames
- Do not use address abbreviations. Spell out words like Avenue, Drive, South, etc.
- Do not include personal information (birth date, marital status, family information, religion, social security number)

Tip # 31

Double-check your contact information to ensure that a scholarship committee could reach you quickly and easily if necessary. Since most programs will communicate with you entirely be e-mail, double check your e-mail address.

Tip # 32

Is your e-mail address professional? You've worked hard to create a specific image throughout the entire application. You certainly don't want an unprofessional e-mail address to undo your efforts.

Education

Detail your education in reverse chronological order (i.e., with your most recent or current place of learning first). Include the following:

- Name of institution
- Location of institution
- Area of study or concentration (major/minor)
- Dates of enrollment (month/year)
- Degree(s)

Include information about any graduate and undergraduate education. High school education is generally omitted.

If you received an honor, you can list it here. If you have multiple awards, you can list them together in an "honors/awards" section. If you have completed a thesis or dissertation for a particular degree, you may wish to include it in this section.

Avoid these mistakes…

- Abbreviations for degrees are the norm. Exceptions to this rule would be unusual degrees or abbreviations not widely known. If this pertains to you, provide the full degree name.
- Institutions do change their names. If your institution has changed its name, record the current name.
- Do not use abbreviations for institution names. Use the full name along with the location (city, state, country).
- The order in which you present the information is up to you but be consistent (i.e., date first, institution first, degree first).

Employment Experience

List jobs you have held, along with the dates of employment. For most applicants who have pursued a traditional path (college to medical school), this is generally not an extensive section.

If you have had extensive work experience prior to starting medical school, you should include these jobs as well. Military service can also be placed in this section. Include your branch of service, number of years served, highest rank achieved, and any awards earned.

For each work experience, list the employer, location (city/state), job title, duties/responsibilities, and dates of employment. Give a brief description of your responsibilities using action verbs. For example, tutoring may have helped you develop skills in directing, guiding, or supervising.

Teaching Experience

For each teaching experience, include your position, subject taught, audience, location, frequency of teaching, and date. Don't forget about tutoring, advising, and mentoring.

Honors and Awards

In this section, the focus should be on awards received during college and medical school. Awards and scholarships earned during the high school years can also be included here, particularly if they are of great significance. You need not limit this section to academic awards. It is appropriate to include organizational, community, institutional, and departmental awards. If the honor is one that you feel a scholarship committee might value, then you should include it.

For awards that are not self-explanatory, include a single-sentence description to ensure that the reader understands the award's significance. Also include the date that you received the award and the bestowing organization.

Professional Memberships/Affiliations

List all professional organizations of which you are, or were, a member, along with the dates of your membership. Leadership or committee positions within an organization are significant. Include appropriate dates for each position listed. When listing the organization's name, do not use the abbreviation.

Research Experience

List all research experience, even if it did not lead to a publication or presentation. Be specific in describing your duties and responsibilities. If your project was funded, list the amount and source of funding. You should always list your research mentor and principal investigator of the project.

Publications

List all abstracts and articles that you have published. The most recent publication is listed first, followed by all others in reverse chronological order. If you have been particularly productive, the section can be subdivided into peer review journal articles, non-peer review journal articles, abstracts, and books/chapters.

Applicants often forget to include articles published in newsletters, newspapers, magazines, or the Internet. Contributions to a book, not just authorship of a book, may be listed as well. List publications in the standard format used by medical journals. Most commonly, citations are listed using the American Psychological Association or American Medical Association format.

Presentations

Although "presentations" can be combined with "publications" in one category, you may wish to create two categories. If you've only given one presentation, however, then use the joint category.

With presentations, it is particularly important to document the title, name of organization, location, and date. Include presentations given to academic societies and professional associations at the regional, national, and international level. Poster presentations should be listed here as well.

Extracurricular activities

Scholarship programs take interest in an applicant's extracurricular activities. They respect the fact that students active in organizations have demonstrated an ability to balance a difficult workload with outside activities.

List activities you were involved in during college and medical school. Avoid listing activities prior to college unless they are of significance. If the type of activity is not obvious, include a description.

Personal Interests

Few applicants give enough thought to this section. Often, two or three hobbies or interests are placed here without any consideration of how best to present the information. However, if done properly, this section can provide readers with insight into your personality and interests.

Scholarship interviews commonly begin with discussion of an applicant's personal interests as a way to break the ice. Applicants have been surprised to learn that they share the same interests as the interviewer.

While this section should not be any longer than a line or two, make every word count.

Did you know...

"You will find you'll need a CV for scholarship, externship, fellowship, and other applications in your medical student years," writes the University of Iowa Carver College of Medicine.[2]

References

[1]Ohio State University College of Medicine. Available at: http://medicine.osu.edu/students/life/career_advising/pages/cv.aspx. Accessed July 2, 2014.
[2]University of Iowa Carver College of Medicine. Available at: http://www.medicine.uiowa.edu/md/cv/. Accessed July 22, 2014.

Chapter 8

Letters of Recommendation

You will recall that letters of recommendation were an important component of the medical school application. How important are letters in the scholarship application process? As you search for medical school scholarships, you will note that most applications ask for one or more letters of recommendation. You will also read language indicating that letters are a key component in the judging or selection process.

If you are able to secure and submit powerful letters of recommendation, you will significantly enhance the strength of your scholarship application. Because so many letters are unremarkable, glowing letters of recommendation will certainly set you apart from other applicants.

Your choice of letter writer can make a major difference in the strength of the letter. Although letter writers are well-intentioned, some produce suboptimal letters. Why does this happen? Most writers have never received instruction on how to write compelling reference letters. Some writers do not have the requisite writing skills to develop a powerful letter. Other factors that may impact letter quality include the writer's time, energy, mood, and desire.

Unlike other components of the scholarship application, letters of recommendation are not under your complete control. Although you cede control to the letter writer, most writers want to write the best letter possible. The good news is that you can do much more than you perhaps realize to make this a reality.

Of key importance is establishing and cultivating strong relationships with potential letter writers. As you progress through medical school, make relationship building a priority. Unfortunately, many students don't make these necessary efforts with the end result being the development of a mediocre or lukewarm letter.

Tip # 33

Find ways to build relationships with potential letter writers. Meet with faculty during office hours. Ask questions if time permits after class or lab. Are you a member of a med school group or organization? If so, interact with the faculty sponsor. Are you meeting with your mentor regularly? Such efforts can deepen your relationships, and provide writers with evidence needed to produce glowing reference letters.

As the deadline for the scholarship approaches, consider whom you will ask to write the letter. Begin the process by making a list of potential letter writers. At this point, do not be restrictive. Simply write down the names of all people who could possibly write you a letter. How well does each writer know you? What is the nature of your relationship? What are the qualities and skills you demonstrated through your interactions with the writer? Take the time to write the answers to these questions for each individual on your list.

Although you do not have to secure letters from everyone on your list, we recommend that you request letters from as many people as possible. Why? There is no way for you to know with certainty which letter or letters will be the strongest. When I was applying for a faculty award at the Baylor College of Medicine, I asked a colleague to write me a letter of recommendation. Since I had worked with her closely as part of an educator group for five years, I felt confident that she would write me a glowing letter of recommendation. You can imagine my surprise when she handed me a letter that was only four lines in length. Needless to say, I did not include this letter in my portfolio. Thankfully, I had requested and received letters from other colleagues. Take heed of my example, and make efforts to secure more letters than you need. After you receive all letters, you will be able to select which ones are best.

Tip # 34

Most scholarship programs ask applicants to include the letter of recommendation with the rest of the application. You will generally not be asked to waive your right to read the letter. This means that you will have the chance to read the letter and evaluate its quality before submission. If you have secured more letters than the number required, you can pick and choose which letter or letters to send.

Did you know…

Securing as many letters as possible also allows you to collect letters that highlight different qualities and strengths. Your writers will have worked with you in a variety of settings, and bring different perspectives.

Your chances of having glowing letters of recommendation increase considerably if you can help the letter writer write the letter. Obviously, you can't and shouldn't tell the writer what to say but most letter writers welcome information that would make it easier for them to draft the letter. The key is to do this tactfully and delicately.

> **Did you know…**
>
> Some scholarship applications ask letter writers to address certain qualities or areas. For example, the Endowment for South Asian Students of Indian Descent Scholarship requires two reference letters. Writers are asked to provide information about the applicant's integrity, interpersonal skills, and potential as a future physician. In order to be seriously considered for this award, you must communicate these instructions to your letter writer.

How should you proceed? A useful approach is to create an information packet containing essential information such as activities, accomplishments, and awards. We have seen some applicants overwhelm letter writers with too much information. Your goal is to provide only the information you would like the writer to address or include.

> **Tip # 35**
>
> Always include a cover letter (see example at end of chapter) with the following information:
>
> - Name of scholarship
> - Focus of the scholarship
> - Date letter is due
> - Instructions for the letter writer from the scholarship program
> - Specific points you hope the writer will include

If you will be applying for other scholarships, you may wish to ask the letter writer to provide you with an electronic unsigned copy of the letter. When you are ready to apply for another scholarship, you can simply replace any mention in the letter of the old scholarship with the new scholarship. After updating the letter, print it out and present it to the writer for his review and signature. This approach saves the writer considerable time and effort. It also ensures that your new letter is accurate with no delays in submission. Keep in mind that not all letter writers will be comfortable with this approach. You will have to decide whether to adopt this approach, taking into account the nature of your relationship. If you do not feel comfortable with this approach or the writer isn't able to accommodate you in this manner, you will need to ask the writer to make changes to the letter each time you decide to apply for a scholarship. Even if a writer provides you with an electronic unsigned copy, scholarships may differ in their instructions or preferences for letter content. If that's the case, the letter writer will have to modify the letter that was written.

Tip # 36

Thank letter writers every time they help you, and let them know when you win an award or scholarship. Although this seems obvious, medical students often don't follow up with letter writers or express appreciation. Since you will likely be applying for other awards, being courteous and appreciative will help you keep writers in your corner.

Since you will usually be able to read your reference letters, you must be able to differentiate between average and superb letters. This will ensure that you submit the most effective letters while avoiding mediocre ones.

What makes a letter strong? Strong letters of recommendation include specifics, the type of details that convince the reader that the praise is true. Stories and examples may be used to highlight certain strengths and qualities. After reading a strong letter of recommendation, the reader is left with the feeling that this letter was written for *you*.

Tip # 37

Among the most common mistakes scholarship applicants make is submitting a letter from a famous figure. Unless you know the writer well, such letters generally lack specifics. It is far better to select an individual who has worked with you closely over a significant period of time.

Tip # 38

Another advantage of securing scholarship letters is that it allows you to plan strategy in the future as it relates to the residency application process. Based on the quality of letters you receive, you will be able to decide which letter writers should remain in this position when it comes time to apply for residency.

Tip # 39

Most scholarship programs ask applicants to include the letter of recommendation with the rest of the application. You will generally not be asked to waive your right to read the letter. This means that you will have the chance to read the letter and evaluate its quality before submission. If you have secured more letters than the number required, you can pick and choose which letter or letters to send.

Sample Cover Letter for Recommendation Letter Writers

Your Name
Address

Date

Name
Title
Address

Dear _____:

I would like to apply for [Scholarship Name] sponsored by [Scholarship Organization]. This [Scholarship Name] is awarded to [Briefly Provide Description of Scholarship], and I believe that I would be eligible for this scholarship because of [Briefly Describe Qualifications or Fit]. To complete the application, I must submit a letter of recommendation. Since you have supervised me closely… [Briefly Describe Relationship], I would like to request a letter of recommendation from you in support of my application. The scholarship committee particularly values letters that address the applicant's leadership abilities and potential.

I have enclosed information to help you develop this letter:

- Curriculum vitae
- Additional information about me and my involvement outside the classroom

I have to include this letter as part of my application packet, and must submit the application on September 20. Upon completion of the letter, I will make arrangements to pick it up from you. If you have any questions or require additional information, please call me at [phone number] or email me at [email address].

Thank you so much for your help.

Sincerely,

Signature/Name

Did you know…

How do scholarship committee members evaluate letters of recommendation? They will look to see if the letter confirms what has been written in the application, and provides specific examples to support the student's characteristics or qualities. Reviewers will also determine if the letter distinguishes the student from others. In other words, the letter should be personalized in such a way that it could not possibly be written for someone else.

Chapter 9

Scholarship Essay

The most dreaded aspect of the scholarship application, for most students, is the essay. However, it should be viewed as a unique opportunity to impress the scholarship committee. In your essay you can showcase your strengths and those qualities that set you apart from other candidates. You can weave in evidence that confirms your qualities. You can use this opportunity to convince the scholarship committee that you would be an ideal candidate for their program.

With sufficient time and effort, you can create an essay that effectively sells yourself to the scholarship program. While a well-written essay can strengthen your application, a poorly written one can eliminate you from further consideration, even if you are a worthy applicant in all other respects.

Recognize the Importance of the Scholarship Essay

An essay is an important part of the application for many scholarship programs. In fact, some awards are bestowed solely on the quality of the essay. The ACLS Healthcare Training Scholarship asks applicants for nothing else but a 500 to 1000-word essay. "Share with us your experience with lifesaving techniques if you have assisted someone in the past, what you did, how you felt and how the situation was resolved. If not, let us know how you will handle being in these lifesaving situations in the future..."[1] Even when the essay is just one component of the scholarship application, don't underestimate its importance. Realize that many scholarship programs will receive applications from a number of qualified applicants with similar backgrounds, activities, and aspirations. An essay that makes you stand out from the field will significantly increase your chances of winning the award.

Tip # 40

A critical component of the scholarship application is the essay. Assuming that the rest of your application is compelling, a thoughtful and interesting essay can help you win the award over other qualified applicants. For scholarship programs that require an interview, an insightful and informative essay can lead the committee to offer you an interview invitation.

Understand the Purpose of the Scholarship Essay

What are your values and passions? What are your interests and ideals? What have your accomplished and achieved? What makes you unique? The answers to these questions are important to scholarship programs, and the essay is an opportunity to reveal who you are, what you have done, and what you have to offer.

Begin by Brainstorming

Writing the essay is a daunting task. Most applicants have no idea where or how to start. Without a plan, you may be stuck waiting for random inspiration. A specific strategy can make this entire process easier by breaking a large task into smaller, more manageable components.

Your first step is to brainstorm. One goal is to pinpoint a unique or distinctive item about you that will pique the scholarship committee's interest. Take a piece of paper or sit in front of your computer, and start writing down everything you can think of, without any editing. It may even be better to record your answers to these questions on a tape recorder, since transcribing the text may provide further inspiration. Now ask yourself the following questions:

- What are my strengths and skills?
- What are my most significant accomplishments?
- What activities am I most proud of?
- What makes me stand out from the rest of the candidates?
- What is unique or distinctive about me or my life story (undergraduate, medical school, personal events, work experience, volunteer experience, teaching experience, research, hobbies, languages, travel, sports, etc.)?
- Why should the scholarship committee be interested in me?
- Was there a challenge or hardship that I had to overcome? How did this experience shape me?
- If I had to write my own letter of recommendation, what are the most important things I would include?
- What are my professional goals and aspirations?

If you find it difficult to answer any of these questions, look over your CV. Discuss your accomplishments and experiences with a friend, family member, or advisor. Those close to you may be able to identify accomplishments which have escaped your attention. Consider polling those close to you while writing your essay. The following questions may be used as springboards for discussion:

- What is it about me that the scholarship committee absolutely needs to know?
- What is about me or my background that you find distinctive?

- Are there any events or experiences in my background that would be of interest to a scholarship committee?
- Which of my qualities or skills should I showcase in my statement? How do you think these qualities or skills have helped me in the past? How might they help me be successful in my career?

Responses to these questions can be used to help you outline your essay.

Tip # 41

Are you having difficulty coming up with a unique characteristic, experience, or subject to write about in your essay? Many students are anxious to complete their essay, and consider sitting around and "reflecting" to be a waste of time. Many therefore skip this critical step.

Consider starting your essay with a hook

Scholarship committees may be reading hundreds of essays. That's why it's often recommended that essays begin with an attention-grabbing statement. You can capture your reader's attention by beginning with a story, question, quote, or even an anecdote. This will help your statement stand out. Does your opening draw the reader into the rest of your essay?

No matter how you choose to hook your audience, make sure that the hook is relevant to the purpose of your essay. Telling a catchy story is only effective if you can tie it in to this point.

Tip # 42

The essay question you are asked to address may have bearing on your decision to use a hook. If the essay question asks you to address a particular issue, you may feel more comfortable starting the essay with a thesis statement which provides the reader with an idea of what's to come.

Tip # 43

Many scholarship applicants find the introduction to be the most difficult part of the essay to write. There's no rule that says you must write the introduction first. If you're having difficulty, move on to the body of the essay. You can come back to the introduction later.

> **Tip # 44**
>
> The body of the essay is what follows the introduction, and is typically 2 – 3 paragraphs in length. In the body, you will develop your main points and ideas. Each paragraph should be devoted to the development of a main point. In evaluating your essay, scholarship committees will see if your points are logically presented with a natural flow from one paragraph to another.

Back statements up with support

In reviewing essays, we've seen how common it is for students to make statements without providing the support that makes the assertions believable. This is a particularly common mistake, one that often leads scholarship committees to remove applications from further consideration. Instead of simply writing that you are resilient, incorporate into the essay a situation or story that demonstrates your resilience. If you've made strong contributions in advocacy through persistence and determination, describe an activity or event in which you've shown these qualities.

Be revealing

To be compelling, your essay must be personal. In other words, it should reveal something about you. Applicants often fail to do this, and the end result is an essay that could have been written by just about anyone. Although others may have been involved in the same activities, you have brought your own thoughts and perspectives to these experiences, and your beliefs have guided, shaped, and stimulated you in different ways. The incorporation of personal details into the essay can make your essay more powerful.

Programs don't always want a generic statement. Read the instructions.

Many scholarship programs ask the applicant to address specific questions or issues. The Buckfire & Buckfire P.C. Medical School Diversity Scholarship asks applicants to submit a personal essay describing how you will utilize your medical degree to promote ethnic diversity. The Polish University Club of New Jersey Scholarship requires a personal statement that addresses the question, "If you were to present a twenty minute talk at a meeting of the Polish University Club of NJ on a topic of your choice, what would it be?" To be considered for the Paul Calebresi Medical Student Research Fellowship, applicants must submit a personal statement describing your plans for the future, synopsis of your career, your interests, and how the fellowship will affect your path.

> **Tip # 45**
>
> Before you write, carefully review any personal statement directions the program may have. Failure to follow the instructions may lead the program to remove your application from further consideration.

Know your audience. Convince them that you embody the qualities that they are seeking.

Before drafting your personal statement, consider your audience. Every scholarship program is searching for a particular type of student. How can you determine what they are looking for?

- Carefully read the criteria used for the selection of scholarship winners
- Research the organization and its mission
- Look closely over the questions you are asked to address in the essay
- Learn about past award recipients

These efforts will help you determine what you should emphasize in the essay. Is the program looking for someone who has demonstrated commitment to community service? Does the award seek to recognize someone who has shown exemplary professionalism? With this information in hand, you'll be ready to tailor your essay in the appropriate way.

Finish your essay early.

It may not take that long to actually crank out a one-page essay. However, we recommend that you start the process a minimum of two months out. Brainstorming and outlining should be done in multiple sessions, especially since you need to provide multiple opportunities for inspiration to hit. You'll also need to give your reviewers sufficient time to complete their work, and to provide yourself enough time to process their comments and make multiple revisions.

Submit a personal essay of the correct length.

Do whatever it takes to create a personal essay that is the "right" length. First, comply with all rules regarding the length of the personal statement. Second, don't go on and on. Your audience includes scholarship committee members who have neither the time nor the patience to read through lengthy tomes.

Tip # 46

Scholarship committees appreciate sentences that are concise and direct. Avoid using extraneous or unnecessary words. Choose your words carefully, using the right word rather than the longest word possible.

Don't submit a personal essay that is too short, either. A short statement suggests that you did not expend much time, energy, and effort in its creation.

Learn the art of effective self-promotion.

Some applicants downplay their successes in the personal essay. They hesitate to make strong statements about their strengths and skills for fear that it might be perceived as self-serving. While humility is an admirable quality, it shouldn't be the aim of your personal essay. You must be able to write about your accomplishments, skills, and strengths in a way that emphasizes that you are a desirable candidate.

Tip # 47

The personal essay is not place to be modest. You have to be comfortable writing about your assets. If you don't, who will?

Leave out your entire life story

In the one page that you have for your personal essay, you cannot, and should not, try to write your life story. Some applicants write about all the experiences and events that they consider significant. It is far better to describe a few events or accomplishments in some detail, and emphasize what these experiences meant to you, and how they reflect upon your individual strengths. A laundry list of experiences, events, and honors in an essay will read like a resume or CV, and it would not reveal anything new about you.

Do not permit even a single spelling or grammatical mistake.

Spelling and grammatical mistakes are glaring errors that can seriously damage your candidacy. "Please check your essays thoroughly as we will not be entertaining entries with grammatical errors and typos," writes ACLS Healthcare.[1]

One of our colleagues in medicine who is involved in the selection of residents reads every personal essay with a red pen in hand. He then proceeds to circle all grammatical, spelling, and punctuation errors. At the end of the statement, if he has more than a few circles, he downgrades the application.

Tip # 48

In reviewing your essay, scholarship committees will look at the quality of your writing, not just its content. While the proper grammar and spelling will not impress them, errors will severely weaken your application. The criteria for evaluation for the New Look Laser Tattoo Removal Semiannual Scholarship include posts that "give clear details, avoid grammatical or spelling errors, demonstrate creativity, and weave in the applicant's personal thoughts."[2]

To catch spelling errors, use the spell check function of your word processor. However, don't rely solely on the spell check. Proofread your work carefully, looking for both typographical and grammatical errors. It can be particularly useful to put aside your essay for a few days. Reading it with a fresh eye may help you spot these mistakes. Reading it out loud or backwards one word at a time are other useful techniques.

Ask others to review your essay.

When your essay is ready for submission, you should seek the feedback of others. When asking others to review your essay, avoid waiting until the last minute. Reviewers can make valuable suggestions, but only if they have sufficient time. Give them at least two to three weeks to read your essay. A hasty review may not be as thorough or helpful.

Your goal is to solicit detailed feedback from others. Note that you are seeking detailed feedback. Comments such as "it's great" are reassuring, but you really need to know how to improve your statement. Ask your reviewers if it holds their interest, if your main points are clear, if it flows smoothly, if it includes enough detail, and if it begins and ends in a compelling fashion.

Consider giving the reviewer an essay review form like the one we have developed on the following page.

Tip # 49

Always seek out several reviewers to read your personal essay before submission. This can be a parent, spouse, teacher, or friend but be sure to select people who write well and are detail-oriented.

Tip # 50

Some reviewers will be superb at spotting grammar and spelling errors. Others may be better or more focused on giving you advice about the essay's content. Aim to find both types of reviewers.

Tip # 51

Don't feel obliged to make every change that is recommended. However, if multiple reviewers make the same point, then give careful thought to their recommendation.

Did you know…

The University of Washington reminds scholarship committee members to assess the following with respect to scholarship essays:

- "Some applicants are fantastic writers who have great things to say on the surface, but no experience to back up their statements. Exceptional applicants will show, rather than tell, about themselves and their ideas.

- Does the applicant simply restate, or even copy wholesale, information from his or her resume/CV? Exceptional applicants will use the essays to provide context for the most pivotal experiences listed on the resume/CV, reflecting on them and going beyond, but not just recreate the list in narrative form."[3]

Scholarship Essay Review Form		
	Yes	No
When held at arm's length, the statement looks pleasing to the eye.		
The font size and type are consistent with essay instructions (or allow for easy reading if no instructions are given).		
Introduction includes an attention-grabber or thesis statement.		
Each paragraph revolves around a main idea or point.		
The paragraphs are too long.		
The ideas flow logically.		
There is good transition between the ideas in each paragraph.		
The word "I" is overused.		
The sentences are short and crisp rather than long and rambling.		
A variety of sentence structures are used to keep the essay interesting.		
Active rather than passive sentences are used.		
Action verbs and words are used.		
There are no unnecessary words.		
Grammatical/spelling errors are not present.		
Jargon and abbreviations are avoided.		
The essay keeps interest throughout.		
The essay revolves around a theme.		
The essay answers the question posed (if applicable).		
The essay establishes a relationship between the scholarship's mission and the applicant's goals or interests.		
The essay is neither too long nor too short.		
The essay is written in a professional, confident, and upbeat tone.		
There are no signs of arrogance.		

References

[1]ACLS Training Association. Available at:
http://www.aclsrecertification.com/scholarship. Accessed July 2, 2014.
[2]New Look Laser Tattoo Removal Semiannual Scholarship. Available at:
http://www.newlookhouston.com/New_Look_Scholarship.html. Accessed June 2, 2014.
[3]University of Washington. Available at:
http://expd.washington.edu/scholarships/common/general-guidelines-for-reviewing-scholarship-applications.html. Accessed July 2, 2014.

Chapter 10

Research Grants, Scholarships, and Fellowships

Medical students at the University of Wisconsin School of Medicine and Public Health are heavily involved in research, with many performing research in the summer between the first and second years of medical school. In fact, over 50% of students in the class of 2009 were awarded summer fellowships to perform research. According to Dr. Patrick McBride, Associate Dean for Students, summer research offers numerous benefits. Students gain a basic understanding of research, and their projects often lead to presentations and published manuscripts.[1]

Research can enhance the residency application. According to Dr. Julie Parsonnet, one positive effect of research is the "possibility that participating in a scholarly activity could result in publications and/or presentations that would improve a student's ability to match into a desired field and/or into a competitive residency program."[2] In a survey of University of Tennessee medical students, 63% reported that research experience was beneficial in helping them secure a residency position.[3]

Although most students secure funding for research through their own institutions, there are numerous grants and fellowships available through national organizations. These are prestigious awards that signal to others that your work is highly valued, and that you have to potential to make important contributions. In this chapter, we describe these awards in further detail and offer profiles of award recipients.

AcademyHealth Student Poster Award

Description: AcademyHealth is an organization that aims to improve health care by generating new knowledge and moving knowledge into action. It is the major forum for health services research. At the Annual Research Meeting in June, attendees discuss health policy and research issues. Medical students are eligible to submit their research for poster presentation. The Student Poster Award is given for outstanding research and quality of presentation.

To Apply: For more information, visit the website below.

Deadline: For information, please visit the following link:

http://www.academyhealth.org/about/content.cfm?ItemNumber=958&navItem Number=2342

American Academy of Neurology Medical Student Summer Research Scholarship (See Chapter 25)

American Association for the Surgery of Trauma Research and Education Foundation Medical Student Scholarship (See Chapter 23)

American College of Sports Medicine Student Awards

Description: The American College of Sports Medicine (ACSM) grants awards to those medical students who are interested in the field. Currently, there are six awards sponsored by the ACSM, and the Research Review Committee determines which grant award an applicant's project falls under:

- *ACSM Foundation Doctoral Student Research Grant*: Ten $5,000 awards are given to doctoral students enrolled in a full-time program to be used to defray costs for experimental purposes.

- *Coca-Cola Company Doctoral Student Research Grant on Behavior Research*: One $5,000 award is given to research that addresses "behavioral strategies and techniques to promote the adoption and maintenance of physical activity/exercise [in a given age group]. Studies that focus on innovative strategies to improve individual-level adoption and/or maintenance of physical activity will be given first priority."[4]

- *Raymond and Rosalee Weiss Research Endowment*: One $1,500 award is given to applied research involving the study of health benefits of physical activity and sports. Psychological and emotional benefits are of particular importance to this award and are, as such, given priority.

- *NASA Space Physiology Research Grant*: $5,000 awards are given to research addressing "exercise, weightlessness, and musculoskeletal physiology."[4]

- *Carl V. Gisolfi Memorial Fund*: One $5,000 award is granted to research involving "thermoregulation, exercise, and hydration."[4]

- *International Student Award*: This $1,000 award helps defray the costs of travel to the ACSM Annual Meeting for students who have been accepted to present research.

To Apply: Candidates must fill out a common ACSM Foundation Research Grant Program application to apply for the aforementioned awards. In addition, the candidate be a member of ACSM at the time of application submission and must have graduate student status by the time of funding. International candidates are welcome to participate in all grants with the exception of the NASA Space Physiology Research Grant, which is open to U.S. residents only. **Deadline:** The deadline for all awards listed is in January except for the International Student Award (February deadline). More information can be found on the award's website:

http://www.acsm.org/find-continuing-education/awards-grants/student-awards

American Dermatological Association Medical Student Fellowship Program (See Chapter 20)

American Heart Association Student Scholarships in Cardiovascular Disease (See Chapter 24)

American Medical Association Seed Grant Research Program

Description: Due to the increasing difficulty of young physician scientists to find adequate resources and support for research, the American Medical Association (AMA) Foundation created the Seed Grant Research Program. This program was founded in 2000 to encourage medical students, physician residents and fellows to enter the research field. The program will provide $2,500 to selected individuals to help them conduct small basic science, applied, or clinical research projects.

To Apply: To be eligible, applicants must be medical students, physician residents or fellows of an accredited United States medical school or institution. Applicants must also be permanent residents or citizens of the United States. AMA membership is not required to apply for this program and does not factor into the grant selection process.

Deadline: The deadline for application is usually in December and recipients are announced in March. For information, please visit the following link:

http://www.ama-assn.org/ama/pub/about-ama/ama-foundation/our-programs/medical-education/seed-grant-research.page

American Medical Association Research Symposium

Description: The American Medical Association (AMA) invites its medical student, resident, fellow, and international medical graduate members to submit abstracts of their scientific research. Abstracts will be reviewed, and considered for poster presentation at the Symposium. A small number will be chosen for participation in the Oral Presentation Competition. The Symposium is held in November. Medical students are eligible to win prizes in eight categories (biochemistry/cell biology, cancer biology, clinical outcomes and healthcare improvement, immunology/infectious disease/inflammation, neurobiology/neuroscience, public health and epidemiology, radiology/imaging, and surgery/biomedical engineering.

To Apply: Visit the website below for more information.
Deadline: The deadline for application is in August. For information, please visit the following link:

http://www.ama-assn.org/ama/pub/about-ama/our-people/member-groups-sections/medical-student-section/news-events/research-symposium.page

---

Profile of a Winner

In 2009, the AMA awarded the Seed Grant to Dr. Ami Raval, a Tufts Medical Center neurosurgery resident. "The seed grant allowed me to form my own niche in the lab and do my own research," said Dr. Raval in an AMA article.[5]

Dr. Raval has been performing research to identify ways to halt or slow down the progression of glioblastoma multiforme (GBM), the most common type of primary brain tumor. In the future, she hopes that her research will not only lead to a better understanding of the genetic component of GBM, but also provide means for a direct-targeted therapy for malignant brain tumors.

In 2014, Rachel Hanke, a second-year medical student at the Oakland University William Beaumont School of Medicine, was one recipient of the AMA Seed Grant. The funding will support her efforts to identify patients at risk for stroke. Her research involves analysis of blood and plaque samples of patients with carotid atherosclerosis. The hope is that the work will allow her research team to identify biological markers linked to plaques that are unstable. This knowledge could then be used to develop blood tests to identify these high-risk patients.

"It's not very common for a second-year medical student to win a grant like this," said her mentor, Dr. Samia Ragheb. "The Seed Grant Research Program from the AMA Foundation is intended to support research by medical students, physician residents and fellows. Rachel was competing with residents and fellows who are more advanced in their studies, and also with students from medical schools all over the country."[6]

American Society of Clinical Nutrition Internship Program

Description: Through the program, medical students have the opportunity to work with a clinical nutrition expert. The internship usually takes place during the summer, and lasts for eight weeks. The award amount is $2,500.
To Apply: The application includes transcript, CV, Dean's letter, and personal statement.
Deadline: The application deadline is in January/February. For more information, visit:

http://www.nutrition.org/education-and-professional-development/graduate-and-professional-development/clinical-nutrition-internship-program/

Profile of a Winner

Gregory Joice, a fourth-year medical student at Columbia University College of Physicians & Surgeons, was the overall winner among medical students at the 2014 AMA Research Symposium. He was recognized for his talk, "Failure to Rescue and Inter-Hospital Transfer after Radical Cystectomy." This was research he performed for his school's Scholarly Project requirement. His work involved studying death in the 30 days following complications of radical cystectomy. He began the research during the summer after his first year of medical school, and worked with faculty members in the Department of Urology. He chose to perform outcomes research because it "gives you results much sooner than clinical trials or basic science, so it made sense for me to work on it as a medical student." Joice is planning to pursue a career in urology.[7]

American Skin Association Medical Student Grants Targeting Melanoma and Skin Cancer (See Chapter 20)

American Society of Colon and Rectal Surgeons Medical Student Research Initiation Grant (See Chapter 23)

American Society of Nephrology Scholar Grants and Funding (See Chapter 24)

Association for Academic Surgery Student Research Award (See Chapter 23)

Baystate Summer Student Scholars Program

Description: Baystate Medical Center, the Western Campus of Tufts University School of Medicine, offers a mentored research program for eligible college and medical students who are exploring the potential of a career in medical, biomedical, public health, or behavioral health research. The 10-week summer program offers the opportunity to participate in a research project from start to finish and present project outcomes to the scientific community. A stipend of $3,500 is awarded to Summer Scholars.

To Apply: Eligible students are limited to local college juniors and senior and medical students (either entering medical school or between the first and second years) who are exploring the potential of a career in medical, biomedical, public health, or behavioral health research.

Deadline: Application materials must be received by February. For more information, visit:

http://baystatehealth.org/AcademicAffairs/Main+Nav/Research/Summer+Student+Scholars

Carolinas HealthCare System Summer Research Scholars Program

Description: Through the Summer Research Scholars Program at Carolinas HealthCare System, medical students can conduct original research under the supervision of faculty mentors. Research can be performed in a variety of disciplines. Scholars receive a stipend of $5,000 for the ten-week experience. At the end of the research period, scholars will present their work at a student research day where prizes will be awarded.
To Apply: Medical students are eligible to apply. An undergraduate overall GPA ≥ 3.5 is required as is an undergraduate math and science GPA ≥ 3.6. The application includes transcripts and three letters of recommendation. Prior interest in and commitment to research is valued.
Deadline: Application materials must be received by February. For more information, visit:

http://www.carolinashealthcare.org/summer-research-scholars#guidelines

Carolyn L. Kuckein Student Research Fellowship

Description: The Alpha Omega Alpha (AΩA) Student Research Fellowship is for clinical investigation, basic laboratory research, epidemiology, social science/health service research, leadership, or professionalism. Research support will be given for a continual period of a minimum of 8 to 10 weeks, 30 hours or more per week, or an average of 4 hours per week for 12 months over 1 to 2 years. Recipients will receive $5,000. Half will be given on announcement of the award. The other half will be released on approval by AΩA of a final report of the research. Up to $ 1,000 will be reimbursed for travel to present research results at a national meeting.
To Apply: Only first-, second-, and third-year students from schools with active AΩA chapters are eligible. Each school may select only one candidate for nomination. See the link below for more information.
Deadline: The proposal to the AΩA councilor is due in December. Applications are then sent by the councilor to the AOA national office in January. Visit the following link for more information:

http://www.alphaomegaalpha.org/student_research.html

Profile of a Winner

Ingrid Wahjudi, a student at the Loma Linda University School of Medicine, was a recent recipient of AΩA Student Research Fellowship. "Personally, the research fellowship was invaluable to my experience in medical school," she wrote in an article published on the AΩA website. "It opened the doors for me to work in the field of medicine that I am interested in. Prior to this, I had never done clinical research. This fellowship enabled me to gain experience in going through the process of clinical research from applying for IRBs, setting up databases, analyzing statistical data, and performing surgery. Through this process I got to know urology attendings and residents and learn more about urology. In addition, this opened the doors for me to publish abstracts and articles in urologic journals and speak at two conferences about my project. These are just a few of the opportunities that I experienced through the generosity of this grant."[8]

Center for Science in the Public Interest Internship Program

Description: The Center for Science in the Public Interest aims to promote national policies responsive to consumers' interests. Its primary focus is on health and nutrition issues. Internships are available for medical students during the summer as well as the school year. Students are paid at a rate of $9.25/hour.
To Apply: The application includes cover letter, resume, and writing sample. Candidates invited for interview may have to submit letters of recommendation.
Deadline: There are three application review periods (February/March, July/August, and December/January for summer, fall, and spring internships, respectively). For more information, visit:

http://www.cspinet.org/about/jobs/200801042.html

Charles S. Houston Award

Description: The Wilderness Medical Society (WMS) is keenly interested in fostering awareness and appreciation among healthcare professionals and scientists for the research of health-related concerns in outdoor and wilderness activities. The Charles S. Houston Award is given annually to one or two students who have submitted research proposals most likely to result in a substantive contribution to the field of wilderness and environmental medicine.
To Apply: The successful applicant will submit a project proposal and conduct a well-defined project during the ensuing year and present an abstract of his/her findings at a future WMS Annual Meeting.
Deadline: Applications are accepted annually at the end of the year. For more information, visit:

http://wms.org/research/default.asp

Chinese American Medical Society Research Scholarship

Description: The Chinese American Medical Society (CAMS) offers scholarships for medical students working on summer research projects. The purpose is to promote and support clinical and basic science research among Chinese American medical and dental students. Students will be paid a stipend of $400 per week for 6 to 10 weeks. Research support and expenses are the responsibility of the sponsor.

To Apply: Projects lasting 6 to 10 weeks can either be in the basic sciences or clinical research. A dentist or a physician must sponsor and supervise the project. For application information, visit the website below.

Deadline: The application deadline is in April. For more information, visit:

http://chineseamericanmedicalsociety.cloverpad.org/Default.aspx?pageId=1070537

Cook/Rutledge Fellowship

Description: The Office of Minority and Multicultural Health at the New Jersey Department of Health and Senior Services offers the Cook/Rutledge Fellowship to medical students interested in gaining a better understanding of the health disparity issues impacting the racial, ethnic minority populations in New Jersey. The award amount is $6,000 for 8 – 10 weeks.

To Apply: The program is only open to residents of New Jersey attending school either in or out of state. The application includes resume, Dean's Letter, and two reference letters. A personal essay describing the applicant's interest and experience relevant to the fellowship is also required.

Deadline: The application deadline is in February. For more information, visit:

http://rwjms.rutgers.edu/education/current_students/research_commexp/research_listing/research_clinical/documents/cr_fellowship2014.pdf

Crohn's & Colitis Foundation Student Research Fellowship Award (See Chapter 24)

Cystic Fibrosis Foundation Student Traineeships (See Chapter 32)

David E Rogers Fellowship Program

Description: The Rogers Fellowship provides research funding to medical and dental students interested in addressing the human needs of underserved or disadvantaged patients or populations. Up to five grants will be awarded with a stipend of $4,000 each for research projects in the summer of the award year. The stipend will be paid directly to the student in two equal installments (at the beginning and end of the grant period).

To Apply: Competition is open to candidates attending medical or dental school in the United States. Funding will be provided for research projects lasting between ten and twelve weeks in the summer of the application year.

Deadline: Generally at the beginning of every year. For more information, visit:

http://www.nyam.org/grants/rogers.html

Profile of a Winner

Edison Tsui is a third-year medical student at The Commonwealth Medical College (TCMC). Initially from Seattle, Washington, Edison was attracted to TCMC based on its mission to train physicians through an innovative community-based curriculum. Edison was one of several recipients of the 2012 David E. Rogers Fellowship bestowed by The New York Academy of Medicine.

His project titled "A Mulitlingual Population Health Management Program" involved studying a health program utilized by the Seattle-based community health center, International Community Health Services (ICHS). The program focuses on the management of chronic disease, and was designed to serve a diverse patient population speaking over a dozen languages. The research project was supported by mentorship from TCMC faculty and ICHS.

The study results were published in the *Journal of Ambulatory Care Management*. In the future, Edison plans on using his experience gained from this fellowship program to provide quality and population-based patient care.[9]

Eastern-Atlantic Student Research Forum

Description: The Eastern-Atlantic Student Research Forum is an international symposium held at the University of Miami Leonard M. Miller School of Medicine. Students and resident physicians have the opportunity to present original basic science and clinical research in a variety of fields. Multiple awards are given at the symposium.
To Apply: The process begins with submission of an abstract. If the abstract is chosen for oral and/or poster presentation, the applicant will then prepare and submit a manuscript. For application information and instructions, contact the organization.
Deadline: The deadline for abstract submission is September. For more information, visit:

http://uresearch.miami.edu/esrf

EMF/SAEM Medical Student Research Grant (See Chapter 21)

EMRA Research Grant (See Chapter 21)

Endocrine Society Summer Research Fellowship (See Chapter 24)

Epilepsy Foundation Student Fellowships (See Chapter 25)

Excellence in Professional Student (MD or DO) Research Travel Award

Description: The Excellence in Professional Student (MD or DO) Research Travel Award provides up to $1,800 in funding to cover the costs associated with travel and registration for the Experimental Biology Meeting. The applicant must be working with a member of the American Physiological Society, and present his research at the meeting.
To Apply: For application information and instructions, contact the organization.
Deadline: For more information, visit:

http://www.the-aps.org/mm/awards/Other-APS-Awards/Graduate-or-Medical-Student

Frontera/Border Health Scholars Program

Description: Through this ten-week summer research experience at the Arizona Health Sciences Center in Tucson, medical students will have the opportunity to explore health inequities.
To Apply: For application information and instructions, contact the organization.
Deadline: The deadline for the application is in March. For more information, contact Kameron Hanson at (520) 626 – 6148 or khanson@azcc.arizona.edu.

Ferdinand C. Valentine Medical Student Research Grant (See Chapter 38)

Fight for Sight Summer Student Scholarship (See Chapter 28)

Gina M. Finzi Memorial Student Summer Fellowship (See Chapter 24)

Glorney-Raisbeck Medical Student Grants in Cardiovascular Research (See Chapter 24)

Grants Targeting Melanoma and Skin Cancer (See Chapter 20)

Gold Student Summer Fellowships

Description: The Student Summer Fellowship program offers opportunities for medical students to complete a research or service project related to community health. Projects are focused on studying cultural competency issues, developing skills to become relationship-centered physicians, and addressing a public health need in an underserved community or population. Forty-one fellowships are awarded for a service or research project. Projects take place in the U.S. or in developing countries with students working on community health issues affecting underserved patient populations.

To Apply: Projects must meet a 10-week requirement. Medical students at an accredited U.S. or Canadian school of medicine or osteopathy may apply for either the Research Fellowship or the Service Fellowship program.

Deadline: Annually in March and notifications of awards are given in May. For more information, visit:

http://www.humanism-in-medicine.org/index.php/programs_grants/gold_foundation_programs/student_summer_fellowships

---

Profile of a Winner

At the University of Virginia School of Medicine, Emily Knudsen, a student in the Class of 2015, is excited about her research linking medical students with underserved diabetes mellitus patients in an effort to improve glucose control. "Students will meet patients in the program face-to-face in clinic and call them on the phone each week to go over their blood glucose readings and adjust patients' insulin dosage," said Knudsen in an article posted on the school's website. Her research is supported by the Arnold P. Gold Foundation, and she is the recipient of the Student Summer Fellowship.[10]

Herbert Brendler, MD Summer Medical Student Fellowship Program (See Chapter 38)

HONORS (Hematology Opportunities for the Next Generation of Research Scientists) Award (See Chapter 24)

Hospital for Special Surgery Medical Student Summer Research Fellowship (See Chapter 29)

Howard Hughes Medical Institute Summer Medical Fellows Program

Description: The Howard Hughes Medical Institute (HHMI) administers the Summer Medical Fellows Program. Through this program, fellows spend 8 to 10 weeks performing research under the supervision of a HHMI investigator, HHMI early career scientist, or Janelia scientist. Up to 20 fellowships are awarded annually. The award amount is $5,000.

To Apply: This program is for medical, dental, and veterinary students attending schools located in the United States. Applicants must be first- or second-year students. For application information, visit the website below.

Deadline: The deadline is in February. For more info, visit:

http://www.hhmi.org/programs/medical-research-fellows-program/summer-program

Howard Hughes Medical Institute Medical Research Fellows Program

Description: The Howard Hughes Medical Institute (HHMI) administers the Medical Research Fellows Program. Through this program, fellows have the opportunity to perform one year of basic, translational, or applied biomedical research at any research institution in the United States or abroad.

To Apply: Key criteria for selection include mentor selection and research project proposal. Medical student applicants are urged to work with an HHMI investigator, early career scientist, or HHMI professor. For application information and information, visit the website below.

Deadline: The deadline is in January. For more info, visit:

http://www.hhmi.org/programs/medical-research-fellows-program/year-long-program

Howard Hughes Medical Institute Year-Long Medical Fellows Program at Janelia and K-RITH

Description: The Howard Hughes Medical Institute (HHMI) administers the Year-Long Medical Fellows Program at Janelia and K-RITH. At the Janelia Farm Research Campus, students interested in neuronal network function or imaging at the cellular and molecular level can perform research. Students interested in researching HIV or TB should consider applying for fellowship positions at K-RITH.

To Apply: For application information and information, visit the website below.

Deadline: The deadline is in January. For more info, visit:

http://www.hhmi.org/programs/medical-research-fellows-program/year-long-program-at-janelia/eligibility-financial-support-and-application-process

Profile of a Winner

David Blauvelt, a student in the class of 2015 at Harvard Medical School, was a HHMI Fellow during the academic year 2012 – 2013. He generated high-resolution, 3-dimensional images of vasculature using light. By color coding individual vessels by velocity, he hopes to use the knowledge and technology to better study tumor angiogenesis and vascular disease. Fellows in the program also benefit from the networking opportunities available at HHMI dinners attended by prominent scientists. "Many fellowship programs give monetary support, but few provide these enrichment experiences," said Blauvelt in an interview with *The Benefactor*. "I want to take advantage of everything thrown my way." His goals as a fellow also include presenting research at major conferences and publishing his work in journals.[11]

Icahn School Environmental and Occupational Health Summer Traineeship

Description: The Division of Environmental and Occupational Medicine of the Department of Community and Preventive Medicine at the Icahn School of Medicine offers NIH-funded summer traineeships to interested medical students to learn more about the field. The traineeships are available for periods of eight to ten weeks during June, July and August. A standard NIH stipend is provided.
To Apply: The student works on a research project under the supervision of experienced faculty in occupational and environmental medicine, epidemiology, or toxicology. Emphasis is on learning methods of research and understanding the context of the research.
Deadline: The application deadline is in February. Applicants will be notified by March or sooner. For more information, visit:

http://icahn.mssm.edu/departments-and-institutes/preventive-medicine/programs-and-services/environmental-and-occupational-health-summer-program

Infectious Disease Society of North American Scholar Program (See Chapter 24)

James Ewing Foundation Summer Fellowships in Oncology (See Chapter 23)

Joan F. Giambalvo Memorial Scholarship

Description: This is a scholarship open to medical students interested in performing research on professional work/practice issues affecting women physicians.

To Apply: To be eligible, the applicant must be performing research alone or in collaboration with others on a project that focuses on professional work/practice issues affecting women physicians. A budget must be submitted.

Deadline: The deadline is in February. For more information, visit:

http://www.ama-assn.org

Joslin Summer Research Student Internship

Description: Through this program, medical students can participate in diabetes-related biomedical research during a 10-12 week summer experience. Two funded positions are available for current medical students, dental students, and graduate students. An additional six positions are available at Joslin through the NIDDK Medical Student Research Program in Diabetes. Students will receive a stipend of $3,000.

To Apply: For application information and instructions, visit the website below.

Deadline: The deadline is in January. For more information, visit:

http://summerstudent.joslinresearch.org/content/2014-joslin-research-summer-student-internship

Lawrence S. Linn Research Grant

Description: Through this Society of General Internal Medicine grant program, young investigators receive funding for HIV or AIDS research. The award amount is up to $5,000. Medical students may apply for the grant.

To Apply: Criteria for evaluation include originality, significance, methodological rigor, and likelihood of being completed. For application information and instructions, visit the website below.

Deadline: The deadline is in January. For more information, visit:

http://www.sgim.org/career-center/awards-and-grants/national-grants/linn-grant

Los Angeles Children's Hospital Summer Oncology Fellowship (See Chapter 32)

M-STREAM Program (See Chapter 35)

Massachusetts General Hospital Division of Thoracic Surgery Summer Scholars Program (See Chapter 23)

Medical Student Anesthesia Research Fellowship Program (See Chapter 19)

Melanoma Research Foundation Grant (See Chapter 20)

Memorial Sloan-Kettering Cancer Center Medical Student Summer Fellowship Research Program (See Chapter 24)

Midwestern Student Biomedical Research Forum

Description: The Midwest Student Biomedical Research Forum is a symposium sponsored by the University of Nebraska Medical Center and Creighton University. Medical students have the opportunity to present their original biomedical research in either an oral or poster format. Multiple awards are given at the symposium.
To Apply: Abstracts for original basic science or clinical science research are accepted. For further application information and instructions, contact the organization.
Deadline: The deadline for abstract submission is December. For more information, visit:

https://unmc.edu/cce/msbrf.htm

Myofascial Trigger Points Research Scholarship (See Chapter 33)

NASPGHAN Foundation Summer Student Mentor Program (See Chapter 32)

National Space Biomedical Research Institute Summer Apprenticeship Program

Description: The summer apprenticeship program provides medical students with the opportunity to gain experience in space biomedical research at the Johnson Space Center in Houston, Glenn Research Center in Cleveland, or Ames Research Center in California. This 11-week program comes with a stipend of $6,600.
To Apply: The application includes CV, letter of interest, and reference letter.
Deadline: The deadline is in December. For more information, visit:

http://www.nsbri.org/summerapprenticeship/

National Student Research Forum

Description: The National Student Research Forum is an international symposium held at the University of Texas Medical Branch in Galveston, Texas. Medical students have the opportunity to present research in the basic sciences, clinical sciences, or medical humanities. The work may not have been published prior to abstract submission. Multiple awards are given at the symposium. Approximately $9,000 in prize money is awarded.

To Apply: The process begins with submission of an abstract. If the abstract is chosen for oral presentation, the applicant will then prepare and submit a manuscript. For further application information and instructions, contact the organization.

Deadline: The deadline for abstract submission is February. For more information, visit:

http://www.utmb.edu/nsrf/

NIH Medical Research Scholars Program

Description: The National Institutes of Health sponsors the Medical Research Scholars Program (MSRP). This is a year-long immersive experience for research-oriented medical students at the NIH campus in Bethesda, Maryland. Scholars perform basic, clinical, or translational research under the supervision of a mentor.

To Apply: Medical students who have completed core clerkships are eligible to apply. However, applications will be accepted from students with strong research interests who have not completed their clinical rotations. For application information and instructions, visit the website below.

Deadline: The deadline is in January. For more information, visit:

http://clinicalcenter.nih.gov/training/mrsp/index.html

New York City Health Department HRTP

Description: The New York City Health Department administers the Public Health Internship Program. Medical students can work closely with professionals with expertise in public health. Interns receive direct hands on experience, attend seminars, and participate in workshops.

To Apply: Medical students who are residents of New York City may apply. The application includes personal statement and letter of recommendation.

Deadline: There are three available sessions with application deadlines in February, August, and November. For more information, visit:

http://www.nyc.gov/html/doh/html/career/hrtp.shtml

Pharmaceutical Research and Manufacturers of America Foundation Paul Calabresi Medical Student Research Fellowship

Description: The Pharmaceutical Research and Manufacturers of America Foundation offers the Paul Calabresi Medical Student Research Fellowship to students with an interest in pursuing research and teaching careers in pharmacology. The fellowship duration must be at least six months, and can last up to 24 months. The stipend is $1,500/month up to a maximum of

$18,000. The research can take place either at the applicant's school or another institution.

To Apply: Medical students who have completed at least one year of school are eligible to apply. Applicants who have demonstrated strong commitments to careers in clinical pharmacology will be given preference. The application includes CV, research plan, research abstract, Dean's Letter, reference letter from faculty sponsor, sponsor's biosketch, budget, and two other reference letters. A personal essay describing your plans for the future, synopsis of your career, your interests, and how the fellowship will affect your path is required.
Deadline: The deadline is in February. For more information, visit:

http://www.phrmafoundation.org/index.php?option=com_award&task=sdetail &id=20

Pine Family Foundation Scholarship

Description: The Pine Family Foundation offers scholarships for students interesting in conducting AIDS or Alzheimer's disease research.
To Apply: For application information and instructions, visit the website below.
Deadline: For more information, visit:

http://www.pinefamilyfoundation.org/

Ragon Institute Outreach, Education and Training Program

Description: The goal of this program is to encourage students to pursue research in HIV. During this 8 – 12 week research experience, students perform research, attend lectures, and participate in departmental events. At the end of the experience, students will have the opportunity to submit a written report, poster, and oral presentation.
To Apply: Medical students are eligible to apply. The application includes CV and personal letter. The letter should describe your motivation for applying to the program and previous research experience.
Deadline: The application deadline is in March. For more information, visit:

http://ragoninstitute.org/education/summer-program/

Reading Hospital and Medical Center Student Summer Training Grant Program

Description: Reading Hospital and Medical Center offers 6-week internships to medical students. Half of the time is spent in research. Seven internships are available in internal medicine (2), family medicine (2), obstetrics & gynecology (2), and infectious disease (1). Interns work closely with faculty members, observe patient care, and participate in research projects that may lead to publication. Interns will receive a stipend of $2,000.

To Apply: The application includes transcript and resume. A personal statement describing area of interest, aptitude in medicine and a description of benefits expected to be gained from the program is also required.
Deadline: The application deadline is in March. For more information, visit:

https://www.readinghealth.org/education-and-research/academic-affairs/students/undergrad-internships/student-summer-training-program/

Rheumatology Research Foundation Medical and Graduate Student Achievement Award (See Chapter 24)

Ross Student Research Fellowship (See Chapter 23)

Sigma Xi Scientific Research Society Grants-in-Aid of Research Program

Description: Through the Sigma Xi Grants-in-Aid of Research Program, medical students can receive up to $1,000 to support research. Grants of up to $2,500 and $5,000 are also available for vision-related and astronomy research, respectively.
To Apply: Students currently enrolled in medical school are eligible to apply. Although membership in Sigma Xi is not required, students who are members or whose project advisor is a member are more likely to receive full funding. For application information and instructions, visit the website below.
Deadline: For more information, visit:

https://sigmaxi.fluidreview.com/

Society for the History of Navy Medicine Graduate and Medical Professional Student Research Grant

Description: An annual grant of $1,500 is available from the Society for the History of Navy Medicine for research in the history of naval or maritime medicine.
To Apply: Although society membership is not required, it is encouraged. The application includes project description and budget.
Deadline: The deadline is in April. For more information, visit:

http://historyofnavymedicine.org/programs/studentresearchgrant/

Society of American Gastrointestinal and Endoscopic Surgeons Medical Student Scholarship Award (See Chapter 23)

Society of Vascular Surgery Student Research Fellowship (See Chapter 23)

Summer Internship Scholarship in Cardiovascular Surgery (See Chapter 23)

Vanderbilt University Research Training Program (See Chapter 24)

Visiting Immunology Scholars Program

Description: Through this program, medical students are able to spend 1 – 2 weeks at another medical institution. The program was established to support the clinical and laboratory training experiences of the awardee. Each awardee will receive $1,000 - $2,000.
To Apply: The application includes CV, letter of support from Department Head, and career statement outlining goals and potential impact of a visiting scholar's experience on attaining those goals.
Deadline: There are three application cycles with deadlines in April, August, and December. For more information, visit:

http://usidnet.org/mentoring/visiting-immunology-scholars-program/

Western Medical Student Research Forum

Description: The Western Medical Student Research Forum is open to medical students, and allows a venue for the presentation of research. The Forum takes place in January. Participants are eligible to win one of the following awards:

- WAFMR Edwin E. Osgood Student Research Award
- WSPR Lowell Glasgow Student Pediatric Research Award
- WCSI Student Subspecialty Awards
- WSMRF Klea D. Bertakis, Dionesia P. Bertakis, Gale Hansen Starich, Clifford Lardinois, Claude Lardinois, and David Lupan Student Awards

Abstracts may be published in the *Journal of Investigative Medicine*.
To Apply: For abstract information and instructions, visit the website below.
Deadline: The application deadline is in October. For more information, visit:

http://www.wsmrf.net/

William B. Bean Student Research Award

Description: The American Osler Society presents this award to medical students to support research in medical history and medical humanities. Selected applicants may be asked to present their research findings at an American Osler Society meeting. The research award stipend is $1,500. An additional $750 may be available for travel to the annual meeting contingent upon submission of a paper acceptable to the Committee at the conclusion of the studentship.

To Apply: Candidates must be current students at an accredited medical school in the United States or Canada. A letter of support from a faculty sponsor must be submitted along with the application form. See the link below for the application form.

Deadline: The application deadline is in March. See the following link for more information:

http://aosler.org/willian-bean-award/

Profile of a Winner

In 2009, for the third time in four years, a University of North Carolina (UNC) medical student won the William B. Bean Research Award. Christopher Dibble, a third-year M.D./Ph.D. student, received the award for his proposal entitled "Osler and Trudeau: The North American Campaign Against Tuberculosis."

The previous two winners from UNC were James Fraser in 2008 and Lee Hampton in 2006. Fraser's proposal was entitled "Molding an Independent Specialty: Plastic Surgery in Postwar America, 1919 – 1941." Lee's proposal was "Albert Sabin and the Western Hemisphere Polio Eradication Campaign."[12]

William J. von Liebig Summer Research Fellowship (See Chapter 23)

References

[1] Universityof Wisconsin School of Medicine and Public Health. Available at: http://www.med.wisc.edu/news-events/news/students-make-an-impact-on-patients-through-research/26401. Accessed July 2, 2014.

[2] Parsonnet J, Gruppuso P, Kanter S, Boninger M. Required vs. elective research and in-depth scholarship programs in the medical student curriculum. *Acad Med* 2010; 85(3): 405-8.

[3] Solomon S, Tom S, Pichert J, Wasserman D, Powers A. Impact of medical student research in the development of physician scientists. *J Investig Med* 2002; 51(30: 149-56.

[4] American College of Sports Medicine. Available at: http://www.acsm.org/find-continuing-education/awards-grants/student-awards. Accessed July 18, 2014.

[5] American Medical Association. Available at: http://www.ama-assn.org/ama/pub/about-ama/ama-foundation/recipient-stories/ami-raval.page?. Accessed January 14, 2013.

[6] Oakland University William Beaumont School of Medicine. Available at: https://www.oakland.edu/?id=31299&sid=340. Accessed July 18, 2014.

[7] Columbia University Medical Center. Available at: http://newsroom.cumc.columbia.edu/blog/2014/02/20/columbia-university-medical-student-receives-top-award-ama-research-symposium/. Accessed July 2, 2014.

[8] Alpha Omega Alpha Honor Medical Society. Available at: http://alphaomegaalpha.org/news_student_research_testimonials.html. Accessed January 20, 2014.

[9] David Rogers Fellowship. Available at: http://www.nyam.org/grants/rogers-prev.html. Accessed June 2, 2014.

[10] University of Virginia School of Medicine. Available at: http://news.med.virginia.edu/medicinematters/uvasomrestriction/public/2014/06/04/gold-foundation-awards-emily-knudsen-summer-fellowship/. Accessed July 2, 2014.

[11] Harvard Medical School. Available at: http://hms.harvard.edu/sites/default/files/Benefactor_Spring2013_0.pdf. Accessed July 2, 2014.

[12] University of North Carolina School of Medicine. Available at: http://news.unchealthcare.org/som-vital-signs/archives/vital-signs-june-26/unc-medical-student-wins-bean-student-research-award#.UZ6DN5UgpxE. Accessed January 20, 2014.

Chapter 11

Scholarships and Awards for Female Medical Students

As recently as the 1960s, women represented only 4% of physician graduates in the United States. Since then, the numbers of women in medicine has climbed significantly. The year 2003 was particularly remarkable. For the first time, over half of U.S. medical school applicants and enrollees were women. Now, women account for over 30% of our physician workforce.

In an effort to encourage women to pursue careers in medicine, a number of scholarship programs were developed. Although the gender disparity in medicine has lessened, these programs continue to provide support to women seeking to become physicians. In this chapter, we list and describe these awards.

AAUW Selected Professions Fellowship

Description: The American Association of University Women Education (AAUW) Foundation offers the Selected Profession Fellowship to female medical students. Medical students who are members of ethnic minorities historically underrepresented in medicine are eligible to apply. The award amount is between $5,000 and $18,000.
To Apply: The application includes career plans, professional goals, narrative autobiography, and letters of recommendation.
Deadline: The deadline is in January. For more information, visit:

http://www.aauw.org/what-we-do/educational-funding-and-awards/selected-professions-fellowships/selected-professions-fellowships-application/

Alpha Epsilon Iota Scholarship

Description: Female medical students attending an accredited U.S. medical school may apply. The award amount is up to $3,500.
To Apply: Criteria for selection include academic merit and financial need.
Deadline: For more information, contact AEI Scholarship Fund, c/o Society Trust Bank Dept. B, Todd Jones, Vice President, 100 South Main St., Ann Arbor, MI 48104 or call (313) 994 – 5555.

AMWA Medical Education Scholarship

Description: The American Medical Women's Association (AMWA) offers this scholarship to women currently enrolled in medical school. Award recipients will receive $1,000.

To Apply: Financial need is a consideration. The application includes letter of recommendation and essay responses. The essay prompts ask applicants to answer the following questions:

- Tell us about a situation in which you demonstrated leadership.
- What year did you join AMWA and what is your current involvement with AMWA? If you have not yet entered medical school, what do you know about the organization?
- In a greater sense, what are your goals for women in medicine? What makes you qualified to assist in realizing these goals?
- What are your plans for future AMWA involvement?
- Do you have any unusual circumstances which you would like to share?

Deadline: There are two application periods during the year. The deadlines are September and January. For more information, visit:

http://www.amwa-doc.org/students/awards/medical-education-scholarship/

AMWA Medical Student Kaplan Scholarship

Description: The American Medical Women's Association (AMWA) offers this scholarship to women to help defray the costs of USMLE/COMLEX test preparation at Kaplan. Two $1,000 scholarships will be given.

To Apply: Applicants must be national AMWA members. Criteria for selection include embodiment of the goals of AMWA. Financial need is a consideration. The application includes essay responses to the following questions:

- What has been your most humbling experience and how will that experience affect your interactions with your peers and patients?
- Describe a situation in which you felt empowered to advocate for women in medicine.
- What is your current involvement with AMWA? What are your plans for future AMWA involvement?
- Do you have any unusual circumstances that you would like to share?

Deadline: There are two application periods during the year. The deadlines are September and January. For more information, visit:

http://www.amwa-doc.org/students/awards/medical-student-kaplan-scholarship/

AMWA Heller Outstanding Branch Award

Description: The American Medical Women's Association (AMWA) offers this award to an AMWA student branch for notable accomplishments in chapter activities, including recruitment and service. Recipients will receive $250, and receive recognition at the Annual Meeting.
To Apply: Branch presidents may self-nominate their branches. For more information about the application process, visit the website below.
Deadline: The deadline is in February. For more information, visit:

http://www.amwa-doc.org/students/awards/heller-outstanding-branch-award/

AMWA Student Poster Presentations

Description: Original research and case studies can be presented as poster presentations at the AMWA Annual Meeting.
To Apply: For more information, visit the website below.
Deadline: The deadline is in January. For more information, visit:

http://www.amwa-doc.org/students/awards/annual-meeting-poster-presentations/

AMWA Service Recognition Award

Description: The American Medical Women's Association (AMWA) offers this award for commitment to service.
To Apply: Criteria for selection includes a minimum of 50 cumulative hours of service with AMWA, participation in a project aligned with AMWA's mission, and recommendation from a supervising AMWA leader.
Deadline: For more information, visit:

http://www.amwa-doc.org/students/awards/service-recognition-award/

AMWA American Women's Hospital Service Overseas Assistance Grant

Description: The American Women's Hospital Service Overseas Assistance Grant is offered to national AMWA members pursuing medical studies abroad to benefit the underserved. Recipients may receive up to $1,000.
To Apply: Applicants must be national AMWA members attending an accredited allopathic or osteopathic medical school. Grants are awarded to students completing their second, third, or fourth year of medical school. A minimum of 4 weeks must be spent abroad. The application includes letter from Dean, letter of recommendation, description of overseas program, personal statement, and travel budget.

Deadline: There are four application cycles per year with deadlines in January, April, July, and October. For more information, visit:

http://www.amwa-doc.org/our-work/american-womens-hospital-services/overseas-assistance-grants/

Anarcha, Betsy and Lucy Memorial Scholarship Award (See Chapter 13)

Anne C. Carter Global Health Fellowship

Description: Four members of the American Medical Women's Association (AMWA) will receive this two-year fellowship. During the first year, fellows explore the global health curriculum, learn about local project development, and benefit from mentorship. In the second year, fellows are involved in a global health project in Uganda.

To Apply: The application includes a letter of recommendation and personal essay responses. Applicants are asked to answer the following questions:

- Please describe your interest and past experiences in global health. Include a timeline with dates or any projects or trips.
- Please describe a problem you saw in your community and what you personally did to address the problem.
- Please write one paragraph describing a project idea for AMWA local or national branches that promotes global health awareness.
- Please describe what you hope to accomplish through this fellowship and how you think it will impact your future path.

For more information about the application process, visit the website below.
Deadline: The deadline is in September. For more information, visit:

http://www.amwa-doc.org/students/awards/anne-c-carter-global-health-fellowship/

Profile of a Winner

Oluwatoni (Toni) Aluko, a medical student at the Meharry Medical College, was an Anne C. Carter Global Health Fellow from 2012 to 2014. She attended the University of Maryland at College Park where she graduated with a degree in Kinesiological Sciences with minors in Spanish and Community Health. As a medical student, she has been actively involved in a variety of activities outside the classroom, serving as the AMWA National Global Health Chair, class liaison to the Family Medicine Interest Group, and volunteer at Meharry's free student-run clinic. In the future, she hopes to encourage other students, particularly those who belong to traditionally underrepresented groups in medicine, to become involved in global health.[1]

Anne C. Carter Leadership Award

Description: A medical student member of the American Medical Women's Association (AMWA) will receive this award for outstanding leadership. The recipient will be given $1,000.
To Apply: The application includes CV, award nomination form, and personal statement.
Deadline: The deadline is in November. For more information, visit:

http://www.amwa-doc.org/students/awards/anne-c-carter-leadership-award/

Profile of a Winner

In 2012, Linda J. Wang, a medical student at Harvard University, was the recipient of the Anne C. Carter Student Leadership Award. She has been actively involved in AMWA from the start of medical school. During her first year, she served as one of the directors of the Harvard AMWA student branch. Through her work as a student liaison for the National AMWA Membership Committee and Women's Health Working Group, she has been able to launch new recruitment initiatives and contribute to efforts for the inclusion of gender- and sex-specific medicine into the curriculum of our nation's medical schools. She will continue to advance the cause of the AMWA during her tenure as AMWA National Student President-Elect.[2]

Dr. Marie E. Zakrewski Medical Scholarship

Description: This scholarship is given to a young woman of Polish ancestry who is attending medical school in an accredited U.S. institution. To be eligible, you must be a female resident of Massachusetts. If no qualified applicants are found in the state, the scholarship committee will consider applicants from other states in New England. The award amount is $3,500.
To Apply: Only students entering their first, second, or third year of medical school may apply. The application includes statement of purpose, transcripts, two letters of reference, and proof of Polish ancestry. Criteria for selection include academic excellence, achievements, interests, motivation, interest in Polish subjects, and involvement in the Polish American community. Financial need is a consideration.
Deadline: The deadline is in January. For more information, visit:

http://www.thekf.org/scholarships/tuition/mzms/

Ethel O. Gardiner Scholarship (See Chapter 43)

Gertrude B. Elion Mentored Medical Student Research Award (See Chapter 71)

Ida Foreman Fleisher Fund (See Chapter 12)

Leah J. Dickstein, M.D. Award (See Chapter 35)

Mary Ball Carrera Scholarship (See Chapter 13)

Patricia Numann Medical Student Award (See Chapter 23)

Rebecca Lee, M.D. Scholarship Award

Description: The Association of Black Women Physicians provides scholarships to female medical students. Students must be residents of Southern California or enrolled in medical school in Southern California. The award amount is between $1,000 and $5,000.
To Apply: Criteria for selection include academic merit, financial need, and commitment to the organization's mission.
Deadline: For more information, visit:

http://www.blackwomenphysicians.org/

RJOS Medical Student Achievement Awards (See Chapter 29)

Ruth G. White Scholarship (See Chapter 43)

S. Evelyn Lewis Memorial Scholarship in Medical Health Sciences

Description: The S. Evelyn Lewis Memorial Scholarship is open to undergraduate and graduate young women enrolled in a health sciences or medical program. The award amount is $500 to $1,000.
To Apply: Women enrolled in medical school are eligible to apply.
Deadline: For more information, visit:

http://www.zphib1920.org/nef/schapp.pdf

Sara's Wish Foundation Scholarship (See Chapter 14)

Scanlan/Women in Thoracic Surgery Traveling Mentorship Program (See Chapter 23)

Soroptimist International of Los Angeles Graduate Student Fellowship Award (See Chapter 43)

Stephen Bufton Memorial Educational Fund Scholarship

Description: This scholarship program is open to female graduate students studying in the fields of science, technology, engineering, or mathematics.
To Apply: Criteria for selection include minimum GPA, biographical sketch, three letters of reference, and transcript. For more information, visit the website below.
Deadline: The deadline is in May. For more information, visit:

https://www.sbmef.org/National/Details.cfm?ScholarshipID=%21%28P%20%20%20%0A

Women in Medicine LGBT Leadership Scholarships

Description: Women in Medicine (WIM) provide three LGBT Leadership Scholarships to medical students. The award amount is $5,000. Winners will receive their awards at the WIM Annual Meeting.
To Apply: Allopathic and osteopathic medical students in the U.S. and Canada are eligible to apply. The application includes CV, Dean's letter, and letter of reference from faculty member. Criteria for judging include demonstrated leadership to the LGBTQ community.
Deadline: The deadline is in April. For more information, visit:

http://womeninmedicine.org

Women's Microsurgery Group Travel Scholarship (See Chapter 34)

Young Women in Science Awards

Description: The Young Women in Science Awards recognizes outstanding student achievement in basic science and research. Three winners are selected based on student poster presentations at the American Medical Women's Association (AMWA) Annual Meeting. Award recipients are recognized at the AMWA Annual Meeting Awards Ceremony.
To Apply: For more information, visit the website below.
Deadline: The deadline is in January. For more information, visit:

http://www.amwa-doc.org/students/awards/young-women-in-science-award/

References

[1]Anne C. Carter Global Health Fellowship. Available at:
http://carterfellows.wordpress.com/current-fellows/. Accessed July 22, 2014.
[2]American Medical Women's Association. Available at:
http://americanmedicalwomensassociation.blogspot.com/2012/03/linda-j-wang-to-receive-amwas-2012-anne.html. Accessed July 12, 2014.

Chapter 12

Ethnicity-Based Awards & Scholarships

Ethnic organizations and groups are an important source of scholarship support. Rola Daher, a medical student of Lebanese descent attending Wayne State University, was the recipient of the Ibn Sina Endowed Scholarship. This is a scholarship that has helped Arab American and Chaldean-American medical students reach their professional goals. "I can't tell you how much it means to me to know that people of my own background and culture are supporting me, sort of as cheerleaders in my efforts," said Daher. "The $20,000 I received was so helpful. I know students who are graduating with a crushing load of debt. My debt is minimal, thanks to the Ibn Sina Scholarship."[1]

In this chapter, we list and describe ethnicity-based awards and scholarships. Note that this chapter does not include awards for groups that have traditionally been underrepresented in medicine (African-American/Black, Hispanic/Latino, American Indian/Alaska Native, or Native Hawaiian/Pacific Islander). These awards and scholarships are presented in chapter 13.

Anna and Ida Reiss Memorial Fund Scholarship

Description: This scholarship is open to Jewish students pursuing a career in medicine. The award amount ranges from $1,000 to $10,000.
To Apply: The applicant will need to submit proof of matriculation in an accredited medical school and proof of Jewish faith. Financial need is a consideration.
Deadline: For more information, email hmiles@greenmiles.com or contact:

Harry Miles, Esq., Trustee
Anna and Ida Reiss Memorial Fund Scholarship
C/O Green, Miles, Lipton, White & Fitz-Gibbon
77 Pleasant St.
PO Box 210
Northampton, MA 01061-0210

Armenian Professional Society Graduate Student Scholarship

Description: The Armenian Professional Society offers scholarships to graduate students.
To Apply: The application includes transcript, essay, financial need, and two letters of reference. The essay should provide the applicant's background information, involvement in the Armenian community, and why the applicant believes he should be the award recipient.
Deadline: The deadline is in September. For more information, visit:

http://www.apsla.org/APS_Website/scholarships_2.html

Chinese American Medical Society Research Scholarship (See Chapter 10)

Chinese American Physician's Society Scholarship

Description: The Chinese American Physician's Society (CAPS) offers scholarships to medical students.
To Apply: Medical students requiring financial assistance are eligible regardless of hometown, sex, race, or color. Criteria for selection include academic achievement, financial need, and community service. The application includes personal essays. Preference is given to applicants who intend to serve the Chinese community following graduation.
Deadline: The deadline is in March. For more information, visit:

http://www.caps-ca.org

Dr. Marie E. Zakrewski Medical Scholarship (See Chapter 11)

Fadel Educational Foundation Scholarship

Description: The Fadel Educational Foundation supports education for Muslim U.S. citizens and permanent residents. Recipients are chosen based on merit and financial need. The award amount is $3,500.
To Apply: For application information and instructions, visit the website below.
Deadline: The deadline is in May. For more information, visit:

http://fadelfoundation.wordpress.com/

Hellenic-American Medical & Dental Society of Southern California S. James Vamvas Scholarship

Description: This scholarship supports medical and dental students attending schools in Southern California.

To Apply: To be eligible, the applicant must be of Hellenic (Greek) descent and enrolled in an accredited institution in California. Criteria for selection include good class standing and financial need.
Deadline: The deadline is in June. For more information, visit:

http://hamds.org/programs/scholarship/

Hellenic Medical Society of New York Scholarship

Description: The Hellenic Medical Society of New York offers this scholarship to medical students of Hellenic heritage who are from the states of New York, Connecticut, New Jersey, or Pennsylvania.
To Apply: To be eligible, the applicant must be of Hellenic (Greek) descent and enrolled in an accredited institution in the U.S. The applicant must have completed the first year. Only applicants who are from New York, New Jersey, Connecticut, or Pennsylvania will be considered. Criteria for judging include academic achievement and/or financial need.
Deadline: The deadline is in July. For more information, visit:

www.hmsny.org

Hellenic University Club of Philadelphia Scholarship

Description: The Hellenic University Club of Philadelphia offers scholarships to medical students of Greek descent who are residents of certain counties in Pennsylvania or New Jersey.
To Apply: To be eligible, the applicant must be a medical student of Greek descent who is a legal resident of Berks, Bucks, Chester, Delaware, Lancaster, Lehigh, Montgomery, or Philadelphia Counties in Pennsylvania or Atlantic, Burlington, Camden, Cape May, Cumberland, Gloucester, or Salem Counties in New Jersey.
Deadline: The deadline is in April. For more information, visit:

http://www.thekf.org

Houtan Scholarship

Description: The Houtan Scholarship Foundation offers this award to students from all origins having an interest in promoting the culture, heritage, language, and civilization of Iran. The award amount is $2,500 per semester.
To Apply: To be eligible, the applicant must write, speak, and read Parsi at an intermediate level. Criteria for selection include academic achievement.
Deadline: There are two application cycles with deadlines in June and October. For more information, visit:

www.houtan.org

Ida Foreman Fleisher Fund

Description: The fund provides scholarships to assist the professional education of Jewish women. The award amount ranges from $2,000 to $8,000.
To Apply: To be eligible, applicants must be from or attend school in the Greater Philadelphia area, including New Jersey and Delaware. The application includes personal mission statement, FAFSA, transcript, and letters of recommendation.
Deadline: The deadline is in May. For more information, visit:

https://www.jewishphilly.org/programs-services/educational-scholarships/educational-loan-and-scholarship-funds

Iranian-American Scholarship

Description: The Iranian-American Scholarship offers support to Iranian American students.
To Apply: To be eligible, the applicant must be a U.S. citizen or permanent resident. The application includes Student Aid Report, two essays, letters of recommendation, and medical school transcript.
Deadline: The deadline is in May. For more information, visit:

http://iasfund.org/applications/.

Japanese American Citizens League Scholarship

Description: The Japanese American Citizens League (JACL) offers scholarships to qualified medical students nationwide.
To Apply: To be eligible, the applicant must be an active member of JACL. JACL membership is open to individuals of every ethnic background. The completed application includes personal statement, letter of recommendation, transcript, work experience, and extracurricular activities.
Deadline: For more information, visit:

http://www.jacl.org/edu/scholar.htm

Japanese Medical Society of America Scholarship

Description: The Japanese Medical Society of America (JMSA) offers these scholarships to support the education of medical professionals. Award winners will be recognized during the organization's annual spring dinner in New York. The award amount is between $2,500 and $20,000.
To Apply: Criteria for selection include strong interest in JMSA and its goals and proposal of a clear, achievable project to benefit JMSA and the Japanese community. The application includes letter of recommendation and transcript. The reference letter should address how you exemplify the goals of the JMSA.

Applicants are also asked to briefly describe a project they would like to complete related to the JMSA mission.
Deadline: The deadline is in December. For more information, visit:

http://jmsa.org/student-members/about-scholarships

Japanese American Medical Association Scholarship

Description: The Japanese American Medical Association (JAMA) offers this scholarship to medical students. The award amount is up to $2,500.
To Apply: To be eligible, the applicant must be in the first, second, or third year of medical school. Criteria for selection include academic achievement, financial need, and desire to serve the Japanese American community.
Deadline: For more information, visit:

http://jamasocal.org/

Knights of Dabrowski Crusade for Education

Description: This is a scholarship for medical students of Polish descent.
To Apply: Criteria for selection include financial need, academic performance, and community involvement. The student must also be a Chicago Metro area resident for at least four years prior to application. An interview is required.
Deadline: The deadline is in May. For more information, contact kofd@sbcglobal.net.

Korean American Medical Association Scholarship

Description: The Korean American Medical Association (KAMA) offers scholarships for basic science/clinical research and community outreach. The award amount is at least $1,000.
To Apply: To be eligible, the applicant must be a member of KAMA. First-, second-, and third-year medical students may apply. The application includes medical school transcript, CV, and letters of recommendation.
Deadline: The deadline is in July. For more information, visit:

http://www.kamaus.org/info/index.php/medical-students/80-scholarship-program

Korean American Scholarship Foundation

Description: The Korean American Scholarship Foundation provides scholarships to full-time students.
To Apply: Koreans (international students) and Korean-Americans are eligible to apply. Criteria for selection include minimum GPA and financial need. The application includes transcript, letters of recommendation, and personal essay.
Deadline: The deadline varies from May to July. For more information, visit:

http://www.kasf.org/application

Kosciuszko Foundation Scholarship

Description: Medical students who are U.S. citizens of Polish descent, or Poles who are permanent residents of the U.S. may apply for this scholarship.
To Apply: Criteria for judging include academic excellence and evidence of identification with the Polish American Community.
Deadline: For more information, contact:

The Kosciuszko Foundation
Domestic Grants Office
15 East 65th Street
New York, NY 10021

Momeni Foundation Financial Assistance Scholarship

Description: The Momeni Foundation Financial Assistance Scholarship is open to students of Iranian descent. The award amount ranges from $500 to $1,000.
To Apply: To be eligible, the applicant must be of Iranian descent.
Deadline: The deadline is in June. For more information, visit:

www.momenifoundation.org

National Italian American Foundation Scholarship Program

Description: The National Italian American Foundation (NIAF) provides scholarships for Italian American students. The award amount ranges from $2,000 to $12,000.
To Apply: To be eligible, the applicant must be an Italian American. Criteria for selection include academic achievement and demonstration of outstanding potential.
Deadline: The deadline is in March. For more information, visit:

www.niaf.org/scholarships

New England Hellenic Medical and Dental Society Scholarship

Description: The New England Hellenic Medical and Dental Society offer scholarships to medical students who are of Greek descent.
To Apply: To be eligible, medical school applicants must be members of the society. Criteria for judging include academic performance and/or need. Students who have demonstrated ongoing interest and commitment to the health field and to Hellenic issues are encouraged to apply. The application includes transcript, letter of recommendation, and personal essay responses to the following questions:

- Why do you consider yourself a worthy candidate for this scholarship?
- What are your long-range goals in the health field?
- How do you embody the Hellenic spirit?
- How do you envision contributing to the society in the future?

Deadline: For more information, visit:

http://www.nehmds.org/

Polish University Club of New Jersey Scholarship

Description: The Polish University Club of New Jersey awards scholarships to deserving medical students.
To Apply: To be eligible, the applicant must be a New Jersey resident of Polish descent. The application includes transcript, student aid report, personal statement, and two reference letters. The personal statement should address the question, "If you were to present a twenty minute talk at a meeting of the Polish University Club of NJ, on a topic of your choice, what would it be?" An interview is required.
Deadline: The application deadline is in March. For more information, visit:

http://www.pucnj.org/scholarships.php

Ryu Family Foundation Scholarship

Description: The Ryu Family Foundation offers scholarships to Korean-American and Korean students.
To Apply: To be eligible, the applicant must be a Korean-American or Korean student attending medical school full-time in one of 10 northeastern states. These include Pennsylvania, New Jersey, New York, Connecticut, Vermont, Rhode Island, New Hampshire, Massachusetts, and Maine. The application includes personal essay, letter of reference, transcript, and FAFSA.
Deadline: For more information, contact the Ryu Family Foundation at (973) 692 – 9696.

Sons of Italy National Leadership Grant

Description: This grant provides support to U.S. citizens of Italian descent enrolled in an undergraduate/graduate program. Medical students are eligible.
To Apply: For application information and instructions, visit the website below.
Deadline: The deadline is in February. For more information, visit:

http://www.osia.org

Swiss Benevolent Society Scholarship

Description: The Swiss Benevolent Society of New York awards scholarships to students who are of Swiss descent. Medical students may apply. To be eligible, the applicant (or parent) must be a Swiss national. For the Pellegrini and Zimmerman scholarships, the applicant must be a permanent resident of New York, New Jersey, Connecticut, Pennsylvania, or Delaware.
To Apply: For application information, visit the website below.
Deadline: For more information, visit:

http://www.sbsny.org/sbs_scholarship_programs.html

Turkish American Doctors Association of Midwest Scholarship

Description: The Turkish American Doctors Association of Midwest offers scholarships to medical students with a Turkish-American heritage. The award amount is $1,000.
To Apply: The application includes Dean's letter, letters of recommendation, personal statement, and CV.
Deadline: The deadline is in February. For more information, visit:

http://www.tadamonline.org/

Vietnamese American Medical Association Scholarship

Description: The Vietnamese American Medical Association offers scholarships to third-year medical students. The award amount is $1,000.
To Apply: The application includes personal essay, medical school transcript, letter from financial aid office, USMLE Step 1 scores, and letter of recommendation.
Deadline: The deadline is in May. For more information, visit:

http://www.vamausa.org/

Vietnamese American Medical Association Memorial Travel Scholarship

Description: The Vietnamese American Medical Association offers scholarships to students rotating in a foreign country during medical school. The award amount is $2,500.
To Apply: Preference is given to students rotating in Vietnam. The application includes personal essay, budget, and written report following rotation.
Deadline: The deadline is in June. For more information, visit:

http://www.vamausa.org/

References

[1]Wayne State University School of Medicine. Available at: http://today.wayne.edu/featured-stories/7312. Accessed July 2, 2014.

Chapter 13

Minority Medical Awards & Scholarships

Although African Americans, Hispanics/Latinos, and Native Americans comprise up to 25% of the U.S. population, only 6% of the physician workforce are members of these groups. There are strong efforts underway to increase the number of physicians from these underrepresented groups, and scholarship support is one way to do so. Medical schools have an Office of Multicultural Affairs, and medical student members of underrepresented groups in medicine are encouraged to visit this office to learn about scholarship opportunities. In this chapter, we list and describe awards for groups that have traditionally been underrepresented in medicine.

AAFP Minority Scholarships Program for Residents and Medical Students (See Chapter 22)

AAUW Selected Professions Fellowship (See Chapter 11)

Aetna Foundation/NMF Healthcare Leadership Program

Description: The Aetna Foundation/NMF Healthcare Leadership Program is available through National Medical Fellowships.
To Apply: Allopathic and osteopathic medical students are eligible to apply. To be eligible, the applicant must be an underrepresented minority medical student in the second or third year of medical school. Criteria for selection include a commitment to serving medically underserved communities, outstanding academic achievement, leadership, and potential for contributions to medicine. Only students attending medical school in California (Los Angeles), Connecticut, Illinois (Chicago), New Jersey, New York (New York City), and Pennsylvania (Philadelphia) may apply.
Deadline: For more information, visit:

http://www.nmfonline.org/programs/general-scholarships-awards#anarcha

American Academy of Child and Adolescent Psychiatry Jeanne Spurlock Research Fellowship in Drug Abuse and Addiction for Minority Medical Students (See Chapter 35)

American Academy of Dermatology Diversity Medical Student Mentorship Program (See Chapter 20)

American Academy of Neurology Minority Scholars Program

Description: The Minority Scholars Program was created by the American Academy of Neurology (AAN) to promote diversity in the field of neurology and to provide medical students with an opportunity to learn more about careers in neurology and neuroscience. Students are selected based on their interest in neurology as a career, their academic achievements and community involvement, as well as their plans to maximize the AAN Annual Meeting opportunity. The recipient will receive airfare and lodging for up to four nights to attend the AAN Annual Meeting. They will also be able to register for educational programs and participate in the Medical Student rush line. See the link below for other benefits.

To Apply: Medical students from underrepresented and underserved groups are eligible to apply for this program. The student must be in good standing at a U.S. medical school. Preference is given to second- and third-year students. Application requirements include a one-page essay, a letter of recommendation, and CV. Visit the link below for more information.

Deadline: The deadline for the application is in October. See the following link for more information:

http://tools.aan.com/science/awards/?fuseaction=home.info&id=25

Profile of a Winner

In 2012, Gabriel Moreno, a third-year medical student at Wayne State University School of Medicine, was one of the eight members of the AAN Minority Scholars Program. His interest in medicine began during his childhood when concern for his father's Parkinson's disease was coupled with fascination of his mother's clinical experiences as a registered nurse.

"Gabriel is very active in his Hispanic community," said Dr. Maher Fakhouri, Assistant Professor of Neurology at Wayne State University, in his nomination letter. "He identified that our medical school has minimal representation from the Hispanic and Latino communities and formed the Latin American and Native American Medical Student Association, the first medical student association at Wayne State University committed to raising awareness of the health issues of Hispanic and Latino Americans and to increasing opportunities in medicine for Hispanic and Latinos in the Detroit area."[1]

American Gastroenterological Association Investing in the Future Student Research Fellowship (See Chapter 24)

American Indian College Fund Scholarship

Description: The American Indian College Fund offers support to students who are registered members (or descendant of a tribe member) of a tribe recognized by the government.
To Apply: The application includes personal essay, transcript, financial aid form, and proof of tribal membership.
Deadline: The deadline is in May. For more information, visit:

http://www.collegefund.org/students_and_alumni/content/graduate_special_sch olarships

American Medical Association Minority Scholars Award

Description: Through this program, the American Medical Association (AMA) Foundation hopes to increase the number of minority physicians to meet the diverse needs of our communities. Each year, approximately seven to twelve medical students are given this award, each in the amount of a $10,000 scholarship.
To Apply: Each medical school may submit up to two nominees for the award. The nominee must be a first- or second-year medical student and a permanent resident or citizen of the United States. Eligible students from traditionally underrepresented groups in the medical profession include African American, American Indian, Native Hawaiian, Alaska Native and Hispanic/Latino. Criteria for selection include commitment to the elimination of healthcare disparities, outstanding academic achievement, leadership activities and community involvement. Contact your medical school if you are interested in being nominated for this award.
Deadline: Nomination forms are usually available in late January to early February and are due in March. Please visit the following link for more information:

http://www.ama-assn.org/ama/pub/about-ama/ama-foundation/our-programs/medical-education/minority-scholars-award.page

American Psychiatric Association Minority Medical Student Summer Mentorship Program (See Chapter 35)

American Psychiatric Association Minority Student Summer Externship in Addiction Psychiatry (See Chapter 35)

American Psychiatric Association Travel Scholarship for Minority Medical Students (See Chapter 35)

Profile of a Winner

Lissette Jimenez, a University of Washington School of Medicine student, was one of thirteen students who received the AMA Minority Scholars Award in 2010. Ms. Jimenez's interest in medicine began when she was interpreting for her Mexican parents during physician visits in rural eastern Washington State. As she witnessed her parents' chronic conditions progress, Ms. Jimenez's heightened awareness for health care disparities convinced her to devote her career to providing culturally competent health care to immigrants.

"Thank you for this opportunity and inspiration. The amount of support I've been given will multiply when I go out into the community to help others. It will extend far beyond the recipient," said Ms. Jimenez in an AMA article.[2]

American Society of Hematology Minority Medical Student Award Program

Description: This award program is an 8 – 12 week research experience for minority students from the United States and Canada who are in their early years of medical school. At the end of the research experience, students are expected to present their findings at the American Society of Hematology (ASH) Annual Meeting. Participants are paired with ASH members who serve as research and career development mentors. The selected participants will receive a $2,000 allowance for travel to the ASH Annual Meeting. Recipients will also be given a $5,000 stipend for research. Complimentary subscriptions to *Blood* and *The Hematologist* are also provided through the end of residency.

To Apply: To participate in this program, students must be minority individuals from racial and ethnic groups that have been underrepresented in health-related sciences in the United States and Canada. Applicants must also be enrolled in M.D., D.O., or M.D./PhD programs and be citizens or permanent residents of the United States or Canada. Three recommendation letters must be submitted as part of the application. Students are evaluated on research, academic potential, leadership, service, and interest in hematology. Visit the link below for more information.

Deadline: Applicants must request a mentor in January, and then submit an application in March. Award winners are usually notified in April. See the following link for more information:

http://www.hematology.org/awards/mmsap/2624.aspx

American Society for Investigative Pathology Summer Research Opportunity Program in Pathology (See Chapter 31)

American Society of Radiation Oncology Minority Summer Fellowship Award (See Chapter 36)

Anarcha, Betsy and Lucy Memorial Scholarship Award

Description: The Anarcha, Betsy and Lucy Memorial Scholarship Award is available through National Medical Fellowships. Allopathic and osteopathic medical students are eligible to apply. To be eligible, the applicant must be an African-American female who is a known descendant of American slaves.
To Apply: The application includes verification of U.S. citizenship, student aid report, documentation of loan history, financial aid transcript, two personal statements, CV, biosketch, medical school transcript, and letters of recommendation.
Deadline: For more information, visit:

http://www.nmfonline.org/programs/general-scholarships-awards#anarcha

Association of American Indian Affairs Scholarship

Description: This scholarship is available to American Indian and Alaskan Natives. The award amount is $1,500.
To Apply: For application information, visit the website below.
Deadline: The deadline is in June. For more information, visit:

www.indian-affairs.org

Association of American Indian Physicians Research Poster Competition

Description: The Association of American Indian Physicians invites undergraduate students, graduate students, medical students, residents, and physicians to submit their research for poster presentation at the Annual Meeting in July. Three winners will be named in each of three categories – undergraduate, graduate/medical student, and professional (residents and physicians).
To Apply: Abstracts must be less than 250 words. Include cover letter and brief biographical sketch. For more information, visit the website below.
Deadline: The deadline is in July. For more information, visit:

https://www.aaip.org/media/news/m.blog/76/aaip-research-poster-announcement

Beca Foundation/Alice Newell Joslyn Medical Scholarship (See Chapter 43)

Buckfire & Buckfire P.C. Medical School Diversity Scholarship

Description: The Diversity Scholarship will be given to a medical student who is either a member of an underrepresented group in medicine or has shown commitment to issues of diversity.
To Apply: To be eligible, the applicant must be a member of a minority group in medicine. Medical students who have shown a commitment to issues of diversity may also apply irrespective of ethnicity. The application includes transcript and personal essay describing how you will utilize your medical degree to promote ethnic diversity.
Deadline: The deadline is in May. For more information, visit:

http://www.buckfirelaw.com/library/buckfire-buckfire-medical-school-diversity-scholarship-application-2014.cfm#top

Case CFAR Minority HIV Research Training Program (MHRTP)

Description: The focus of this program is to encourage interest in HIV/AIDS research among minority research trainees. Participants will receive a $3,500 stipend to conduct research for a period of 8 weeks under the supervision of a research mentor.
To Apply: To be eligible, the applicant must be a member of a minority group in medicine (African American, American Indian, Alaskan Native, Hispanic/Latino, Native Hawaiian, or Pacific Islander). The application includes CV, transcript, and two letters of reference.
Deadline: The deadline is in February. For more information, visit:

http://cfar.case.edu/mhrtp_program.htm

Case Western Reserve University Heart, Lung and Blood Summer Research Program

Description: This program is administered by the Case Western Reserve University School of Medicine. It offers medical students an opportunity to participate in biomedical research in the areas of cardiovascular, pulmonary, hematological, and sleep medicine. The award amount is $1,750 per month. Recipients must commit to an experience of at least two months.
To Apply: Medical students who are members of underrepresented groups (African American, Latino, Puerto Rican, Pacific Islanders, students from low-income families, or those with disabilities) in the biomedical sciences are eligible to apply. The application includes letters of recommendation and transcripts.
Deadline: The deadline is in March. For more information, visit:

http://casemed.case.edu/gradprog/summer.cfm

CDC Experience Applied Epidemiology Fellowship

Description: Through this fellowship, medical students have the opportunity to develop skills and knowledge of applied epidemiology and the role of physicians in the public health system. Fellows spend up to one year at the CDC working with experts on current public health issues. Fellows can participate in seminars, lead journal clubs, perform epidemiologic analyses and research, and report results of their work through written and oral scientific presentations.
To Apply: Medical students can apply in their second or third year. For application information and instructions, visit the website below.
Deadline: For more information, visit:

http://www.cdc.gov/CDCExperienceFellowship/More.html

Congressional Hispanic Caucus Institute Scholarship

Description: The Congressional Hispanic Caucus Institute provides scholarships to Latino medical students. The award amount is $5,000.
To Apply: Latino medical students who have demonstrated commitment to public service-oriented activities in their communities and a desire to continue such efforts in the future are encouraged to apply.
Deadline: For more information, visit:

http://www.chci.org/scholarships/page/chci-scholarship-program

Conquer Cancer Foundation of the American Society of Clinical Oncology Medical Student Rotation

Description: The Conquer Cancer Foundation of the American Society of Clinical Oncology (ASCO) established this program to encourage individuals from underrepresented populations in medicine to explore a career in oncology. This is an 8- to 10-week clinical or clinical research rotation. Award recipients are given a $5,000 stipend for the rotation along with $1,500 to defray the costs associated with travel to the ASCO Annual Meeting.
To Apply: Eligible applicants include those enrolled in M.D. or D.O schools. Although the summer between the first and second year of medical school is an ideal time for the rotation, students beyond their first year may also apply if their schedule allows for the time commitment. Individuals must be members of an underrepresented population. Criteria for judging include interest in oncology as a career and demonstration of leadership, volunteerism, and commitment to underserved populations. Applicants must submit a resume, personal statement, transcript, and letter of recommendation.
Deadline: The application deadline is in December. For more information, visit:

http://www.conquercancerfoundation.org/cancer-professionals/funding-opportunities/medical-student-rotation-underrepresented-populations

---

Profile of a Winner

Imoh Ikpot, a first-year medical student at the Cooper Medical School of Rowan University, is a recent winner of the Medical School Rotation Award for Underrepresented Populations from the Conquer Cancer Foundation and American Society of Clinical Oncology. He was one of only ten medical students nationwide to receive this award.

After receiving his education in biomedical engineering at the University of Rochester, Ikpot completed a two-year post-baccalaureate fellowship at the National Institutes of Health. Although he entered Cooper Medical School with a background in cancer research, it was his hematology/oncology course that really spurred him to seriously consider a career in oncology.

Ikpot will be working with Dr. Gregory Kubicek, a radiation oncologist at Cooper Medical School. "Imoh is very bright and very self-motivated," said Dr. Kubicek. "He was very industrious in finding this particular project. He spoke with multiple faculty members, hoping to find a project that was both challenging and important. I'm pleased that he has chosen to dedicate his efforts toward this significant research."[3]

Dr. David Monash/John Caldwell Scott Medical Student Scholarship

Description: The Chicago Community Trust and National Medical Fellowships offer this award to medical students who are committed to community service in Chicago.

To Apply: To be eligible, students must have completed their first year in an allopathic or osteopathic Chicago medical school. Criteria for judging include outstanding academic achievement, leadership, and potential for distinguished contributions. For application information and instructions, visit the website below.

Deadline: For more information, visit:

http://www.nmfonline.org/monash-scott

Dr. James A. Ferguson Emerging Infectious Diseases Fellowship Program (See Chapter 24)

Profile of a Winner

Wanda Averheart, a medical student at the University of Illinois College of Medicine, received the Monash Scholarship in 2012. After receiving her Bachelor's in Molecular and Cellular Biology degree from the University of Illinois Urbana Champaign, she has remained active in a variety of efforts to improve the health of uninsured and underserved populations. Averheart has cared for patients in local free clinics, tutored high school and college students, and performed research. Her research has centered on children and obesity in underserved populations. In the future, she hopes to practice primary care medicine.[4]

Dr. Richard Allen Williams & Genita Evangelista Johnson/Association of Black Cardiologists Scholarship

Description: This scholarship program is administered by the AMA Foundation and the Association of Black Cardiologists. Its mission is to promote diversity in medicine, encourage efforts to eliminate health care disparities, and support future cardiologists. The award amount is $5,000.
To Apply: First- and second-year African-American medical students with an interest in cardiology are encouraged to apply. Each medical school may nominate one student for this scholarship.
Deadline: For more information, visit:

http://www.ama-assn.org//ama/pub/about-ama/ama-foundation/our-programs/medical-education/minority-scholars-award.page

GEMS for Health Professional Students

Description: The GEMS for Health Professional Students is a program that provides medical students with summer research opportunities at the University of Colorado. The award amount is $711 per week. The costs of air travel for out-of-state students to and from Denver will be covered.
To Apply: Underrepresented minority medical students are eligible to apply. These include individuals with low-income and financial need, first-generation college attendees, and members of underrepresented groups (African American, Hispanic, American Indian, Alaska Native, Southeast Asian, or Pacific Islander). For application information and instructions, visit the website below.
Deadline: For more information, visit:

http://www.ucdenver.edu/academics/colleges/medicalschool/programs/GEMS/Pages/GEMS-for-Health-Professional-Students-(GEMS-HP).aspx

GE/NMF International Medical Scholars Program

Description: Through this scholarship program, medical students can participate in a two-month mentored clinical experience in Ghana and Kenya. Osteopathic and allopathic medical students may apply. To be eligible, the applicant must be an underrepresented minority student.
To Apply: For application information and instructions, visit the website below.
Deadline: For more information, visit:

http://www.nmfonline.org/ge-international

Hispanic Health Professional Student Scholarship

Description: The National Hispanic Health Foundation (NHHF) offers this scholarship to Hispanic students dedicated to pursuing health care careers. Twenty scholarships will be awarded to health professions students. Eighty percent will receive $5,000 with the remainder receiving $2,000.
To Apply: Applicants need not be Hispanic but should have a deep interest in the health of Hispanic communities. To be considered, applicants must submit the application form, CV, one letter of recommendation, school transcript, and a personal statement with career goals. Criteria for judging include academic performance, leadership, and commitment to Hispanic communities.
Deadline: The application deadline is in September – October. For more information, visit:

http://www.nhmafoundation.org/scholarshipprogram.html

Hispanic Scholarship Fund

Description: The Hispanic Scholarship Fund is available to students of Hispanic heritage. The award amount ranges from $1,000 to $15,000.
To Apply: To be eligible, the applicant must be a United States citizen or permanent legal resident. Criteria for selection include financial aid and minimum GPA.
Deadline: The deadline is in December. For more information, visit:

http://hsf.net/en/scholarships

HTVN Research and Mentorship Program Scholar Grants

Description: The Research and Mentorship Program (RAMP) is sponsored by the HIV Vaccine Trial Network (HVTN) and provides support for HIV vaccine development research. Grant recipients will conduct research in the areas of basic, clinical, behavioral and social science. Short-term (2-4 months) and long-term (9-12 months) opportunities are available. The award amount varies depending on duration.
To Apply: African American and Hispanic medical students are eligible to apply. For application information and instructions, visit the website below.

Deadline: The application deadline is in February. For more information, visit:

http://www.hvtn.org/ramp/

Profile of a Winner

In 2010, Oliva Campa, a first-year student at the University of California Davis School of Medicine, was one of the award recipients of the Hispanic Health Professional Student Scholarship. In medical school, she has been actively involved in efforts to reduce health disparities. She has also made it a priority to increase awareness of health care career opportunities for underserved populations.

Despite the demands of her coursework, Oliva was able to organize a free health fair. Held at the state Capitol, the fair offered Spanish-speaking participants the opportunity to receive important information about diabetes, hypertension, and obesity. Participants had their blood pressure, blood sugar, and body mass index measured.

"Olivia is an inspiration," said Darin Latimore, Director of the Medical Student Diversity Office. "She has been in medical school less than three months and has already displayed the desire and dedication it takes to be a health leader in the community."[5]

Hugh J. Anderson Memorial Scholarship

Description: The Hugh J. Anderson Memorial Scholarship is available through National Medical Fellowships. Allopathic and osteopathic medical students are eligible to apply. To be eligible, the applicant must be an underrepresented minority medical student in Minnesota. Only second- and third-year students are eligible.

To Apply: The application includes verification of U.S. citizenship, student aid report, documentation of loan history, financial aid transcript, two personal statements, CV, biosketch, medical school transcript, and letters of recommendation.

Deadline: For more information, visit:

http://www.nmfonline.org/programs/general-scholarships-awards#anarcha

Indian Health Services – Health Professions Scholarship Program

Description: These scholarships are available to American Indian and Alaska Native students who are enrolled in health professions programs. There is a service obligation that comes with this scholarship.
To Apply: For application information and instructions, see website below.
Deadline: For more information, visit:

http://www.ihs.gov/scholarship/

John Cuckler Senior Orthopaedic Visiting Medical Student Scholarship (See Chapter 29)

Johns Hopkins Department of Otolaryngology – Head and Neck Surgery Clerkship Program for Underrepresented Minority Students (See Chapter 30)

Josiah Macy Jr. Foundation Scholarship

Description: The Josiah Macy Jr. Foundation Scholarship is available through National Medical Fellowships. Allopathic and osteopathic medical students are eligible to apply. To be eligible, the applicant must be an underrepresented minority medical student in the second or third year of medical school.
To Apply: The application includes verification of U.S. citizenship, student aid report, documentation of loan history, financial aid transcript, two personal statements, CV, biosketch, medical school transcript, and letters of recommendation.
Deadline: For more information, visit:

http://www.nmfonline.org/programs/general-scholarships-awards#anarcha

La Unidad Latina Foundation Scholarship

Description: The La Unidad Latina Foundation offers scholarships to Hispanic medical students.
To Apply: The applicant must be a Hispanic medical student who has completed at least one semester of a graduate program. Criteria for judging include academic excellence, extracurricular activities, and financial need.
Deadline: The application deadline is in March. For more information, visit:

http://www.lulfoundation.org/Apply/tabid/60/Default.aspx

Mary Ball Carrera Scholarship

Description: The Mary Ball Carrera Scholarship is available through National Medical Fellowships. Allopathic and osteopathic medical students are eligible to apply. To be eligible, the applicant must be a Native American female medical student.

To Apply: The application includes verification of U.S. citizenship, student aid report, documentation of loan history, financial aid transcript, two personal statements, CV, biosketch, medical school transcript, and letters of recommendation.

Deadline: For more information, visit:

http://www.nmfonline.org/programs/general-scholarships-awards#anarcha

Massachusetts General Hospital Summer Research Trainee Program

Description: Through the Summer Research Trainee Program, trainees are linked with a preceptor at the Massachusetts General Hospital who will supervise a chosen project. A stipend of $4,000 will be given for the 8-week experience. At the end of the program, trainees will prepare an oral presentation of their work and write an abstract.

To Apply: First-year medical students who are members of groups that are underrepresented in medicine are eligible to apply. These groups include Latino/Hispanic, African-American/Black, American Indian, Native Hawaiian, and Alaska Native. The application includes resume, personal statement, photo, three letters of recommendation, and official transcripts. The personal statement should describe your educational and professional goals and how involvement in the program will help you reach your goals. The statement must not exceed 750 words.

Deadline: The application deadline is in February. For more information, visit:

http://www.massgeneral.org/education/internship.aspx?id=5

Mayo Clinic Summer Research Fellowship

Description: Through the Summer Research Fellowship, students will be prepared for careers in clinical care and patient-oriented research. Fellows are matched with Mayo faculty, and supervised during the fellowship. The award amount is up to $6,180. The student must devote a minimum of 8 weeks.

To Apply: The fellowship is open to minority allopathic medical students who seek research experience during the summer between the first and second year of medical school. Members of the following underrepresented groups are eligible: African American/Black, Hispanic/Latino, American Indian/Alaska Native, Native Hawaiian/U.S. Pacific Islander, and persons with life-altering disabilities.

Deadline: The application deadline is in March. For more information, visit:

http://www.mayo.edu/msgme/diversity-programs/summer-research-fellowship

National Association of Medical Minority Educators Scholarship

Description: The National Association of Medical Minority Educators (NAMME) established this scholarship in 1995 to support underrepresented minority students who have completed the first year of health professions training. Each year, eight $1,000 scholarships are awarded.

To Apply: Students must be nominated for the award. Nominated students are then judged on their academic record, community service, financial need, and personal statement. For application information and instructions, visit the website below.

Deadline: The organization begins accepting nominations in the Spring. For more information, visit:

http://www.nammenational.org/scholarships.html

Profile of a Winner

In 2009, Josepha Iluonakhamhe, a second-year medical student at the Medical College of Georgia, was one recipient of the National Association of Medical Minority Educators scholarship. She received the award for her academic standing and contributions to community service. She has been actively involved in mentoring and teaching through the MCG Student Educational Enrichment Program (SEEP). This is a summer program that provides high school and college students with opportunities to explore the health sciences. Josepha's interest in serving as a SEEP assistant stems from her participation in SEEP prior to medical school. "It made me want to give back and help other students," said Iluonakhamhe. "I had mentors who really inspired me and introduced me to different things, and I wanted to do the same."[6]

NMF Emergency Scholarship

Description: The NMF Emergency Scholarship is available through National Medical Fellowships. Allopathic and osteopathic medical students are eligible to apply. To be eligible, the applicant must be a third- or fourth-year underrepresented minority medical student who requires financial assistance because of emergency.

To Apply: For application information, visit the website below.

Deadline: For more information, visit:

http://www.nmfonline.org/programs/general-scholarships-awards#anarcha

NMF California Community-Service Learning Program

Description: This program was established to improve access to quality healthcare in underserved communities in California. Scholars will conduct a self-directed community health project under the guidance of a mentor. Recipients will receive a $5,000 scholarship award. Fourteen awards will be given.

To Apply: Criteria for selection include demonstrated leadership at an early stage of their career and commitment to serving medically underserved communities. Only medical students who are attending school in California and are members of minority groups (African American, Latino, or Native American) are eligible. For application information and instructions, visit the website below.

Deadline: For more information, visit:

http://www.nmfonline.org/ccslp

Rebecca Lee, M.D. Scholarship Award (See Chapter 11)

Sherry R. Arnstein Minority Student Scholarship

Description: The American Association of Colleges of Osteopathic Medicine (AACOM) offers this award to osteopathic underrepresented minority students. Two students (one newly accepted and one continuing) at each osteopathic school will receive the award.

To Apply: To be considered, the applicant must be a member an underrepresented minority group (African American, Native American, Alaska Native, Native Hawaiian, Hispanic, or mainland Puerto Rican). Applicants must be in good standing and enrolled as a first-, second-, or third-year student at an osteopathic medical school. The award is also open to applicants who have been accepted but not yet matriculated. An essay must be submitted as part of the application. In the essay, applicants should describe the reasons that led them to osteopathic medicine, their thoughts on how schools can increase the number of underrepresented minority medical students, and the contributions they can make to facilitate this.

Deadline: The application deadline is in March. For more information, visit:

http://www.aacom.org/InfoFor/students/finaid/Pages/ArnsteinScholarship.aspx

Society of Vascular Surgery Minority Medical Student Travel Scholarship (See Chapter 23)

Texas Medical Association Minority Scholarship (See Chapter 81)

United Health Foundation/NMF Diverse Medical Scholars Program

Description: The United Health Foundation/NMF Diverse Medical Scholars Program is available through National Medical Fellowships. Awardees will complete a community health project of 150 hours in an underserved area. The amount of the award is $7,000.

To Apply: Allopathic and osteopathic underrepresented minority medical students are eligible to apply. To be eligible, the applicant must be attending an accredited medical school in New York (greater metropolitan New York City), Florida (Orlando and Greater Miami), Louisiana (New Orleans, Baton Rouge, and Shreveport), or Georgia (Atlanta). Criteria for selection include demonstrated leadership and commitment to serving medically underserved communities.

Deadline: For more information, visit:

http://www.nmfonline.org/programs/general-scholarships-awards#anarcha

University of Michigan Health Disparities Summer Program

Description: The Health Disparities Summer Program at the University of Michigan supports the research efforts of up to eight students. This is a 10-week summer program where students work closely with a research mentor to design and conduct studies to address health disparities.

To Apply: Medical students who are members of underrepresented groups are given preference. For application information and instructions, visit the website below.

Deadline: For more information, visit:

http://www.michr.umich.edu/education/predoctoral/hdsummer

Victor Grifols Roura Scholarship

Description: The Victor Grifols Roura Scholarship is available through National Medical Fellowships. Allopathic and osteopathic medical students are eligible to apply. To be eligible, the applicant must be a second- or third-year Latino medical student with an interest in hematology. The applicant must be a student at an accredited medical institution in the Los Angeles metropolitan area.

To Apply: The application includes verification of U.S. citizenship, student aid report, documentation of loan history, financial aid transcript, two personal statements, CV, biosketch, medical school transcript, and letters of recommendation.

Deadline: For more information, visit:

http://www.nmfonline.org/programs/general-scholarships-awards#anarcha

Visiting Research Internship Program

Description: This program takes place at Harvard University. Interns conduct summer research over a period of 8 weeks under the mentorship of faculty.
To Apply: First- and second-year medical students who are members of underrepresented or disadvantaged groups are given preference. For application information and instructions, visit the website below.
Deadline: For more information, visit:

https://mfdp.med.harvard.edu/dcp-programs/medicalgraduate/visiting-research-internship-program-vrip

Wayne Anthony Butts Scholarship

Description: The Wayne Anthony Butts Scholarship is available through National Medical Fellowships.
To Apply: Allopathic and osteopathic medical students are eligible to apply. The applicant must be an underrepresented minority medical student attending school in New York City. The completed application includes verification of U.S. citizenship, student aid report, loan history, financial aid transcript, personal statements, CV, biosketch, medical school transcript, and letters of recommendation.
Deadline: For more information, visit:

http://www.nmfonline.org/programs/general-scholarships-awards#anarcha

William and Charlotte Cadbury Award

Description: The National Medical Foundation administers the Cadbury Award. It is presented annually to a senior medical student. The recipient receives a certificate of merit and $2,000 stipend.
To Apply: Allopathic and osteopathic medical students who are members of underrepresented groups (African-American, mainland Puerto Rican, Mexican-American, Native Hawaiians, Alaska Natives, or American Indian) are eligible to apply. To be considered, you must be nominated by your medical school. Criteria for judging include academic achievement, leadership, and community service.
Deadline: The deadline is in July. For more information, visit:

http://www.nmf-online.org/Programs/MeritAwards/Cadbury/Overview.htm

William G. Anderson, DO, Minority Scholarship (See Chapter 17)

Profile of a Winner

Alia Sommerville, a medical student at Touro College of Osteopathic Medicine, was awarded a $5,000 scholarship from National Medical Fellowships. The organization's mission is to increase the number of underrepresented minority physicians. Among Alia's notable accomplishments:

- Minority Services Coordinator for AMA
- Touro College of Medicine Liaison to the Student National Medical Association (SNMA)
- Launched program to retain minorities in medicine through SNMA
- Mentored Harlem youth interested in pursuing health science careers
- Started Black Student Health Alliance at Touro
- Medical mission trip to Haiti following earthquake
- International health experience in Ghana

Following graduation, she will be an obstetrics and gynecology resident at York Hospital in Pennsylvania.[7]

References

[1]Wayne State University School of Medicine. Available at: http://prognosis.med.wayne.edu/article/som-student-one-of-eight-nationwide-selected-for-aan-foundations-minority-scholars-program. Accessed January 20, 2014.

[2]American Medical Association. Available at: http://www.ama-assn.org/ama/pub/about-ama/ama-foundation/recipient-stories/lissette-jimenez.page. Accessed January 14, 2014.

[3]Cooper Medical School of Rowan University. Available at: http://www.rowan.edu/coopermed/about/news/ikpot.php. Accessed January 20, 2014.

[4]National Medical Fellowships. Available at: http://www.nmfonline.org/monash-scott/scholar-bios-2012. Accessed June 23, 2014.

[5]University of California Davis School of Medicine. Available at: http://www.ucdmc.ucdavis.edu/medalumni/newsflash/news/nsa.html. Accessed January 20, 2014.

[6]University System of Georgia. Available at: http://www.usg.edu/system. Accessed January 20, 2014.

[7]Touro College of Osteopathic Medicine. Available at: http://www.touro.edu/news/press-releases/tourocom-student-wins-fellowship.php. Accessed June 3, 2014.

Chapter 14

Global/International Health Scholarships, Awards, and Grants

In 1979, approximately 6% of graduating medical students reported participation in a clinical overseas elective. In 2007, nearly thirty years later, over 27% of all medical students in the U.S. had taken part in an international health experience. The cost of participating in a global health rotation or experience can be significant, and may prevent students from pursuing such opportunities. Fortunately, there are sources of support in the form of scholarships or grants. You are encouraged to seek support from religious organizations, ethnic organizations, local and regional chapters of professional organizations, foundations, civic organizations, and alumni associations. Because funding from these sources is not often publicized, it's well worth the effort to make inquiries. Inquiries should also be made with your Dean's office and faculty members actively involved in global health. Below we have compiled a list of global health scholarships and grants. Note that some listings are opportunities rather than awards but we have found that the sponsoring organizations often work with students to identify sources of funding.

Albert Schweitzer Fellowship

Description: Through this program, students can develop service projects to address the root causes of health disparities in underserved communities.
To Apply: For more information, contact the program below.
Deadline: For more information, visit:

http://www.schweitzerfellowship.org/news/category/press-releases/2014-15-columbus-athens-schweitzer-fellows-named/

Amazon Promise

Description: Amazon Promise invites medical students to consider joining professionals on 3-week medical expeditions. Trips take place from July through October. Participants will work in impoverished neighborhoods of Iquitos and remote jungle communities.
To Apply: For application information, visit the website below. The organization has helped students find scholarships and raise funds.
Deadline: For more information, visit:

http://www.amazonpromise.org/

American Institute for Maghrib Studies Saharan Crossroads Fellowship

Description: This fellowship program offers medical students the opportunity to conduct research in any part of North or West Africa. The award amount is up to $3,000 for three months.
To Apply: Priority is given to applicants with an interest in conducting fieldwork in Algeria, Morocco, Tunisia, or anywhere in West Africa. For more information, contact the program below.
Deadline: For more information, visit:

http://aimsnorthafrica.org/fellowships/lstuscitz_grants.cfm

American Jewish World Service

Description: American Jewish World Service is an organization committed to alleviating poverty, hunger and disease in the developing world. The organization has a presence in a number of countries, including Cambodia, El Salvador, Ghana, Guatemala, Honduras, India, Mexico, Nicaragua, Senegal, South Africa, Thailand, and Uganda.
To Apply: Opportunities for medical student involvement are available. For more information, contact the organization.
Deadline: For more information, contact volunteer@ajws.org.

American Society of Tropical Medicine and Hygiene Fellowship

Description: Through this program, medical students can receive support to perform research on the transmission dynamics of Shigella. The minimum research period is four months.
To Apply: The program is open to third- and fourth-year medical students. For more information, contact the program below.
Deadline: For more information, contact Margaret Kosek at mkosek@jhsph.edu.

AMSA Clinical Exchange

Description: Through the AMSA Clinical Exchange Program, students are able to complete a clinical rotation in a foreign country. Participants agree to provide the same opportunity for foreign students at their school.
To Apply: The exchange program is generally limited to AMSA chapters that also accept incoming international students. For application information, visit the website below.
Deadline: For more information, visit:

http://www.amsa.org/AMSA/Homepage/EducationCareerDevelopment/International Exchanges/Clinical.aspx

AMSA Research Exchange

Description: Through the AMSA Research Exchange Program, students are able to conduct research in a foreign country. Participants travel to a foreign country where they perform basic or clinical research under the supervision of a faculty member. During the period of research, students have the opportunity to interact with medical students in other countries. Participants agree to provide the same opportunity for foreign students at their school.
To Apply: For application information and instructions, visit the website below.
Deadline: For more information, visit:

http://www.amsa.org/AMSA/Homepage/EducationCareerDevelopment/Internat
ionalExchanges/Research.aspx

AMWA American Women's Hospital Service Overseas Assistance Grant (See Chapter 11)

Anne C. Carter Global Health Fellowship (See Chapter 11)

Baptist Mid-Missions

Description: Baptist Mid-Missions has opportunities for medical student involvement in short-term medical missions.
To Apply: For more information, contact the organization.
Deadline: For more information, contact Steve Fulks at sfulks@bmm.org.

Benjamin H. Kean Travel Fellowship in Tropical Medicine

Description: Through the American Society of Tropical Medicine and Hygiene (ASTMH), students can receive support to complete an elective overseas. The award amount is up to $1,000.
To Apply: Full-time medical students in the U.S. or Canada are eligible to apply. Applicants must propose an elective conducting research or clinical training in tropical medicine or global health. Preference is given to students seeking experiences lasting longer than one month. Proposals that involve study of disease common in the tropics other than HIV/AIDS are preferred. Although membership in ASTMH is not required, members will be given priority. The application includes CV, letter of recommendation, overseas mentor approval letter, and elective proposal.
Deadline: For more information, visit:

http://www.astmh.org/AM/Template.cfm?Section=ASTMH_Sponsored_Fello
wships&Template=/CM/ContentDisplay.cfm&ContentID=5513

Profile of a Winner

In 2013, Christian Parobek and Seth Congdon were two of the 22 recipients chosen by the American Society of Tropical Medicine and Hygiene to receive the Benjamin Kean Travel Fellowship in Tropical Medicine. Parobek is a M.D./Ph.D. student at the University of North Carolina. His fellowship will support a six-week period of malaria research in Thailand and Cambodia. Following residency and fellowship training, he hopes to continue clinical work and research in infectious diseases and global health. "My experiences will give me a better understanding of malaria research in Southeast Asia and of global public health research in general," said Parobek in an article published on the University of North Carolina School of Medicine website.[1]

Seth Congdon is also a medical student at the University of North Carolina. The funds he received from the fellowship allowed him to complete his research project in Zambia. Congdon investigated factors contributing to rotavirus vaccine failure in Zambian infants. "I am strongly interested in making clinical research in this region of Africa part of my career as a doctor," said Congdon.[1]

Beyond the Biologic Basis of Disease: The Social and Economic Causation of Illness

Description: This is a social medicine immersion experience in northern Uganda.
To Apply: The program is open to third- and fourth-year medical students from across the world. Scholarship support is available to offset some of the cost associated with the experience.
Deadline: For more information, visit:

http://www.socmedglobal.org/uganda-course.html

Boehringer Ingelheim Fonds Award

Description: This award provides funding to medical students to conduct basic biomedical research in Germany for 10 – 12 months.
To Apply: For application information and instructions, visit the website below.
Deadline: For more information, visit:

http://www.bifonds.de/fellowships-grants/md-fellowships.html

Boren Fellowship

Description: This fellowship provides support for study and research in areas of the world that are critical to U.S. interests. These areas include Africa, Asia, Central & Eastern Europe, Eurasia, Latin America, and the Middle East. The emphasis is on the acquisition of an important international and language component to the student's education. The award amount is up to $30,000.
To Apply: For application information and instructions, visit the website below.
Deadline: For more information, visit:

http://www.borenawards.org/boren_fellowship

Botswana USA Partnership Student Fellowship

Description: The Botswana USA (BOTUSA) Partnership sponsors a medical student fellowship program for students to participate in CDC research in Botswana.
To Apply: Third- and fourth-year medical students are eligible to apply. For application information and instructions, visit the website below.
Deadline: For more information, visit:

http://www.cdc.gov/botusa/TB-HIVResearch.htm#student

Bridges to Community

Description: Bridges to Community is a community development organization which relies on volunteers to live and work with local communities around the world. Volunteers participate in construction, health, and environmental projects.
To Apply: Opportunities for medical student involvement are available. For more information, contact the organization.
Deadline: For more information, visit:

http://www.bridgestocommunity.org/

Caring Partners International

Description: Caring Partners International is a Christian ministry which sponsors and organizes medical mission teams to provide service in countries such as Cuba, Guatemala, Nicaragua, Ecuador, and Ukraine.
To Apply: Opportunities for medical student involvement are available. For more information, contact the organization.
Deadline: For more information, visit:

http://www.caringpartners.org/

Catholic Medical Mission Board

Description: The Catholic Medical Mission Board recruits and places volunteers at healthcare facilities across the world. Among the countries requiring assistance include Armenia, Belarus, Belize, Chad, Dominican Republic, Ecuador, Ethiopia, Ghana, Guatemala, Honduras, Kenya, Jamaica, Malawi, Mexico, Paraguay, Peru, South Africa, Sudan, Zambia, and Zimbabwe.
To Apply: Opportunities for medical student involvement are available. For more information, visit the website below.
Deadline: For more information, contact info@cmmb.org.

Center for Personal Restoration

Description: The Center for Personal Restoration believes in personal renewal of healthcare professionals through volunteer service abroad.
To Apply: Opportunities for medical student involvement are available. For more information, contact the organization.
Deadline: For more information, contact Dr. David Krier at dbkmd@earthlink.net.

Children of Peace International

Description: The mission of Children of Peace International is to help the people of Vietnam. The organization offers support to hospitals, clinic, and orphanages in Vietnam. Volunteers can participate in two medical missions each year.
To Apply: Opportunities for medical student involvement are available. For more information, contact the organization.
Deadline: For more information, visit:

http://www.childrenofpeace.org/

Concern America

Description: Concern America allows medical students and other professionals to participate in a hands-on learning experience abroad.
To Apply: Opportunities for medical student involvement are available. For more information, contact the organization.
Deadline: For more information, visit:

http://www.concernamerica.org/

Carole M. Davis Scholarship

Description: The Carole M. Davis scholarship is given annually to a medical student seeking funds to support an international health activity. The award amount is $1,000.

To Apply: To be eligible, the applicant must attend a school that is an institutional member of IHMEC. The application includes CV, letter from supervising faculty member, and personal statement. The statement should be no more than 1,000 words, and indicate how the funds will be used during the international health activity.

Deadline: The deadline is in December. For more information, visit:

http://depts.washington.edu/ihg/funding.htm#Carole

Centro de Salud Santa Clotilde

Description: Centro de Salud Santa Clotilde serves thousands of patients in rural Peru. Opportunities for clinical medical students are available. Typical problems seen in the inpatient setting include pneumonia, trauma, snake bites, dengue, malaria, dehydration, and diarrhea. Room and board is provided at a cost of $5/day. Students are responsible for the cost of travel.

To Apply: To be eligible, fluency in Spanish is required since no translators are available.

Deadline: For more information, contact Antoinette Lullo at alullo@hotmail.com.

Chateaubriand Fellowship Program

Description: The Chateaubriand Fellowship Program is administered by the Office for Science and Technology of the Embassy of France in the United States. It provides support for about 20 students to conduct research in a French laboratory over a 6 to 12-month period.

To Apply: To be eligible, the applicant must be a Ph.D. candidate (M.D./Ph.D. applicants are eligible). Prior to applying for the program, the applicant must secure an agreement from a hosting laboratory.

Deadline: For more information, visit:

http://depts.washington.edu/ihg/funding.htm#Carole

CDC – Hubert Global Health Fellowship

Description: The Centers for Disease Control established the Hubert Global Health Fellowship to provide medical students with a population health experience in an international setting. Through this fellowship program, participants attend a Fellowship Short Course in Atlanta and take part in a field assignment. The assignment is a hands-on experience working on a health problem in a developing country under the supervision of CDC staff. Past projects have included health outcome evaluation of home drinking water treatment and storage methods in Guatemala, review of antiretroviral therapy in Kenya, and study of Lassa Fever epidemiology in West Africa. The award amount for this year-long fellowship is $4,000.

To Apply: For application information, visit the website below.

Deadline: For more information, visit:

http://www.cdc.gov/hubertfellowship/More.html

Charles H. Houston Award (See Chapter 10)

Child Family Health International Scholarship

Description: Child Family Health International (CFHI) offers scholarships to medical students to participate in CFHI programs abroad. Programs run on a monthly basis, and last 4 – 8 weeks. The award amount is $500 to $1,000.

To Apply: Medical students are eligible to apply. Preference will be given to students who have demonstrated commitment to their communities and have an interest in exchanging ideas and sharing experiences with people in Bolivia, Ecuador, India, Mexico, and South Africa. CFHI recommends applying 3 months prior to your desired arrival date.

Deadline: For more information, visit:

http://www.cfhi.org/web/index.php/xcms/showpage/page/Scholarships

David E. Rogers Fellowship Program (See Chapter 10)

Doris Duke International Clinical Research Fellowship

Description: The Doris Duke International Clinical Research Fellowship provides support to medical students interested in conducting clinical research in developing countries. The goal of the program is to help develop clinical investigators in the area of global health. Fellows receive a stipend for one year of research.

To Apply: Allopathic and osteopathic medical students are eligible to apply. For application information and instructions, visit the website below.

Deadline: The application deadline is in January. For more information, visit:

http://www.ddcf.org/Programs/Medical-Research/Goals-and-Strategies/Build-the-Clinical-Research-Career-Ladder/International-Clinical-Research-Fellowship/

DOCARE International

Description: DOCARE has global health rotation opportunities for students in Nicaragua and Guatemala. Participants will be involved in providing medical assistance to underserved populations.

To Apply: To be eligible, applicants must be active DOCARE members. Permission from your medical school is required as is the completion of an application packet at least 60 days prior to the trip. Medical students must be in good academic standing.

Deadline: For more information, visit:

http://docare.osteopathic.org/web/Resident%20Rotations.aspx

Fellowships at Auschwitz for the Study of Professional Ethics

Description: The Fellowships at Auschwitz for the Study of Professional Ethics is a unique program that allows students to immerse themselves in contemporary ethical issues through a historical context. This is a two-week intensive course in New York, Germany, and Poland.

To Apply: For application information and instructions, visit the website below.

Deadline: For more information, visit:

http://www.mjhnyc.org/faspe/index.html

Fogarty International Clinical Research Scholar Program

Description: Through this program, medical students perform clinical research in a developing country under the supervision of a mentor. The amount of the award is $25,000 for one year of research.

To Apply: For application information and instructions, visit the website below.

Deadline: For more information, visit:

http://www.fic.nih.gov/programs/pages/scholars-fellows.aspx

Foundation for Sustainable Development

Description: Through this program, medical students can participate in immersive and hands-on community-driven projects in Asia, Africa and Latin America.

To Apply: Opportunities for medical student involvement are available. For more information, contact the organization.

Deadline: For more information, visit:

http://www.fsdinternational.org/

Fulbright Scholarship

Description: Through the Fulbright Program, over 1,000 Americans study or conduct research in other nations each year. Most awards are for one academic year.

To Apply: There are two types of awards – Study/Research Grants and English Teaching Assistantships. Medical students interested in study/research grants must plan their own programs. The application includes project proposal, personal statement, three letters of recommendation, and transcript.
Deadline: For more information, visit:

http://us.fulbrightonline.org/getting-started

Fulbright Travel Grant

Description: This grant provides funding to medical students involved in study or research in Germany, Hungary, or Italy. It serves as a supplement to an award from any source that does not cover costs associated with international travel.
To Apply: For application information and instructions, visit the website below.
Deadline: The deadline is in October. For more information, visit:

https://us.fulbrightonline.org/getting-started

GE/NMF International Medical Scholars Program (See Chapter 13)

Global Health Corps Fellowship

Description: Global Health Corps fellows are able to work at health organizations and government agencies across the world to promote global health equity. This is a one-year fellowship program.
To Apply: For application information and instructions, visit the website below.
Deadline: For more information, visit:

http://ghcorps.org/program/overview/

Global Medical Brigades

Description: Global Medical Brigades aims to provide communities in developing countries with sustainable health care solutions.
To Apply: Opportunities for medical student involvement are available. For more information, contact the organization.
Deadline: For more information, contact Sophia Fang at sophia@medicalbrigades.com.

Global Service Corps

Description: Global Service Corps is an international service-learning organization involved in activities throughout the developed and developing world.
To Apply: Opportunities for medical student involvement are available. For more information, contact the organization.
Deadline: For more information, visit:

http://www.globalservicecorps.org/

Global Volunteers

Description: Global Volunteers seeks short-term volunteers to assist with microeconomic and human development programs worldwide.
To Apply: Opportunities for medical student involvement are available. For more information, contact the organization.
Deadline: For more information, visit:

http://www.globalvolunteers.org/

Gold Student Summer Fellowship (See Chapter 10)

Haiti Mission Trip Scholarship (See Chapter 65)

Health Education & Advocacy Liaisons

Description: Through Health Education & Advocacy Liaisons, clinical medical students can work with physicians at a pediatric clinic in Honduras. The organization does not provide funds but does indicate that many of their interns have been able to keep their month-long internship costs down to $1,500.
To Apply: Opportunities for medical student involvement are available. Fluency in Spanish is required. For more information, contact the organization.
Deadline: For more information, contact healinternship@gmail.com.

Health Horizons International

Description: Health Horizons International strives to deliver quality primary health care to the underserved in the Dominican Republic.
To Apply: Opportunities for medical student involvement are available. For more information, contact the organization.
Deadline: For more information, contact Laura McNulty at lmcnulty@hhidr.org.

HealthCare Nepal

Description: The organization provides free care in rural Nepal by sponsoring and organizing short-term health "camps."
To Apply: Opportunities for medical student involvement are available. For more information, contact the organization.
Deadline: For more information, visit:

http://www.healthcarenepal.org/

Helen Hay Whitney Foundation

Description: The Helen Hay Whitney Foundation grants fellowships to medical students interested in performing research in the U.S., Canada, and elsewhere.
To Apply: For application information, visit the website below.
Deadline: For more information, visit:

http://www.hhwf.org/HTMLSrc/ResearchFellowships.html

Helping Hands Health Education

Description: The aim of this organization is to deliver low-cost quality medical relief services to rural parts of Nepal and Vietnam.
To Apply: Opportunities for medical student involvement are available. For more information, contact the organization.
Deadline: For more information, visit:

http://www.helpinghandsusa.org/

HELPS International

Description: HELPS International works closely with individuals, businesses, and governments to alleviate poverty in Latin America.
To Apply: Opportunities for medical student involvement are available. For more information, contact the organization.
Deadline: For more information, visit:

http://helpsintl.org/

Himalayan Health Exchange

Description: Himalayan Health Exchange provides care to the underserved areas in the Indo-Tibetan Borderlands.
To Apply: Opportunities for medical student involvement are available. For more information, contact the organization.
Deadline: For more information, visit:

http://www.himalayanhealth.com/

Hope Through Healing Hands Frist Global Health Leaders Program

Description: The Frist Global Health Leaders Program offers grants to medical students interested in service and training around the world. Funding helps support training abroad in underserved communities for up to one semester.
To Apply: For application information and instructions, visit the website below.
Deadline: For more information, visit:

http://www.hopethroughhealinghands.org/frist-global-health-leaders

Indicorps

Description: Indicorps annually selects young professionals of Indian origin for one- and two-year service fellowships. Fellows will work with grassroots service organizations in India.
To Apply: To be eligible, the applicant must be of Indian origin and have at minimum a university degree or five years of work experience.
Deadline: The deadline is in January. For more information, visit:

http://www.indicorps.org/.

Infectious Disease Society of American Medical Scholars Summer Program (See Chapter 24)

Naomi Kim Medical Missions Scholarship

Description: The scholarship supports medical students in their first short-term medical missions experience serving the underserved abroad. The award amount will be up to $500.
To Apply: To be eligible, the applicant must be a member of the Christian Medical & Dental Association. The applicant must be new to medical missions. The application includes a letter of no more than 300 words describing their current course of education and motivation for serving in medical missions. The letter should also address what the applicant hopes to learn from the experience.
Deadline: For more information, visit:

https://www.cmda.org/missions/page/naomi-kim-medical-missions-scholarship-fund

Institute for International Medicine

Description: The Institute for International Medicine administers clinical rotations in developing nations with instruction in international medicine, HIV medicine, and public health.
To Apply: Opportunities for medical student involvement are available. For more information, contact the organization.
Deadline: For more information, visit:

http://www.inmed.us/

International Medical Relief/Medical Mission Scholarship (See Chapter 17)

International Rescue Committee

Description: International Rescue Committee provides much needed services, including health care, during humanitarian emergencies.
To Apply: Opportunities for medical student involvement are available. For more information, contact the organization.
Deadline: For more information, visit:

http://www.rescue.org/

International Service Learning

Description: International Service Learning offers medical students the opportunity to be part of an international health team. The organization provides care to the underserved in Central America, South America, Mexico, and Africa.
To Apply: Opportunities for medical student involvement are available. For more information, contact the organization.
Deadline: For more information, visit:

http://www.islonline.org/

LIG Global Foundation

Description: LIG Global Foundation provides medical students with the opportunity to participate in global health throughout the world, including the Dominican Republic, Haiti, Philippines, Tanzania, Uganda, India, and Grenada. Trips are typically 5-12 days in duration. LIG Global Foundation works closely with volunteers to bring down the costs associated with the experience.
To Apply: Opportunities for medical student involvement are available. There are no language requirements because translators are available. However, fluency in Spanish, Hindi, Creole, or Kiswahili is a plus. For more information, contact the organization.

Deadline: For more information, contact Dr. Sarah Timmapuri at Sarah@LIGglobal.org.

Mayan Medical Aid

Description: Mayan Medical Aid offers medical students the opportunity to provide medical care to the underserved in Guatemala. Participants learn Spanish and cultural skills during the experience. Scholarships in the form of matching grants are provided to students who participate in the program for at least two weeks.
To Apply: Opportunities for medical student involvement are available. For more information, contact the organization.
Deadline: For more information, visit the following website:

http://www.mayanmedicalaid.org/project_global_programs.htm

MedSpanish

Description: Through MedSpanish, medical students can participate in a language and cultural immersion program.
To Apply: Opportunities for medical student involvement are available. For more information, contact the organization.
Deadline: For more information, contact Dr. Haywood Hall at haywood@pacemd.org.

Medical Mission Trip Educational Grant (See Chapter 65)

Medical Missions Kenya and Hunger Relief

Description: Medical Missions Kenya and Hunger Relief provide medical students with the opportunity to participate in the delivery of health care to remote villages in Kenya. The typical cost of the experience is $2,500.
To Apply: Opportunities for medical student involvement are available. There is no language requirement. For more information, contact the organization.
Deadline: For more information, visit:

http://medicalmissionskenya.org/

Mission Doctors Association

Description: The organization recruits, trains, and sends Catholic doctors and professionals to serve in mission hospitals and clinics around the world.
To Apply: Opportunities for medical student involvement are available. For more information, contact the organization.
Deadline: For more information, visit:

http://missiondoctors.org/

Mountain Medics International

Description: The organization aims to improve health in mountain communities where underserved populations reside.
To Apply: Opportunities for medical student involvement are available. For more information, contact the organization.
Deadline: For more information, visit:

http://mountainmedics.org/

Multidisciplinary International Research Training Program

Description: The Multidisciplinary International Research Training Program provides opportunities for underrepresented students to participate in short-term global research training in public health. This program is administered by the Harvard School of Public Health which has developed training sites around the world, including Chile, Ecuador, Georgia, Peru, Malaysia, Thailand, and Zimbabwe.
To Apply: For application information, visit the website below.
Deadline: For more information, visit:

http://www.hsph.harvard.edu/mirt/

Physicians for Peace

Description: The organization trains and educates health care professionals around the world.
To Apply: Opportunities for medical student involvement are available. For more information, contact the organization.
Deadline: For more information, visit:

http://physiciansforpeace.org/

Project HOPE

Description: Project HOPE sends health care volunteers at all levels, from birth attendants to cardiac surgeons, to areas of the world lacking resources.
To Apply: Opportunities for medical student involvement are available. For more information, contact the organization.
Deadline: For more information, visit:

http://www.projecthope.org/

Project Hope Northwest

Description: The scholarship supports medical students in their efforts to serve the underserved abroad during 4 – 8 week mission trips. The average award amount is $1,500.

To Apply: Medical students in the Pacific Northwest are given preference. Allopathic and osteopathic medical students may apply.
Deadline: There are two application cycles with deadlines in September and January. For more information, visit:

http://www.projecthopenorthwest.org/apply-for-support.html

Project Vietnam

Description: Project Vietnam provides health care assistance to children living in rural Vietnam.
To Apply: Opportunities for medical student involvement are available. For more information, contact the organization.
Deadline: For more information, contact Dr. Quynh Kieu at qkieu@projectvietnam.net.

Riken Brain Science Institute Summer Program

Description: The Riken Brain Science Institute Summer Program was developed to further the education of young neuroscientists. The Institute is based outside Tokyo, and offers students the choice of either a two-month laboratory internship or an intensive 7-day lecture course. Every year, 45 international students are accepted.
To Apply: For application information, visit the website below.
Deadline: For more information, visit:

http://www.brain.riken.jp/en/summer/index.html

RISE Global Health Initiative

Description: RISE Global Health Initiative provides medical students with the opportunity to participate in an international health experience in Nigeria. Participants must agree to at least 2 weeks of involvement. Food, housing, ground transportation, and security is provided by the organization. Students must play for the cost of air travel.
To Apply: There is no language requirement. Contact the organization for more information.
Deadline: For more information, visit:

http://www.riseghi.org/

Saint Francis Hospital

Description: Saint Francis Hospital is a large rural hospital serving an underserved population in Zambia.
To Apply: Opportunities for medical student involvement are available. For more information, contact the organization.
Deadline: For more information, contact Dr. Richard Newell at richard@saintfrancishospital.net.

Sara's Wish Foundation Scholarship

Description: Sarah's Wish Foundation provides scholarships to women who are committed to making the world a better place. With the support of the foundation, women have made remarkable contributions in all areas of the globe.

To Apply: Criteria for judging include a commitment to public service, strong record of scholarship, history of leadership experience, and a sincere interest in the work of Sara's Wish Foundation. For application information and instructions, visit the website below.

Deadline: For more information, visit:

http://www.saraswish.org/scholarships/

SOMA's International Health Program Scholarship (See Chapter 17)

Steury Scholarship

Description: The Christian Medical & Dental Association sponsors the Steury Scholarship. The scholarship provides tuition support to medical students who are committed to careers in foreign or domestic medical missions. Applicants must be willing to serve for an extended period of time. The award amount is up to $25,000. The scholarship becomes an interest-bearing loan if the student withdraws from medical school or fails to enter the mission field or serve for the required period of time.

To Apply: To be eligible, the applicant must be a CMDA member who is beginning their first or second year of medical school. Osteopathic and allopathic medical students are invited to apply. Criteria for judging include academic record, cross culture experience, leadership ability, spiritual maturity, references, and extracurricular activities.

Deadline: For more information, visit:

https://www.cmda.org/missions/page/steury-scholarship-information

Timmy High Impact Volunteer

Description: Current students or alumni of Timmy Global Health university chapters may apply to become a Timmy High Impact Volunteer. Volunteers receive financial support to volunteer in one of Timmy's program sites on a long-term basis. Participants submit a project proposal describing the contributions they would like to make at a specific Timmy site in Ecuador, Guatemala, or the Dominican Republic. The award amount is $500 to $2,000.

To Apply: Medical students who are alumni of Timmy Global Health university chapters may apply. Preference is given to those who have "demonstrated outstanding dedication and passion toward tackling global health disparities, and are committed to future careers and personal efforts to promote health equity."[2] To be eligible, the applicant must initially be approved as a Long Term Volunteer by Timmy's Global Health LTV Coordinator. Criteria for judging include merit, commitment to service, reference letter, region specific language proficiency, and proposal form.

Deadline: There are three application cycles with deadlines in February, May, and November. For more information, visit:

http://www.timmyglobalhealth.org/?page_id=4063

Timmy Social Entrepreneur Volunteer

Description: Current students or alumni of Timmy Global Health university chapters may apply to become a Timmy Social Entrepreneur Volunteer. Through this program, volunteers receive financial support to implement a self-initiated and self-designed solution to a global health problem.

To Apply: Medical students who are alumni of Timmy Global Health university chapters may apply. To be eligible, applicants must submit a project proposal describing how funds will be used to advance global health equity in innovative ways. The applicant must initially be approved as a Long Term Volunteer by Timmy's Global Health LTV Coordinator. Criteria for judging include merit, commitment to service, reference letter, region specific language proficiency, and proposal form.

Deadline: There are three application cycles with deadlines in February, May, and November. For more information, visit:

http://www.timmyglobalhealth.org/?page_id=4067

Tropical Disease Research Program in Ecuador

Description: Since 2000, the Ohio University Tropical Disease Institute and the Center for Infectious Diseases Research in Quito have partnered together to help control the transmission of Chagas disease in Ecuador.

To Apply: Medical students are eligible to apply. Admission to the program is determined by Dr. Mario Grijalva at Ohio University. Applicants should e-mail (grijalva@ohio.edu) their interest in participating. "Since this is a research training project, admissions will be based on the interface between the applicant's interest and expertise, and the specific needs of the project."[3]

Deadline: The application deadline is in February. For more information, visit:

http://www.oucom.ohiou.edu/tdi/InternationalResearch/InternationalResearch.htm

Unite for Sight Global Impact Corps

Description: Unite for Sight supports eye clinics in Ghana, India and Honduras. Medical students can serve as Global Impact Fellows, and work closely with local doctors to assist with global health delivery. Fellows also have the opportunity to design and pursue a global health research study.

To Apply: For application information, visit the website below.

Deadline: For more information, visit:

http://www.uniteforsight.org/volunteer-abroad/faqs

USAID Internship Program

Description: Through the USAID Internship Program, interns are able to work in a variety of programs in such fields as economic growth, agriculture, education, health, environment, governance, conflict prevention, and humanitarian assistance. Paid and unpaid opportunities are available.
To Apply: For application information and instructions, visit the website below.
Deadline: For more information, visit:

http://www.usaid.gov/work-usaid/careers/student-internships

Vietnamese American Medical Association Memorial Travel Scholarship (See Chapter 12)

Volunteers in Medical Missions

Description: Volunteers in Medical Missions sends teams of Christian health care professionals and volunteers around the world to participate in medical missions.
To Apply: Opportunities for medical student involvement are available. For more information, contact the organization.
Deadline: For more information, visit:

http://www.vimm.org/

Westra Short-Term Mission Scholarship

Description: The Christian Medical & Dental Association sponsors the Westra Short-Term Mission Scholarship. The scholarship supports medical students in their efforts to serve the underserved abroad. The award amount is up to $500.
To Apply: To be eligible, the applicant must be a CMDA member. Only third- and fourth-year medical students may apply. Financial need will be considered. The application includes a letter of recommendation from a pastor which describes the applicant's spiritual maturity and involvement in ministry.
Deadline: Applications are reviewed quarterly with deadlines in April, August, and December. For more information, visit:

http://www.cmdahome.org/missions/page/westra-short-term-mission-scholarship-information

William J. Clinton Fellowship for Service in India

Description: The William J. Clinton Fellowship for Service in India allows young professionals to work with NGOs and social enterprises in India over a ten-month period.

To Apply: To be eligible, the applicant must be a citizen or permanent resident of the U.S. or citizen of India. Only applicants between the ages of 21 and 34 may apply. Selection criteria includes general knowledge of development issues in India, ability to demonstrate appreciation of other cultures, willingness to independently and creatively find ways to be helpful at host organization, and adaptability to challenging living and working conditions. For application information and instructions, visit the website below.
Deadline: For more information, visit:

http://aif.org/investment-area/leadership/

Yale/Stanford Johnson & Johnson Global Health Scholars Program

Description: Through the Global Health Scholars Program, medical students at Yale, Stanford, and other institutions can participate in global health activities in such places as South Africa, Uganda, Liberia, Indonesia, and Rwanda.
To Apply: For application information and instructions, visit the website below.
Deadline: For more information, visit:

http://medicine.yale.edu/intmed/globalhealthscholars/index.aspx

References

[1]University of North Carolina School of Medicine. Available at:
http://news.unchealthcare.org/som-vital-signs/2013/september-26/two-medical-students-awarded-the-benjamin-h-kean-travel-fellows-in-tropical-medicine. Accessed July 22, 2014.
[2]Timmy Global Health. Available at:
http://timmyglobalhealth.org/index.php/timmy-global-health-high-impact-volunteers/. Accessed July 22, 2014.
[3]Ohio University Tropical Disease Institute. Available at:
http://www.oucom.ohiou.edu/tdi/InternationalResearch/InternationalResearch.htm. Accessed July 24, 2014.

Chapter 15

Writing Awards

As a medical student, you are privileged to intimately experience healing and dying from a unique perspective. In developing your clinical skills, you will care for patients at vulnerable times in their lives, and these encounters will often be personal and powerful. If shared, these stories can educate and inspire others. In this chapter, we list writing contests and awards that allow you to tell your stories.

ACLS Recertification Healthcare Training Scholarship

Description: The ACLS Healthcare Training Scholarship Plan offers a $2,000 scholarship to the author of the winning essay. Two runners-up will receive complimentary passes for registration to the ACLS Recertification program of their choice (ACLS, BLS, PALS). The winning essays will be featured on the organization's website.
To Apply: Contestants must submit a 500 – 1000 word essay. The essay should tell the judges "how you feel about providing emergency medical care wherein you shall be called to provide life support from the basic to the more advanced cardiac or pediatric life support."[1] Criteria for judging include sincerity, persuasiveness, and overall cohesion and effectiveness.
Deadline: The deadline is in December. For more information, visit:

http://www.aclsrecertification.com/scholarship

American Academy of Pediatrics Ethics Essay Contest

Description: The American Academy of Pediatrics (AAP) offers the Pediatrics Ethics Essay Contest for medical students. The winner will be recognized at the AAP National Conference and Exhibition. The essay will be published in the Section of Bioethics Newsletter. The award amount is $300.
To Apply: For more information, including the essays of previous award recipients, visit the website below.
Deadline: For more information, visit:

http://www2.aap.org/sections/bioethics/EssayContest.cfm

AMA Virtual Mentor John Conley Ethics Essay Contest for Medical Students

Description: Developed by the American Medical Association *Virtual Mentor*, the John Conley Ethics Essay Contest for Medical Students asks students to submit an essay addressing a question in medical ethics or professionalism. The winner will receive an award of $5,000. The authors of up to three runner-up essays will each receive $1,000. Winning essays will be published in the *Virtual Mentor*.

To Apply: Current osteopathic and allopathic medical students are eligible to enter the contest. An essay up to 2,000 words will be accepted. Criteria for judging include presentation, writing style, and applicability of the argument to actual decision making.

Deadline: The deadline for the contest is in July. See the following link for more information:

http://virtualmentor.ama-assn.org/site/aboutconley.html

AMWA Linda Brodsky MD Essay Award

Description: The American Medical Women's Association (AMWA) offers this award to a student for an essay that honors a female physician who has been a significant mentor or role model. The award recipient will receive $500 and be recognized at the Annual Meeting. The essay will be published at the AMWA website.

To Apply: Essays should be kept under 1000 words. Applicants should discuss the impact the female mentor or role model had on their decision to become physicians.

Deadline: The deadline is in March. For more information, visit:

http://www.amwa-doc.org/students/awards/linda-brodsky-md-essay-award/

American Osteopathic Association History Essay Contest

Description: The American Osteopathic Association (AOA) encourages osteopathic medical students to enter the History Essay Contest. The mission of the contest is to promote awareness of the profession's history, struggles, and achievement. Three winners will receive awards of $5,000, $3,000, and $2,000.

To Apply: The essay should be no longer than 3,000 words. For more information, visit the website below.

Deadline: The deadline is in August. For more information, visit:

http://thedo.osteopathic.org/?p=170941

AMN/HCC Healthcare Scholarship Essay Contest

Description: AMN Healthcare and Health Care Communicators of San Diego (HCC) encourage San Diego County high school and undergraduate students to enter the Healthcare Scholarship Essay Contest.
To Apply: Students should submit an essay addressing the topic "Why I Plan to Enter the Field of Health Care After College Graduation." A letter of recommendation is also required.
Deadline: The deadline is in March. For more information, visit:

http://www.hccsd.org/amn/hcc-scholarship/

Annals Poetry Prize

Description: The *Annals of Internal Medicine* offers a prize for the best poem published annually. The award amount is $500.
To apply: Visit the website below.
Deadline: For more information, visit:

http://annals.org/public/poetryprize.aspx

Ascona Prize for Students

Description: The Foundation for Psychosomatic and Social Medicine invites medical students to apply for the Ascona Prize. Three award winners are chosen for essays describing a student-patient relationship or experience. Winners will be expected to attend the International Balint Congress where they will give a short presentation of their essay. Winning essays will be published in Balint journals. Winners will receive free accommodation and monetary support to defray the cost of travel to the meeting.
To Apply: The paper must be written in English, and should describe a student-patient relationship or experience. Submissions should be between 3,000 and 10,000 words. Criteria used for judging include exposition (presentation of a truly personal experience of a student-patient relationship), reflection, action, and progression. For more information, visit the link below.
Deadline: The application deadline is in December. For more information, visit:

http://www.balintinternational.com/asconaprize.html

Association for Academic Psychiatry Medical Student on *Becoming a Doctor* Essay Contest

Description: The Association for Academic Psychiatry (AAP) sponsors the Medical Student on *Becoming a Doctor* Essay Contest. The winner will receive up to $1,000 to defray the costs of travel to attend the AAP Annual Meeting. The winner will present the essay at the meeting.

To Apply: Medical students in the U.S. and Canada are eligible to enter the contest. The essay will be 2,000 words or less. Criteria for judging include originality, uniqueness, flow of thought, and appropriateness to theme.
Deadline: The deadline is in June. For more information, visit:

https://netforum.avectra.com/eweb/DynamicPage.aspx?Site=aap&WebCode=A wardsDetails#med_stu

BLR Prize

Description: The BLR Prizes recognize outstanding writing in the areas of health, healing, illness, the mind, and the body. The winner in each genre will receive $ 1,000. Contestants who receive honorable mention will receive $250. These works will be published in an issue of BLR.
To Apply: There is an entry fee of $20. Prose should be less than 5,000 words. No more than 3 poems should be submitted. Work that is submitted should not have been previously published.
Deadline: For more information, visit:

http://blr.med.nyu.edu/submissions/BLRPrizes/guidelines#sthash.kRfq38nM.d puf

C. Ronald Stephen, M.D. Anesthesia History Essay Contest

Description: The Anesthesia History Association (AHA) offers this essay contest to medical students, residents, and fellows. Acceptable topics include history of anesthesia, pain medicine, or critical care. The winner will receive $1,000, and the opportunity to deliver an oral presentation of his or her work at the AHA Annual Spring Meeting. The essay will also be considered for publication in the *Bulletin of Anesthesia History.*
To Apply: The essay must be less than 3,500 words. Criteria for judging include originality and appropriateness of topic, quality of research, composition, and bibliography. For more information, visit the website below.
Deadline: The deadline is in September. For more information, visit:

http://ahahq.org/Essay.php

David R. Cox Prize for Rare Compassion

Description: Rare diseases are generally not given high priority or attention from people and organizations. This prize was developed to foster interest and caring among future physicians for patients and families affected by such illnesses. The award amount is $1,000.
Applying for the Award: Applicants are asked to develop a relationship with a patient, family, or advocate affected by a neglected disease. Based on the experience, applicants should write and submit an essay conveying the scope and significance of the disease's impact on the patient, student, and society.

Deadline: For more information, visit:

https://globalgenes.org/david-r-cox-prize-for-rare-compassion/

Ethics and the Physician-Patient Relationship Essay Contest

Description: The contest is administered by the Dr. Shoshanah Trachtenberg Frackman Program in Biomedical Ethics at the Albert Einstein College of Medicine. The winner will receive $1,000 for the best essay devoted to the physician-patient relationship.
To Apply: Medical students in the U.S. and Canada are eligible to enter the contest. The essay will be 2,500 words or less.
Deadline: The deadline is in December. Essays may be mailed or emailed to the following address:

Dr. Ruth Macklin, Professor of Bioethics
Department of Epidemiology and Population Health
Albert Einstein College of Medicine
1300 Morris Park Avenue
Bronx, New York 10461
ruth.macklin@einstein.yu.edu

Giva Semi-Annual Student Scholarship Award

Description: Giva offers this award to help undergraduate and graduate students further their education. Medical students are eligible.
To Apply: To be eligible, the student must submit an essay that answers the following questions:

- How will you use your talents and education to make the world a better place for future generations?
- What are your career and personal goals and why?

A resume must also be included.
Deadline: There are two award cycles each year with deadlines in June and December. See the following link for more information:

http://www.givainc.com/scholarships/

Gold – Hope Tang, MD 2014 Humanism in Medicine Essay Contest

Description: Developed by the Gold Foundation, the Humanism in Medicine Essay Contest asks medical students to submit an essay around a topical theme or quote related to humanism in medicine. Three winners are selected, and their essays are published in *Academic Medicine* and on the Gold Foundation website. Ten others will receive honorable mention.

To Apply: Current osteopathic and allopathic medical students in the U.S. and Canada are eligible to enter the contest. Applicants must submit an essay of 1,000 words or less.

Deadline: The deadline for the contest is in April. See the following link for more information:

http://www.humanism-in-medicine.org/index.php/programs_grants/gold_foundation_programs/essay_contest

Hektoen Essay Contest

Description: Hektoen International invites applicants over the age of 18 to submit essays on a subject related to medicine and culture. The award amount is $1,500 for the winner and $1,000 for the runner-up. The winning essay will be published in an issue of Hektoen International: Journal of the Humanities. Several others will be published as well.

To Apply: The essay must be 1,500 to 2,000 words. Criteria for judging include originality and appropriateness of topic, quality of research, composition, and bibliography. For more information, visit the website below.

Deadline: The deadline is in March. For more information, visit:

http://www.hektoeninternational.org/hektoen-essay-contest-2014.html

Helen H. Glaser Student Essay Awards

Description: The Alpha Omega Alpha (AΩA) Honor Medical Society developed the Student Essay Award to encourage medical students to write creative narratives and scholarly essays relevant to medicine. The essay may be on any nontechnical subject related to medicine. The first prize award winner will receive $2,000. Second and third place winners will receive $750 and $500, respectively. Honorable mention awards of $250 will also be given. Winning essays will be published in future issues of *The Pharos*.

To Apply: Authors must be enrolled at a medical school with an active AΩA chapter but do not have to be members. Each student may submit only one essay, and its length should not exceed 15 pages. The essay must be sent through the online form or by email. Visit the link below for further requirements and application directions.

Deadline: The deadline is in January, and winners are announced by the following May. Visit the link for further information:

http://www.alphaomegaalpha.org/student_essay.html

Profile of a Winner

In 2011, the first prizewinner of the Helen H. Glaser Student Essay Award was Courtney Pendleton, a fourth-year medical student at the Johns Hopkins University School of Medicine. Her essay, "'My life, my soul, my body I owe to you and God': Harvey Cushing and the Patient-Physician Relationship as Seen through Written Correspondence," was featured in the winter 2012 issue of *The Pharos*.

"I studied studio art and English literature at New York University, graduating in 2004, and am currently a fourth-year student at the Johns Hopkins School of Medicine," stated Ms. Pendleton when describing herself in *The Pharos*. In the future, she plans to pursue a career in the field of neurosurgery.[2]

Intima Essay Contest

Description: Intima is an electronic journal created by several University of Columbia students to promote the theory and practice of Narrative Medicine. It sponsors an essay contest "to bridge the alleged gap between the patient's medical history and his or her narrative."[3] The five best essays/poems will be published in Intima.
To Apply: The essay should be no longer than 3,000 words. For more information, visit the website below.
Deadline: The deadline is in December. For more information, visit:

http://www.theintima.org/essay-contest.html

Pharos Poetry Competition

Description: The Alpha Omega Alpha (AΩA) Honor Medical Society created the *Pharos* Poetry Competition to encourage medical students to write effective poetry using imagery and rhythm or rhyme to structure the poem. The poem may be on any subject related to medicine. The first prize award winner will receive $500. Second and third place winners will receive $250 and $100, respectively. Honorable mention awards of $75 will also be given. Winning poems will be published in the future issues of *The Pharos*.
To Apply: Authors must be enrolled at a medical school with an active AΩA chapter but do not have to be members. The poem must be single spaced, single column, and not exceed two pages. Poems must be sent through the online form or by email. Visit the link below for further requirements and application directions.
Deadline: The deadline for entries is in November, and winners are announced by the following April. See the link for further information:

http://www.alphaomegaalpha.org/poetry_competition.html

Profile of a Winner

In 2010, the first prizewinner of the *Pharos* Poetry Competition was Jenna Le, a student at the Columbia University College of Physicians and Surgeons. Her poem, "Sestina on Limb-Lengthening Surgery," was featured in the winter 2011 edition of *The Pharos*.

Ms. Le has always shown a strong talent in writing. Along with winning the *Pharos* Poetry Competition, she has also won the Minnetonka Review Editors Prize, has been nominated for a Pushcart Prize and the PEN Emerging Writers Award, and has also authored a Small Press Poetry Bestseller book titled *Six Rivers*.[4-5]

Major C. W. Offutt Award

Description: The VA encourages medical students to apply for this award by submitting an essay. Three winners will receive a monetary award.
To Apply: The contest is open to third- and fourth-year medical students. Applicants are asked to submit an essay describing their experience of "Caring for America's Heroes" while rotating through the VA Medical Center.
Deadline: The deadline for this award is in April. For more information, contact:

D. Robert McCaffree, M.D.
Chief of Staff
Oklahoma City VA Medical Center
921 N.E. 13th Street
Oklahoma City, OK 73104-5028
(405) 270-5135
robert.mccaffree@va.gov

Medical Student Essay Award – Extended Neuroscience Award

Description: The American Academy of Neurology (AAN) gives this award for the best essay written in Neuroscience. The essay must be suitable for an audience of general neurologists. Recipients are expected to give a poster presentation at the AAN Annual Meeting. The recipient of the award will receive a $1,000 prize, a one-year complimentary subscription to the journal *Neurology*, and recognition at the annual meeting. All expenses for attending the annual meeting will be reimbursed.
To Apply: To be eligible, the student must be enrolled in medical school and in good standing. The applicant must submit an original, lucid essay targeted to general neurologists. The student must also have spent more than one year on a

project leading to the submitted essay. See the link below for further application information.

Deadline: The deadline for this award is in October. Award recipients are notified in January. See the following link for more information:

http://tools.aan.com/science/awards/

Medical Student Essay Award – G. Milton Shy Award

Description: The American Academy of Neurology (AAN) bestows this award to the student who has written the best essay in clinical neurology. The essay must be suitable for an audience of general neurologists. Recipients are expected to give a poster presentation at the AAN Annual Meeting. The recipient of the award will receive a $350 prize, a one-year complimentary subscription to the journal *Neurology*, and recognition at the annual meeting. All expenses for attending the annual meeting will be reimbursed.

To Apply: To be eligible, the student must be enrolled and in good standing in medical school. The applicant must submit an original, lucid essay targeted to general neurologists. The student must also have spent less than one year on a project leading to the submitted essay. See the link below for further application information.

Deadline: The deadline for this award is in October, and award recipients are notified in January. See the following link for more information:

http://tools.aan.com/science/awards/

Profile of a Winner

In 2009, the AAN awarded the Extended Neuroscience Award to Cyrus Raji, a medical student at the University of Pittsburgh. Mr. Raji has shown a commitment to the field of neurology and has been actively involved in research. His research, "Independent Effects of Age and Alzheimer's on Gray Matter in a Community Cohort," focuses on how both normal aging and Alzheimer's disease affect certain regions of the brain.

"By identifying which regions of the brain are most affected by aging and Alzheimer's disease, this research can help us understand why age is such a powerful risk factor for the disorder," said Mr. Raji in an article published by AAN. "I am honored to be the recipient of this award and want to thank my research mentors for their skillful guidance during this project." Mr. Raji received the award at the AAN's 61st Annual Meeting in Seattle.[6]

Profile of a Winner

The 2012 recipient of the G. Milton Shy Award was Tenneille Loo, a medical student from Toronto, Canada. "The Shy award was given to Tenneille Loo for her study of the pharmacogenetics of vincristine induced neuropathy," wrote the Medical Student Essay Award Subcommittee in the AAN Journal. "The awards committee felt that this work nicely combined the clinical area of adverse drug reactions with the developing field of pharmacogenetics, specifically looking at genetic predisposition of ill-effects of medications."[7]

Medical Student Essay Award – Roland P. Mackay Award

Description: The American Academy of Neurology (AAN) created the Medical Student Essay Award to stimulate interest in the field of neurology. This award will be given for the best essay in historical aspects. The essay must be suitable for an audience of general neurologists. Recipients are expected to give a poster presentation at the AAN Annual Meeting. The recipient of the award will receive a $350 prize, a one-year complimentary subscription to the journal *Neurology*, and recognition at the annual meeting. All expenses for attending the annual meeting will be reimbursed.

To Apply: To be eligible, the student must be enrolled and in good standing in medical school. The applicant must submit an original, lucid essay targeted to general neurologists. The student must also have spent less than one year on a project leading to the submitted essay. See the link below for further application information.

Deadline: The deadline for this scientific award is in October. Award recipients are notified in January. See the following link for more information:

http://tools.aan.com/science/awards/

Profile of a Winner

Jessica Shields, a medical student from New Orleans, received the Roland P. Mackay Award in 2012. "Jessica Shields' essay on Native American ethno-botany in the treatment of neurological disease was awarded the Roland P. Mackay Award," wrote the Medical Student Essay Award Subcommittee in the AAN Journal. "The committee felt that this essay captured both an important historical component of certain therapeutic strategies but also touched on the importance of cultural awareness in our field."[8]

Medical Student Essay Award – Saul R. Korey Award

Description: Developed by the American Academy of Neurology (AAN) to stimulate interest in the field, the Medical Student Essay Award is given for the best essay written in experimental neurology. The essays are judged on suitability for an audience of general neurologists. Students are expected to give a poster presentation at the AAN Annual Meeting. The recipient of the award will receive a $350 prize, a one-year complimentary subscription to the journal *Neurology*, and recognition at the annual meeting. All expenses for attending the national meeting will be reimbursed.

To Apply: To be eligible, the student must be enrolled an in good standing in medical school. The applicant must submit an original, lucid essay targeted to general neurologists. The student must also have spent less than one year on a project leading to the submitted essay. See the link below for further application information.

Deadline: The deadline for the award is in October, and the award winner is announced in January. See the following link for more information:

http://tools.aan.com/science/awards/

Profile of a Winner

The 2012 recipient of the Saul R. Korey Award was Mark Ziats, a medical student from Houston, Texas. "Dr. Ziats was awarded the Korey Award for his essay on the genetics that may underlie autism spectrum disorders," wrote the Medical Student Essay Award Subcommittee. "His study provides support to the idea that genetic abnormalities may, in part, be responsible for the molecular abnormalities that help define the pathology of these neuropsychiatric disorders."[9]

Michael E. DeBakey Medical Student Poetry Awards

Description: The Baylor College of Medicine sponsors the Michael E. DeBakey Medical Student Poetry Awards. The award amount is $1,000 for first prize, $500 for second price, and $250 for third prize. The winning poem will be submitted to a major journal for consideration of publication.

To Apply: Original poetry on a medical subject written by current medical students will be considered for awards.

Deadline: For more information, visit:

https://www.bcm.edu/news/awards-honors-students/bcm-11th-debakey-medical-student-poetry-award

Stanley M. Kaplan, MD Medical Student Essay Contest

Description: U.S. medical students are encouraged to submit original written work for this contest. Acceptable entries include topical essays, case reports, review articles or original research. The winner will receive $500. Two runners-up will receive $250.
To Apply: Criteria for judging include creativity, knowledge of psychiatry, style, and contribution to understanding important problems in any of the biological, psychological, or social dimensions of psychiatry. For more information, visit the website below.
Deadline: The deadline is in June. For more information, visit:

http://psychiatry.uc.edu/Libraries/Education_Documents/Flyer_-_Kaplan_Essay_Award_2014.sflb.ashx

Texas Health Resources Literature & Medicine Writing Contest

Description: Texas Health Resources encourages applicants to submit a creative poem, short story, or poetry. Writers may choose to write about working with patients, delivering difficult news to family members, and balancing work and personal life. The grand prize is $500. The first place prize winner in each category (essay, short story, poem) will receive $250.
To Apply: Contestants may submit an essay (5000 words maximum), poetry (42 lines maximum), or short story (5,000 words maximum).
Deadline: The deadline is in September. For more information, visit:

http://www.texashealth.org/workfiles/PHD/Foundation/Lit_Med/2013_Writing_Contest.pdf

William Carlos Williams Poetry Competition

Description: The Department of Family and Community Medicine at Northeast Ohio Medical University sponsors the William Carlos Williams Poetry Competition. Three winners will be selected, and invited to read their poems at an award ceremony. Winning poems will be considered for publication in the *Journal of Medical Humanities*. The award amount is $300 for first place, $200 for second place, and $100 for third place.
To Apply: Allopathic and osteopathic medical students in the U.S. and Canada are eligible to enter the contest. The essay will be 2,500 words or less.
Deadline: The deadline is in March. For more information, visit:

http://www.neomed.edu/academics/medicine/departments/family-medicine/education-and-faculty-development/william-carlos-williams-poetry-competition

William Osler Medal

Description: The William Osler Medal is given to the best essay on a medical historical topic. The winner will be invited to attend the American Association for the History of Medicine (AAHM) meeting where the medal will be given. A travel stipend will also be given to defray the costs associated with attending the conference. At the discretion of the Osler Medical Committee, another applicant may be awarded with honorable mention.

To Apply: Osteopathic and allopathic medical students are eligible to enter. The essay has a maximum of 9,000 words. "Essays may pertain to the historical development of a contemporary medical problem, or to a topic within the health sciences related to a discrete period in the past and should demonstrate either original research or an unusual appreciation and understanding of the problems discussed," writes AAHM.[10]

Deadline: For more information, visit

http://www.histmed.org/about/awards/william-osler-medal

Young Physicians Patient Safety Award

Description: In partnership with the Lucian Leape Institute of the National Patient Safety Foundation (NPSF), the Doctors Company Foundation offers the Young Physicians Patient Safety Award. Recipients are honored at the Annual NPSF Patient Safety Congress. A monetary award of $5,000 is presented to each winner along with reimbursement to cover the cost of registration and travel to the meeting.

To Apply: Medical students and residents are eligible to apply for this award. Six winners are selected. Applicants must submit an essay expressing "their deep personal insights into the significance of patient safety work."[11] Essays must be between 500 and 1,000 words.

Deadline: For more information, visit

http://npsfcongress.org/about-2/young-physicians-award/

References

[1]ACLS Training Association. Available at:
http://www.aclsrecertification.com/scholarship. Accessed June 23, 2014.
[2]Alpha Omega Alpha Honor Medical Society. Available at:
http://www.alphaomegaalpha.org/pharos/AOA-ThePharos-Winter2012.pdf.
Accessed January 20, 2014.
[3]Intima Essay Contest. Available at: http://www.theintima.org/essay-contest.html. Accessed July 2, 2014.
[4]Alpha Omega Alpha Honor Medical Society. Available at:
http://www.alphaomegaalpha.org/news_2010PharosPoetryCompetition.
Accessed January 20, 2014.
[5]The New York Quarterly Foundation. Available at:
http://nyqpoets.net/poet/jennale. Accessed January 20. 2014.
[6]American Academy of Neurology. Available at:
https://www.aan.com/press/?fuseaction=release.view&release=715. Accessed January 20, 2014.
[7]American Academy of Neurology. Available at:
http://tools.aan.com/globals/axon/assets/6168.pdf. Accessed January 20, 2014.
[8]American Academy of Neurology. Available at:
http://www.aan.com/globals/axon/assets/6168.pdf. Accessed January 20, 2014.
[9]American Academy of Neurology. Available at:
http://www.aan.com/globals/axon/assets/6168.pdf. Accessed January 20, 2014.
[10]American Association for the History of Medicine. Available at:
http://www.histmed.org/about/awards/william-osler-medal. Accessed June 23, 2014.
[11]Young Physicians Patient Safety Award. Available at:
http://npsfcongress.org/about-2/young-physicians-award/. Accessed July 2, 2014.

Chapter 16

Leadership Awards & Scholarships

Students who have been heavily involved in student organizations as leaders may be recognized for their contributions with awards. National organizations and medical schools have established awards recognizing exceptional leadership. Leadership awards are described in this chapter.

Alpha Omega Alpha Medical Student Service Leadership Project Award

Description: The Alpha Omega Alpha (AΩA) Honor Medical Society created this award program to support leadership development for medical students through mentoring, observation and service learning. Recipients are awarded $5,000 for the first year, $3,000 for the second year and $1,000 for the third year. Funding for the second and third years is contingent on acceptance of the progress report for the previous year's work.

To Apply: To be eligible, the team of students must be from a school with an AΩA chapter. Priority will be given to AΩA members serving as team leaders and to proposals with matching institutional or dean's funds. Applications must be for new projects that will have potential to generate future support from the medical school or other sources. A new component of an existing program may also be eligible. Visit the link below for further requirements.

Deadline: The application to the AΩA councilor is due in December. Following this, the councilor sends the application to the AΩA national office in January. Visit the following link for further information:

http://www.alphaomegaalpha.org/student_service_leadership.html

American Medical Association Foundation Leadership Award

Description: The American Medical Association (AMA) Foundation's Leadership awards honor medical students, physician residents, fellows, and young physicians who have demonstrated exceptional leadership skills within organized medicine. This award's primary objective is to encourage non-clinical leadership skills in medicine or community affairs, which will positively influence health care. The leadership awards are distributed to approximately 30 medical students, residents/fellows and early career physicians in recognition of their nonclinical leadership skills in advocacy, community service, public health and/or education.

To Apply: These awards are self-nominated. The applicants are responsible for submitting all appropriate materials and documentation. Application materials include the application form, curriculum vitae and a recommendation form.

Deadline: The application deadline is usually in November. For further information, visit:

http://www.ama-assn.org/ama/pub/about-ama/ama-foundation/our-programs/public-health/excellence-medicine-awards.page

---

Profile of a Winner

In 2012, Alpha Omega Alpha bestowed the Service Leadership Project Award to students at the University of Michigan Medical School for AffordCare, Mapping the Road between Uninsured Patients and the Clinics that Serve Them. The AffordCare organization was created to help connect millions of uninsured Americans to free and sliding-scale clinics across the United States.

These innovative students are creating a Google Maps-like website that lists all free and sliding-scale clinics within close proximity to any location. Through this website, the patient or referring clinician can enter his or her address. Within seconds, users can view a list of nearby clinics. The site will also have a list of searchable $4 medications and links to medical education videos and pamphlets.[1]

Profile of a Winner

In 2013, Laura Stone, a third-year medical student from the University of Miami Miller School of Medicine, was one of the twenty AMA Foundation Leadership Award winners. Ms. Stone has been actively involved through her work with the College Republicans and Young Democrats at the University of Georgia, and the Florida Medical Association Medical Student Section Governing Council where she has been serving as the board's Interim Chair. She also has an interest in public service and volunteers with various community outreach initiatives.

"It is such an honor to be recognized for the work I have done both within and outside of the American Medical Association," said Stone in an article published by the Miller School of Medicine at University of Miami. "Political advocacy, civic engagement, and community service represent an important part of my life, and receiving recognition for my involvement in these activities propels me forward as I enter my future career as a physician."[2]

In the future, Ms. Stone is interested in pursuing a career in general or neurological surgery.

Profile of a Winner

In 2014, Nadine Kaskas, a medical student at the LSU Shreveport School of Medicine, was one recipient of the AMA Foundation Leadership Award. Among her notable accomplishments:

- Instrumental in starting the *American Medical Student Research Journal*
- Editor-in-Chief of the *American Medical Student Research Journal*
- Helped establish the Research Distinction Track at the medical school
- Served as representative on the institution's Quality Enhancement Plan Committee for accreditation
- Heavily involved in starting Empathy in Medicine elective for first-year medical students
- Awarded first place in Cancer Biology category at AMA Research Symposium[3]

Herbert W. Nickens Medical Student Scholarship

Description: The Association of American Medical Colleges (AAMC) awards five scholarships to exceptional students entering their third year of medical school who have shown leadership efforts in medical education and health care and in addressing educational, societal, and health care needs of racial and ethnic minorities in the United States. Each recipient receives a $5,000 scholarship and must be nominated by their medical school.

To Apply: A medical school may nominate one student per year for this scholarship. The nominee must be a U.S. citizen or permanent resident and must be entering their third year of study in an LCME-accredited U.S. medical school. See the link below for the required nomination packet materials.

Deadline: The nomination packets are usually due in May. See the following link for more information:

https://www.aamc.org/initiatives/awards/nickens-student/

Profile of a Winner

In 2012, Ndang Azang-Njaah, a third-year medical student at the University of Chicago, was awarded the Herbert W. Nickens Medical Student Scholarship. Mr. Azang-Njaah pursued a career in medicine because it provided him with the opportunity to combine his interests in the biological sciences with his commitment to public service.

Mr. Azang-Njaah has shown his dedication to social justice by being actively involved in several public service activities. During a summer study abroad, he participated in a service-learning program with Education Fights AIDS International, a nonprofit organization in Maroua, Cameroon. When he was a first-year medical student, he led nutrition sessions for local middle school students and conducted blood sugar testing to promote diabetes education and awareness at several health fairs in the Chicago area for the Diabetes Prevention and Management Group. Mr. Azang-Njaah was also involved in providing education about HIV/AIDS to youth in the Chicago Public Schools.[4]

PHR Emerging Leader Award

Description: Physicians for Human Rights (PHR) annually bestows the Emerging Leader Award to a student member who shows commitment to the field of health and human rights and the most promise of making contributions in the future as a leader.
To Apply: Visit the PHR website for more information below.
Deadline: For more information, visit:

http://physiciansforhumanrights.org/press/news/?topics=general&country=

Profile of a Winner

Anna Huh, a student at Dartmouth's Geisel School of Medicine, is a recent winner of this award. As one of the leaders of Geisel PHR chapter, Anna oversees an organization with about 70 active members. The chapter held a three-day symposium delving into issues related to poverty in the Upper Valley, and over 300 people attended. Anna is also working the Dartmouth Center for Health Care Delivery Science on a health-care project in Peru. The project's goal is to establish primary care health clinics in underserved areas of Peru.[5]

References

[1] Alpha Omega Alpha Honor Medical Society. Available at: http://alphaomegaalpha.org/news_2012_MSSLP.html#AffordCare. Accessed January 20, 2014.

[2] University of Miami Miller School of Medicine. Available at: http://med.miami.edu/news/ama-foundation-honors-miller-school-student-with-national-leadership-award/. Accessed January 14, 2013.

[3] Metro Leader Newspaper. Available at: http://www.sbmetroleader.com/news/local/lsu-health-shreveport-med-student-honored-by-ama-foundation/. Accessed July 2, 2014.

[4] Association of American Medical Colleges. Available at: https://www.aamc.org/download/323222/data/2012nickensstudentwinners.pdf. Accessed January 13, 2014.

[5] Geisel School of Medicine. Available at: http://geiselmed.dartmouth.edu/news/2013/03/07_phr/. Accessed January 20, 2014.

Chapter 17

Osteopathic Awards & Scholarships

Osteopathic physicians have had a vital role in meeting the medical manpower needs of the United States, and have made valuable contributions in leadership, research, and teaching. Over 25% of all medical students graduating from U.S. schools are DOs, and many of these students are making their mark in different areas. If you are an osteopathic student, you can be recognized for your contributions and accomplishments through a variety of awards and scholarships. In this chapter, our focus is on awards and scholarships available only to osteopathic students. Awards available to both osteopathic and allopathic students can be found in other chapters.

A Archie Feinstein Scholarship (See Chapter 76)

Alabama College of Osteopathic Medicine Blumberg Scholars

Description: The Blumberg Family Jewish Community Services of Dothan ACOM Scholarship Program offers scholarships to Jewish students attending the Alabama College of Osteopathic Medicine (ACOM).
To Apply: The application includes CV, essay, letters of recommendation, and interview. The essay should describe your background and experiences, focusing on your proven commitment to medical education, service, volunteerism and leadership in the community.
Deadline: For more information, visit:

http://www.samcfoundation.org/wp-content/uploads/2014/04/ACOMBlumbergScholarshipApplication.pdf

Alabama Osteopathic Medical Association Scholarship

Description: The Alabama Osteopathic Medical Association offers this scholarship to osteopathic students from Alabama. The award amount is up to $5,000.
To Apply: Applicants must be in good standing at an AOA-accredited medical school, and have successfully completed their first year. Applicants from Alabama who intend to practice medicine in the state are preferred. Financial need is also a consideration. The application includes a biographical letter

detailing the applicant's background and reasons for selecting osteopathic medicine as a career.
Deadline: The application deadline is in June. For more information, visit:

http://aloma.org/aloma/scholarships/

Alfred A. Grilli Scholarship (See Chapter 76)

ACOFP Emerging Osteopathic Leader Student Scholarship

Description: The American College of Osteopathic Family Physicians (ACOFP) offers this scholarship to emerging student leaders in family medicine. Two osteopathic medical students will be selected as recipients of this award. Winners will receive $2,500.
To Apply: Applicants must be enrolled in an accredited osteopathic medical school, and attend one or more state osteopathic association, ACOFP, or AOA conferences. The application includes CV, letters of recommendation, and an essay. In the essay, applicants are asked to describe goals and aspirations related to the osteopathic profession and family medicine. Applicants are also asked to explain why they feel they are qualified for the scholarship.
Deadline: The deadline is in January. For more information, visit:

http://www.acofp.org/About_ACOFP/Scholarships/

ACOFP Marie Wiseman Memorial Student Scholarship

Description: The American College of Osteopathic Family Physicians (ACOFP) offers this award to one osteopathic medical student for involvement and leadership within the association. The winner will receive $5,000.
To Apply: Applicants must be serving as current committee chairs or in other leadership positions in the ACOFP. Attendance at one or more state osteopathic association, ACOFP, or AOA conferences is required. The application includes CV, letters of recommendation, and an essay. In the essay, applicants are asked to describe goals and aspirations related to the osteopathic profession and family medicine. Applicants are also asked to explain why they feel they are qualified for the scholarship.
Deadline: The deadline is in January. For more information, visit:

http://www.acofp.org/About_ACOFP/Scholarships/

ACOFP Osteopathic Family Medicine Student Scholarship

Description: The American College of Osteopathic Family Physicians (ACOFP) offers this award to 20 osteopathic medical students for involvement and interest in family medicine and the ACOFP. Winners will receive $1,000.
To Apply: Applicants must be currently enrolled in an accredited osteopathic medical school, and a member of the ACOFP. The application includes CV, letters of recommendation, and an essay. In the essay, applicants are asked to

describe goals and aspirations related to the osteopathic profession and family medicine. Applicants are also asked to explain why they feel they are qualified for the scholarship.

Deadline: The deadline is in January. For more information, visit:

http://www.acofp.org/About_ACOFP/Scholarships/

Andrew Taylor Still Memorial Scholarship

Description: The Student Osteopathic Medical Association (SOMA) offers this award to students to encourage utilization of osteopathic manipulative treatment (OMT) in clinical practice. Winners will receive $500.

To Apply: Applicants must be active members of SOMA in their third or fourth year of medical school. The application includes personal essay response, CV, medical school transcript, and a Supervising Physician Form. In the essay, applicants are asked to describe an experience where OMT was utilized during their academic year.

Deadline: The deadline is in February. For more information, visit:

http://www.somafoundation.org/at-still-memorial-scholarship.html

AOF Presidential Memorial Leadership Award

Description: The American Osteopathic Foundation offers this award to an osteopathic medical student leader who is committed to the principles of osteopathic medicine. One award in the amount of $ 5,000 is available. The award is presented to the recipient during the AOF Honors Ceremony. The recipient will receive a travel grant to offset the cost of airfare/lodging.

To Apply: Current members of the Student Osteopathic Medical Association who have completed their first year of medical school are eligible to apply. Criteria for the award include demonstrated commitment to the profession, strong leadership skills, and noteworthy accomplishments, awards, and extracurricular activities. The application includes completed nomination form, letters of recommendation, personal statement, CV, letter from Dean, and medical school transcript.

Deadline: The application deadline is in April. For more information, visit:

https://aof.org/grants-awards/students/aoa-presidential-memorial-leadership-award

Beale Family Memorial Scholarship (See Chapter 57)

Burnett Osteopathic Student Researcher Award

Description: The recipient of this award has shown true dedication to osteopathic-oriented research. The winner will receive $2,000. The award is presented to the recipient during the American Osteopathic Foundation (AOF) Honors Ceremony. The recipient will receive a travel grant to offset the cost of airfare and hotel accommodations.
To Apply: Applicants must be enrolled in an AOA-accredited COM. Criteria for the award include demonstrated commitment to the science and practice of osteopathic medicine, interest in research pertaining to osteopathic medicine and manipulative treatment, outstanding academic achievement, and noteworthy accomplishments in research. The application includes concept paper, letters of recommendation, CV, letter from Dean, and medical school transcript.
Deadline: The application deadline is in April. For more information, visit:

https://aof.org/grants-awards/students/burnett-osteopathic-student-researcher-award

Colorado Society of Osteopathic Medicine Scholarship (See Chapter 44)

Colorado Springs Osteopathic Foundation Scholarship (See Chapter 44)

Commitment to Diversity in Medical Education Scholarship

Description: The Student Osteopathic Medical Association (SOMA) Minority Affairs Director bestows this award to two osteopathic students who have made efforts to target the awareness of multiculturalism and diversity in medical education. Winners will receive $350.
To Apply: Applicants must be entering their second, third, or fourth year of osteopathic medical school. The application includes personal essay response, CV, and medical school transcript. In the essay, the applicant is asked to explain why he or she believes diversity in medical education is important and how one can promote multiculturalism awareness.
Deadline: The application deadline is in February. For more information, visit:

http://www.somafoundation.org/commitment-to-diversity-in-medicine-scholarship.html

Community & Preventive Medicine Scholarship

Description: The Student Osteopathic Medical Association (SOMA) bestows this award to an osteopathic student who demonstrates commitment to community medicine. The winner will receive $1,000.
To Apply: The application includes letter of recommendation, personal essay response, CV, and medical school transcript. In the essay, applicants are asked to describe the work they have done in the field of community medicine and their future career plans.

Deadline: The application deadline is in July. For more information, visit:

http://www.somafoundation.org/community--preventive-medicine-scholarship.html

Denver Osteopathic Foundation Scholarship (See Chapter 44)

Ed and Melissa Loniewski Medically Underserved Scholarship

Description: The Student Osteopathic Medical Association (SOMA) offers this award to students doing an elective rotation in a medically underserved area.

To Apply: Applicants must be in their third or fourth year of osteopathic medical school. The application includes a verification form that the rotation has been approved, proof that the rotation will take place in an underserved area, and demonstrated commitment to the underserved with interest in practicing in such areas following graduation.

Deadline: For more information, visit:

http://www.somafoundation.org/ed-and-melissa-loniewski-medically-underserved-scholarship.html

Georgia Osteopathic Medical Loan (See Chapter 48)

Humanism in Medicine Scholarship

Description: The Student Osteopathic Medical Association (SOMA) bestows this award to an osteopathic student who has demonstrated an unconditional love for their community and peers, leadership, and compassion. The winner will receive $1,000.

To Apply: Applicants must be in their third year of osteopathic medical school. The application includes personal essay response, CV, and medical school transcript. In the essay section, applicants are asked to provide a formal response to one of the following questions:

- Do you desire to be a leader in the osteopathic profession? Why?
- How have your involvements and/or projects affected your academic and/or local community?

Applicants must also provide a creative response to one of the following questions:

- You, as a physician, are presented with a group of your colleagues who have fallen into a routine of trying to see as many patients in a short period of time and "just prescribing medications." How would you mentor them in providing more patient-centered care?
- You, as a physician, are presented with a new medical school of students who have few club involvements. How would you counsel

them that club involvement is essential to their medical education, perhaps, providing strong advice as to how this will affect their interaction with patients?

Deadline: The application deadline is in September. For more information, visit:

http://www.somafoundation.org/humanism-in-medicine-scholarship.html

Indiana Association of Osteopathic Physicians and Surgeons Scholarship (See Chapter 52)

International Medical Relief/Medical Mission Scholarship

Description: The Student Osteopathic Medical Association (SOMA) offers this award to students participating in international medical missions and relief trips. Short-term trips (> 2 weeks) are given preference. Winners will receive $250 to cover costs associated with travel.

To Apply: Applicants must be an active member of SOMA with demonstrated interest in international medicine. Applications are accepted on a rolling basis, and may be submitted by students in all four years of medical school. Of note, you can receive this award even if you have completed the international experience. The application includes personal essay response, CV, and medical school transcript. In the essay, applicants are asked to describe the experiences during the trip (to be completed following the trip).

Deadline: The deadline is in February. For more information, visit:

http://www.somafoundation.org/international-medical-reliefmedical-mission-scholarship.html

John Shonerd, DO Osteopathic Student Leadership Award (See Chapter 75)

Kansas Osteopathic Medicine Service Scholarship (See Chapter 54)

Marvin H. and Kathleen G. Teget Leadership Scholarship

Description: The Student Osteopathic Medical Association (SOMA) bestows this award to two osteopathic students pursuing careers in specialty medicine. Winners will receive $2,000.

To Apply: The application includes personal statement, CV, and medical school transcript. In the essay, the applicant is asked to explain why he or she has chosen a specialty medical career. The statement should also describe his or her role as a leader.

Deadline: The application deadline is in February. For more information, visit:

http://www.somafoundation.org/marvin-h-and-kathleen-g-teget-leadership-scholarship.html

McCaughan Heritage Scholarship

Description: The recipient of this award will have demonstrated commitment to the science, art, and philosophy of osteopathic medicine at an early point in his or her career. An emphasis on the integration of osteopathic principles, practice, and treatment in patient care is sought. The winner will receive $5,000. The award is presented to the recipient during the American Osteopathic Foundation (AOF) Honors Ceremony. The recipient will receive a travel grant to offset the cost of airfare and hotel accommodations.
To Apply: Applicants must be enrolled in the last year of studies in an AOA-accredited COM. Criteria for the award include demonstrated commitment to osteopathic medicine, promotion of osteopathic ideals, participation in extracurricular activities to promote the profession, and professionalism. The application includes letters of recommendation, personal statement, CV, letter from Dean, and medical school transcript.
Deadline: The application deadline is in April. For more information, visit:

https://aof.org/grants-awards/students/mccaughan-heritage-scholarship

Michiana Osteopathic Medicine Foundation Loan (See Chapter 52)

Muskegon General Osteopathic Foundation Loan (See Chapter 60)

Motyka Dannin Osteopathic Educational Foundation Loan (See Chapter 52)

National SOMA Research Symposium Awards

Description: The National SOMA Research Symposium takes place during the AOA Annual Research Conference in October. Osteopathic students are invited to submit abstracts. Approved abstracts will be presented at the symposium and published in the *Journal of the American Osteopathic Association*. Three first place prizes of $500 and six second place prizes of $250 will be given.
To Apply: Criteria for selection include conciseness, content, form and significance.
Deadline: The deadline is in August. For more information, visit:

http://www.osteopathic.org/inside-aoa/development/quality/research-and-grants/Pages/soma-poster-presentation-letter.aspx

New Jersey Osteopathic Education Scholarship

Description: The New Jersey Osteopathic Education Foundation Scholarship Program offers scholarships to first-year osteopathic medical students.
To Apply: Osteopathic applicants must be residents of New Jersey. The application includes reference evaluation forms, MCAT scores, undergraduate transcript, essay, and tax return. In the essay, the applicant should explain why he or she has chosen osteopathic medicine. Semifinalists are invited for an interview. Criteria for selection include undergraduate academic achievement, motivation, financial need, and professional promise as an osteopathic physician.
Deadline: The deadline is in April. For more information, visit:

http://www.njosteo.com/displaycommon.cfm?an=1&subarticlenbr=82

New York State Osteopathic Medicine Society Poster Competition (See Chapter 70)

Nichols LEAD Scholar Award

Description: This award is given to an osteopathic medical student for **L**eadership, **E**xcellence, **A**chievement, and **D**edication. The winner will receive $1,000.
To Apply: Applicants must have completed their first year in an AOA-accredited COM. Criteria for the award includes commitment to leadership and ongoing development of leadership skills that will benefit communities now and in the future.
Deadline: For more information, visit:

https://aof.org/node/224

Northwest Osteopathic Medical Association Scholarships

Description: The Northwest Osteopathic Medical Association Scholarships are awarded to medical students from Alaska, Idaho, Montana, Oregon, and Washington.
To Apply: Osteopathic medical students from Alaska, Idaho, Montana, Oregon, and Washington are eligible to apply. Applicants must be in their second, third, or fourth year of medical school. Priority is given to applicants who are committed to practicing primary care medicine in the Northwest.
Deadline: The application deadline is in May. Please see the following link for further information:

http://www.nwosteo.org/scholarship/

Oklahoma Education Foundation for Osteopathic Medicine Scholarship (See Chapter 74)

Osteopathic Foundation of Central Washington Scholarship

Description: The Osteopathic Foundation of Central Washington awards scholarships to medical students. Preference is given to residents of the Pacific Northwest (Alaska, Idaho, Montana, Oregon, or Washington) who have a commitment to practicing medicine in the region.

To Apply: Students in their second, third, or fourth year of medical school are eligible. Criteria for selection include intention to practice in the region, academic work, and community involvement.

Deadline: For more information, visit:

www.ofcw.org

Osteopathic Foundation of West Michigan Scholarship

Description: The Osteopathic Foundation of West Michigan offers medical education scholarships to osteopathic medical students.

To Apply: Osteopathic applicants must be residents of West Michigan (Muskegon County, Oceana County, and northern Ottawa County).

Deadline: The deadline is in May. For more information, visit:

http://osteopathicfoundation.org/pg/Scholarships/medical_education.htmla

Osteopathic Foundation of Yakima Scholarship

Description: The Osteopathic Foundation of Yakima awards scholarships to medical students. To be eligible, applicants must be residents of the Pacific Northwest (Alaska, Idaho, Oregon, or Washington). Only applicants who are at least second-year students will be considered.

To Apply: For application information and instructions, contact the organization below.

Deadline: For more information, contact:

Osteopathic Foundation of Yakima
Attn: Scholarship Program
P.O. Box 681-147
Yakima, Washington 98907

Osteopathic Medical Student Loan for Service Program (See Chapter 69)

Rossnick Humanitarian Grants

Description: The American Osteopathic Foundation awards this grant to members of the osteopathic profession who travel to disaster stricken or underserved areas to provide medical care.
To Apply: Osteopathic medical students are eligible to apply. Visit the website below for more information.
Deadline: For more information, visit:

https://aof.org/grants-awards/grant-request-special-projects-and-programs/rossnick-humanitarian-grants

Sherry R. Arnstein Minority Student Scholarship (See Chapter 13)

Student Osteopathic Medical Association New Member Scholarship

Description: New members of the Student Osteopathic Medical Association (SOMA) may apply for this award. Winners will receive $500.
To Apply: To be considered, you must be a new member who has joined during the SOMA fall membership drive. Applicants must submit an essay on the topic, "Vision of Osteopathic Medicine."
Deadline: For more information, visit:

http://www.somafoundation.org/new-member-scholarship.html

SOMA's International Health Program Scholarship

Description: The Student Osteopathic Medical Association (SOMA) offers this award to students to promote international medicine. The hope is that through these experiences students will develop an awareness of other cultures' medical practices. Winners will receive $500 to cover the costs associated with travel and lodging during the international elective (> 1 month experience).
To Apply: Applicants must be an active member of SOMA in their third or fourth year of medical school. Applicants must have demonstrated interest in international medicine. The application includes personal essay response, CV, and medical school transcript. In the essay, applicants are asked to describe the experiences during the trip (to be completed following the trip).
Deadline: The deadline is in February. For more information, visit:

http://www.somafoundation.org/international-health-program-scholarship.html

SREB Osteopathy Loan/Scholarship (See Chapter 62)

Washington Osteopathic Foundation Scholarship (See Chapter 85)

Welch Scholars Grant

Description: This award is given to one student from each college of osteopathic medicine. Winners will receive $2,000. Although financial need is a major consideration, also important are academic achievement, involvement in extracurricular activities, and commitment toward osteopathic medicine.

To Apply: Applicants must have completed their first year in an AOA-accredited COM. The Director of Financial Aid at each osteopathic medical school is asked to submit the name of the candidate that meets award eligibility criteria. The application includes letter from the Dean, letter from the Director of Financial Aid, letters of recommendation, personal statement, personal financial need statement, and medical school transcript.

Deadline: The application deadline is in May. For more information, visit:

https://aof.org/grants-awards/students/welch-scholars-grant

Western New York Osteopathic Medical Society Scholarship (See Chapter 70)

William G. Anderson, DO, Minority Scholarship

Description: The recipient of this award will be a minority medical student who is committed to osteopathic principles and practice. Academic excellence and leadership are other important criteria. The winner will receive $5,000. The award is presented to the recipient during the American Osteopathic Foundation (AOF) Honors Ceremony. The recipient will receive a travel grant to offset the cost of airfare and hotel accommodations.

To Apply: Applicants must have completed their first year of studies in an AOA-accredited COM. Criteria for the award include demonstrated commitment to osteopathic medicine, excellent academic achievement, demonstrated leadership efforts addressing the needs of minorities and inequities in health care, noteworthy accomplishments, extracurricular activities, leadership, and financial need. The application includes letters of recommendation, personal statement, personal financial need statement, CV, letter from Dean, letter from the Director of Financial Aid, and medical school transcript.

Deadline: The application deadline is in April. For more information, visit:

https://aof.org/grants-awards/students/william-g-anderson-do-minority-scholarship

Chapter 18

Miscellaneous Scholarships, Awards, & Grants

A Place for Mom Senior Care Innovation Scholarship

Description: A Place for Mom offers this scholarship to students interested in the fields of aging and gerontology. Recipients will receive $1,000. Five winners will be selected.

To Apply: Award winners are chosen based on the quality of essay submitted. A letter of introduction describing your history working or volunteering with seniors, why you're seeking a degree in your field, and why you feel you would be a good candidate for the award is also required. Candidates must be seeking a career that involves working with senior citizens.

Deadline: The deadline is in April. For more information, visit:

http://www.aplaceformom.com/scholarship

AMA Section Involvement Grant

Description: The Section Involvement Grant (SIG) of the American Medical Association (AMA) is designed for local AMA medical student sections (MSS) to educate students about the AMA, provide opportunities for students to get more involved, render services to medical school campuses or communities to help put AMA policies into action, and to engage in AMA's top priority activities. Local sections may receive up to $1,000 per academic year, with a maximum of $500 to support recruitment and $500 to support community service and education events. Grant awards range from $150 to $500 per event. Each event will be evaluated on an individual basis. These grants are intended to support and strengthen AMA-MSS local sections. See the link below for the different types of SIGs.

To Apply: Students are strongly encouraged to involve their medical school staff and faculty as well as state/county medical society staff in medical student projects. You must be an AMA member to apply. To submit a Section Involvement Grant application, see the link below.

Deadline: The online SIG application must be completed at least 30 days before the scheduled event. All local sections receiving SIG funding are required to complete a follow-up SIG Evaluation Form within 30 days of the event. For further information, contact the Medical Students Section at mss@ama-assn.org, or see the link below:

http://www.ama-assn.org/ama/pub/about-ama/our-people/member-groups-sections/medical-student-section/community-service/frequently-asked-questions-about-chapter-involvement.page

---

Did you know...

The AMA SIG program will select one medical student section every month to receive the "Event of the Month" award. A follow-up form and photos must be submitted within 30 days of the event to be eligible for this award. All awards will be showcased at the AMA Annual Meeting at the end of the school year. Students will vote on the monthly awards to elect one "Event of the Year" winner.

AMA Physicians of Tomorrow Scholarship

Description: The American Medical Association (AMA) Foundation created the Physicians of Tomorrow Award program in 2004 to provide financial assistance to medical students facing excessive medical school debt. Over one million dollars has been granted to exceptional medical students across the United States. The scholarship consists of a $10,000 award for current third-year medical students who are approaching their final year of medical school. Each medical school can nominate one person for each of the different scholarship opportunities. Factors taken into consideration are academic excellence, financial need and community involvement. See below to view the different scholarship categories.

To Apply: Contact your medical school if interested in being nominated for the scholarship. The dean or dean's designate chooses scholarship nominees. If nominated, they will provide you with the application form. Required materials include letters of recommendation, transcript/scores and a personal statement.

Type of Award	Selection Factors
Physicians of Tomorrow Award	Based on academic excellence and financial need
Physicians of Tomorrow Award (supported by Johnson F. Hammond, MD, Fund)	Based on commitment to career in medical journalism
Physicians of Tomorrow Fund (supported by Dr. Lin and Minta Hill Alexander Fund)	Recipient must attend medical school in Oklahoma
Physicians of Tomorrow Award for Chicago – area students	Recipient must attend one of six Chicago – area medical schools

Deadline: Nomination materials usually become available in February and the nomination deadline is in May. Visit the link for more information:

http://www.ama-assn.org/ama/pub/about-ama/ama-foundation/our-programs/medical-education/physicians-tomorrow-scholarships.page

---

Profile of a Winner

In 2012, Colleen McCormick from Wright State University Boonshoft School of Medicine was one of eighteen medical students to receive the Physicians of Tomorrow scholarship. Colleen is in a dual degree program, and will receive Doctor of Medicine and Master of Public Health degrees. Colleen is president of the Alpha Omega Alpha Honor Medical Society and a member of the Gold Humanism Honor society.

"Colleen has excelled in medical school. She has always ranked among the top in her class," said Dr. Gary LeRoy, Associate Dean for Student Affairs and Admissions. McCormick plans to be actively involved in academic medicine, quality improvement initiatives and community-based health care interventions. "As physicians, we have a responsibility to improve our world," stated McCormick in a recent article published by the Boonshoft School of Medicine. "As a future physician-leader, I plan to educate, promote behavior change and help improve the health of our population." McCormick is interested in pursuing residency training in pediatrics.[1]

AMA Scholars Fund Awards

Description: The American Medical Association's (AMA) largest volunteer group, the AMA Alliance, has worked with the AMA Foundation since 1950 to raise money for medical schools to distribute to deserving students. The AMA Alliance has provided more than $ 60 million in scholarships to students. The AMA Alliance Scholars Fund, now called the Grassroots Honor Fund, will provide $10,000 scholarships to medical students with a commitment to address the needs of women and children. Find more information at http://www.ama-assn.org/ama/pub/about-ama/ama-foundation/our-programs/medical-education/scholars-fund.page

To Apply: Student applications are not required for this award. Your medical school must submit a Scholars Fund recipient information form to the AMA Foundation. After this form has been received, the AMA Foundation will send the funds to the medical school. Please contact your Dean or Dean's designate if seeking this scholarship fund.

Deadline: On December 31, 2013, the new vehicle for the Alliance's scholarship fundraising efforts became the AMA Alliance Grassroots Honor Fund. For more information about this fund, contact Anne Smith at (312) 464-5852 or anne.smith@ama-assn.org.

Profile of a Winner

Deanna Shoup, a student at University of Minnesota Medical School in Duluth, was a recent winner of the Scholars Fund. "My transition to medical school has been filled with amazing opportunities and trying circumstances," stated Deanna in an article published by the AMA. "My husband and our five children have made this move together and we are all willing to sacrifice, but having this scholarship means that we will not have to sacrifice the important things. It is truly a blessing that the AMA considers this an important investment."[2]

Another recipient of the award is Jay Patel, a student at the University of Alabama School of Medicine. In the same AMA article, Jay expressed his gratitude. "Your support and dedication to my medical education will never be forgotten. Because of your generous gift, I have been able to choose a specialty based on my interests, instead of compensation. Thank you for contributing to the future – and present – of health care."[2]

AAMC Medicine in the Community Grant Program

Description: The Association of American Medical Colleges (AAMC) has developed the Medicine in the Community Grant Program (formerly Caring for Community) to help medical students increase their involvement in community service efforts. The three types of grants offered include New Project Grants, Supplemental Grants and Non-continuous Grants with a maximum grant amount of $30,000, $20,000, and $15,000, respectively. Monetary support for each grant will be provided on a sliding scale in decreasing increments. Visit the link below for more information on the different types of grants.

To Apply: AAMC member schools are eligible to receive support for student-initiated community service projects that help fulfill unmet needs within their local community. Visit the link below to see the application requirements.

Deadline: The grant is currently on hold while seeking more funding, but one grant award cycle is normally held during each calendar year. See the following link for more information:

https://www.aamc.org/initiatives/awards/medicine_community_grant/

Arnold P. Gold Foundation Leonard Tow Humanism in Medicine Award

Description: The Arnold P. Gold Foundation bestows the Leonard Tow Humanism in Medicine Award to a graduating medical student at every school having partnership with the organization. The award recognizes clinical excellence, outstanding compassion, and respect for patients, their families, and healthcare colleagues.
To Apply: Recipients are nominated by medical schools.
Deadline: For more information, visit:

http://humanism-in-medicine.org/programs/awards/leonard-tow-humanism-in-medicine-award/

Profile of a Winner

In 2009, Howard University College of Medicine's New Freedmen's Clinic (NFC) was one of seven recipients of the AAMC Medicine in the Community Grant. NFC is a student-run clinic dedicated to serving the uninsured and underinsured residents of the District of Columbia. The clinic serves their community by providing primary and preventable care services, as well as teaching classes on disease prevention.[3]

Stanford University School of Medicine's Santa Clara Hep B Free Campaign was also awarded this grant in 2009. This outreach and education program helps eliminate the threat of chronic hepatitis B virus infection and liver cancer in Asian and Pacific Islander Americans by creating awareness, screening for disease and vaccinating high-risk populations.[3]

Profile of a Winner

In 2012, Ricardy Rimpel received the Leonard Tow Humanism in Medicine Award from the University of Florida School of Medicine and the Arnold P. Gold Foundation. As a medical student, Rimpel was heavily involved in activities outside the classroom. He volunteered at student-run free health clinics, and participated in several international outreach trips to Haiti and the Dominican Republic. For his contributions in the Florida community and elsewhere along with his dedication to medicine, he was awarded this prestigious honor. He is now a resident in family medicine at the Halifax Health Medical Center.[4]

American Association of Clinical Anatomists Predoctoral Student Presentation Awards

Description: The American Association of Clinical Anatomists (AACA) honors at least two students every year for the best platform and poster presentations at the AACA Annual Meeting. A monetary award of $600 is given to cover the cost associated with travel to the meeting.

To Apply: The awards are open to medical students, graduate students, interns, and residents. The Ralph Ger Student Platform Presentation Award is given to the student with the best platform presentation at an American Association of Clinical Anatomists (AACA) Annual Meeting. The Sandy C. Marks, Jr. Student Poster Presentation Award is given to the student with the best poster presentation.

Deadline: For more information, visit:

http://clinical-anatomy.org/content.php?page=Awards

Dr. Alma S. Adams Scholarship for Outreach and Health Communications to Reduce Tobacco Use Among Priority Populations

Description: Two scholarships will be given to undergraduate or graduate students who have shown commitment to reducing tobacco use among priority populations. These populations include residents of low-income communities, U.S. racial/ethnic minorities, and the Gay/Lesbian/Bisexual/Transgender community. The award amount is $5,000.

To Apply: Criteria for selection include:

- Record of commitment to community service on behalf of an underserved community, preferably related to tobacco prevention and/or control
- Best use of the visual arts, media, creative writing or other creative endeavor to convey culturally appropriate health messages aimed at raising awareness of tobacco's harmful impact

Deadline: The deadline is in April. For more information, visit:

http://www.legacyforhealth.org/get-involved/awards-scholarships/dr.-alma-s.-adams-scholarships/?o=3571

Golden Key Scholar Awards

Description: The Golden Key International Honor Society offers a variety of scholarships to undergraduate and graduate students who are members of the society. Medical students are eligible for these awards.
To Apply: For application information and instructions, visit the website below.
Deadline: For more information, visit:

https://www.goldenkey.org/scholarships-awards/overview/

Jayne M. Perkins Memorial Scholarship

Description: This scholarship is sponsored by the Jayne M. Perkins Foundation, and is offered to medical students. Preference is given to students whose interests include cancer research, dementia, heart disease, and skin disorders. Only students enrolled at one of the following universities are eligible: St. Louis University, Stanford University, University of California San Francisco, University of Washington, and Washington University. The award amount is $10,000. Up to ten awards will be given.
To Apply: For application information and instructions, contact the organization below.
Deadline: The deadline is in April. For more information, visit:

http://foundgroup.com/perkins/PERKINS-gln.pdf

Joseph Collins Foundation Scholarship

Description: Scholarships are available for medical students attending schools located east of or contiguous to the Mississippi River. The maximum amount of the award is $10,000.
To Apply: To be eligible, applicants must be attending an accredited medical school, be in the upper half of their class, and show interest in the arts or other cultural pursuits outside of medicine (e.g., music, theatre, writing). Preference will be given to those interested in pursuing careers as a general practitioner, neurologist, or psychiatrist.
Deadline: The application deadline is in March. For more information, contact Joseph Collins Foundation, 787 Seventh Avenue, Room 3950, New York, NY 10019-6099.

JustHomeMedical.com Health Care Leaders Scholarship

Description: Just Home Medical awards a $1,000 scholarship to one health care student for the best video answering the question "What are your long and short term goals as a future health care leader?" Criteria for evaluation include creativity and thoughtfulness.
To Apply: For more information, visit the website below.

Deadline: The application deadline is in December. For more information, visit:

http://justhomemedical.com/health-care-leaders-scholarship

Keith and Marion Moore Blue Box Award

Description: This award is named after Dr. Keith Moore, the author of a widely used anatomy textbook. It is given to the student who is judged to have written the best student paper published in Clinical Anatomy. The winner receives a certificate and a $500 monetary award.

To Apply: The award is open to medical students and graduate students worldwide. An American Association of Clinical Anatomists (AACA) committee is charged with selecting the award recipient, and the award is presented at the Annual AACA Meeting Banquet.

Deadline: For more information, visit:

http://www.clinical-anatomy.org/honoredmembers.html#adkins

Profile of a Winner

In 2012, St. George's University in Grenada was the host of the 29th Annual American Association of Clinical Anatomists Conference. Zacharcy Klaassen, a medical student at St. George's University, was the recipient of the Marion Moore Blue Box Award for his paper, "Anatomy of the ilioinguinal and iliohypogastric nerves with observations of their spinal nerve contributions."[5]

International Order of the King's Daughters & Sons Health Career Scholarship

Description: This scholarship program is open to medical students. To be eligible, the applicant must be a U.S. or Canadian citizen enrolled full-time in an accredited school in one of these two countries. The application must be for at least the second year of medical school.

To Apply: For application information and instructions, visit the website below.

Deadline: For more information, visit:

http://www.iokds.org/scholarship.html

Leopold Schepp Foundation Scholarship

Description: The Leopold Schepp Foundation provides scholarships to undergraduate and graduate students. Graduate students must be under 40 years of age at the time of application. The award amount is up to $8,500.
To Apply: For application information and instructions, visit the website below.
Deadline: For more information, visit:

http://www.scheppfoundation.org/wp/eligibility-guidelines/

LGBT Heart Scholarship Fund for the Graduate Health Professions

Description: Outstanding LGBT HEART graduate-level students are eligible to receive the LGBT HEART scholarship.
To Apply: Applicants must be enrolled in a health professions program at an accredited U.S. school or university. To be considered, applicants must be "out" as members of the LGBT community. Criteria for judging also include favorable academic record, financial hardship, and commitment or contribution to LGBT community health.
Deadline: The application deadline is in June. For more information, visit:

http://www.aphalgbt.org/resources/Y2009/09_HEART_Application.pdf

McGraw-Hill/Lange Student Award

Description: The McGraw-Hill Medical Publishing division bestows student awards to two outstanding first-year medical students at each medical school. Recipients receive $150 worth of McGraw-Hill books.
To Apply: No application is necessary as these awards are designated by the Dean of your medical school.
Deadline: For more information, visit:

http://www.mhprofessional.com/sites/lange/2010bart.html. Accessed

---

Profile of a Winner

In 2010, the University of Oklahoma College of Medicine presented the McGraw-Hill/Lange Student Award to Bart Blackorby. Bart has developed important leadership skills through his work as class president and service as Second Lieutenant in the U.S. Army. "I feel that volunteering at clinics is important but I also feel that being a leader in the field of medicine can have an even larger impact," said Bart. "Throughout school I plan to build my medical knowledge to directly care for others and develop my leadership skills to direct projects towards helping the community."[6]

Medical Professionals of Tomorrow Scholarship

Description: This scholarship is sponsored by US Medical Supplies. To be eligible, the applicant must be pursuing a health-care related degree. The award amount is $1,000.

To Apply: The application includes an essay describing who or what inspired them to seek out a career in healthcare.

Deadline: For more information, visit:

www.usmedicalsupplies.com/scholarship

MENSA Foundation Scholarship

Description: This scholarship is administered by the MENSA Foundation. The program receives 4,000 to 6,000 applications per year.

To Apply: Criteria for selection include quality of essays submitted. Grades, academic program, and financial need are not considerations in the selection process.

Deadline: The deadline is in January. For more information, visit:

http://www.mensafoundation.org/what-we-do/scholarships/

National Health Services Corps Scholarship Program

Description: The National Health Services Corps Scholarship Program (NHSC SP) offers scholarships to students in return for a commitment to practice medicine in underserved areas following completion of residency training. The student is expected to provide care for one year at an NHSC-approved site for each year of financial support offered. There is a minimum 2-year service commitment. The scholarship covers tuition, fees, and other reasonable costs. Recipients also receive a monthly living stipend.

To Apply: For more information about the program, visit the website below.

Deadline: For more information, visit:

http://nhsc.hrsa.gov/scholarships/overview/index.html

National Rural Institute on Alcohol and Drug Abuse Scholarships

Description: The National Rural Institute on Alcohol and Drug Abuse offers scholarships to medical students seeking training in alcohol and other drug abuse treatments. Training takes place at the National Rural Institute on Alcohol and Drug Abuse Conference. Award recipients receive a scholarship to cover tuition, room and board, and travel expenses.

To Apply: The application includes a brief personal statement and registration form.

Deadline: The deadline is in March. For more information, visit:

http://www.uwstout.edu/profed/nri/scholarships.cfm

National Society Daughters of the American Revolution

Description: This scholarship program is open to medical students. The award amount is up to $5,000, and is renewable for up to four years.
To Apply: The application includes transcript, letters of recommendation, list of achievements/activities/honors, personal statement, and financial need form. The statement should describe the applicant's career objectives.
Deadline: The application deadline is in February. For more information, visit:

http://www.dar.org/national-society/scholarships

New Look Laser Tattoo Removal Semiannual Scholarship

Description: This is a merit-based scholarship that is awarded twice each year to students pursuing a career in nursing, medicine, natural or applied sciences, or engineering. The award amount is $1,000.
To Apply: The application includes small writing project and copy of transcript.
Deadline: There are two application cycles with deadlines in November and June. For more information, visit:

http://www.newlookhouston.com/New_Look_Scholarship.html

Nicholas Skala Student Activist Award

Description: This award is offered by Physicians for a National Health Program (PNHP). It was named in honor of Nicholas Skala who demonstrated tremendous dedication and commitment for a single-payer national health insurance.
To Apply: Visit the PNHP website for more information.
Deadline: For more information, visit:

http://www.pnhp.org/

Profile of a Winner

James Besante, a second-year student at the University of New Mexico School of Medicine, was a recent recipient of the Nicholas Skala Student Activist Award. For several years, he has been advocating for a state constitutional amendment that would recognize health care as a fundamental right. He has attended hearings at the State Capitol where he served as an expert witness, and worked tirelessly to advance the bill through legislative committees.

His advocacy efforts have led to endorsements by numerous organizations, including the New Mexico Public Health Association, Network of Health Professionals for a National Health Program, and the New Mexico Health Equity Working Group.

He received his award at the PNHP Annual Meeting.[7]

Paul Ambrose Scholars Program

Description: Through this program, allopathic and osteopathic medical students are prepared to become leaders in addressing population health challenges at the community and national level. Scholars attend a four-day symposium in Washington D.C., and participate in a community-based health education project at their institution. Students enrolled in a public health program and graduates of public health programs are not eligible.
To Apply: For application information and instructions, visit the website below.
Deadline: For more information, visit:

http://www.aptrweb.org/?page=pasp

Paul & Daisy Soros Fellowships for New Americans

Description: Through this fellowship program, medical students receive grants of $20,000 plus $16,000 for graduate study tuition in the United States.
To Apply: Applicants must be resident aliens (holding a Green Card), naturalized U.S. citizens, or native-born U.S. citizens with both parents being naturalized U.S. citizens. The application includes documentation of "New American" status, personal essays, resume, letters of recommendation, undergraduate and graduate school transcripts, and MCAT scores.
Deadline: The deadline is in November. For more information, visit:

http://www.pdsoros.org/forms/fullapp.pdf

Profile of a Winner

In 2013, Sejal Hathi, a medical student at the Stanford School of Medicine, was one of thirty recipients of the Paul & Daisy Soros Fellowship for New Americans.

Sejal showed tremendous initiative and drive from a relatively young age. At the age of 15, she founded the nonprofit organization Girls Helping Girls. Later, she launched girltank. The mission of these organizations is to train and empower young women to create social change. The scope of these organizations has grown over time to reach more than 30,000 young women in over 100 countries.

Sejal has spoken about gender inequality nationally, and was recognized by *Newsweek* and *Forbes* for her efforts and potential.[8]

Phi Kappa Phi Honor Society Scholarships & Awards

Description: The Phi Kappa Phi Honor Society offers a number of scholarships and awards to members. Medical students are eligible for these awards.
To Apply: For application information and instructions, visit the website below.
Deadline: For more information, visit:

http://www.phikappaphi.org/awards/awardandgrants_2014.pdf

Students to Service Loan Repayment Program

Description: The Students to Service Loan Repayment Program is administered by the National Health Service Corps (NHSC). Allopathic and osteopathic students in their last year of school are eligible to apply. The program provides up to $120,000 to students. In return, students commit to practicing primary health care full time for at least 3 years at an NHSC-approved underserved site.
To Apply: For application information and instructions, visit the website below.
Deadline: For more information, visit:

http://nhsc.hrsa.gov/loanrepayment/studentstoserviceprogram/index.html

Tillman Military Scholars

Description: This is a scholarship administered by the Pat Tillman Foundation to support veterans, active service members, and their dependents.
To Apply: To be eligible, the medical school applicant must be a service member or spouse seeking assistance to pursue a degree as a full-time student.
Deadline: The deadline is in March. For more information, visit:

http://www.pattillmanfoundation.org/tillman-military-scholars/apply/

Tylenol Future Care Scholarship

Description: This scholarship program bestows $250,000 total in scholarships. Ten applicants will receive $10,000. Thirty will receive $5,000. Students pursuing careers in the healthcare industry are eligible to apply. The program is very competitive with over 25,000 applications submitted per year.
To Apply: Applicants must have completed at least one year of undergraduate or graduate study. Criteria for selection include leadership qualities, community involvement, and academic performance. Two 500-word essays and a resume must be submitted.
Deadline: For more information, visit:

http://www.tylenol.com/news/scholarship

Waechter Medical-Legal Scholarhsip

Description: This scholarship program bestows two $1,000 scholarships. One award is given to a medical student.

To Apply: There is no minimum GPA. Creativity in the application is the major criteria used to identify award winners. The applicant must submit a 150-word essay about any of the following:

- How the Medical & Legal Community can work more easily together
- How to reduce medical mistakes
- What lawyers don't know about medicine, but should
- Any other novel topic mixing law and medicine

Deadline: The deadline is in September. For more information, visit:

http://www.birthlaw.com/34.html

Willens Anything But Law School Graduate Scholarship

Description: This scholarship is offered by Willens Law Offices. The award amount is $1,000. To be eligible, you must be an undergraduate entering graduate school. This is not a scholarship for law students, and medical students are encouraged to apply.

To Apply: The application includes transcript, proof of acceptance to graduate school, and one page essay. The essay should describe your reason for choosing your particular program of study and why job prospects appear to be good after graduation.

Deadline: The application deadline is in July. For more information, visit:

http://www.willenslaw.com/anything-but-law-school-graduate-scholarship/

References

[1]Wright State University Boonshoft School of Medicine. Available at: http://www.med.wright.edu/whatsnew/2012/mccormick. Accessed January 14, 2014.

[2]American Medical Association. Available at http://www.ama-assn.org/ama/pub/about-ama/ama-foundation/our-programs/medical-education/scholars-fund.page. Accessed January 14, 2013.

[3]Association of American Medical Colleges. Available at: https://www.aamc.org/initiatives/awards/medicine_community_grant/101720/cfc_2009.html. Accessed January 14, 2013.

[4]University of Florida College of Medicine. Available at: http://humanism.med.ufl.edu/selection-process/the-leonard-tow-humanism-in-medicine-award/. Accessed June 22, 2014.

[5]St. George's University. Available at: http://www.sgu.edu/news-events/news-archives12-sgu-students-sweep-clinical-awards-29th-aaca.html. Accessed January 20, 2014.

[6]McGraw-Hill. Available at: http://www.mhprofessional.com/sites/lange/2010bart.html. Accessed January 20, 2014.

[7]University of New Mexico School of Medicine. Available at: http://news.unm.edu/news/unm-medical-student-receives-national-award-for-health-activism. Accessed January 20, 2014.

[8]Stanford School of Medicine. Available at: http://news.stanford.edu/news/2013/june/soros-award-winners-062713.html. Accessed April 4, 2014.

Chapter 19

Anesthesiology Awards, Scholarships, & Grants

For medical students interested in receiving a scholarship, award, or grant in anesthesiology, begin by researching opportunities at your own institution. The Department of Anesthesiology and Pain Management at UT Southwestern bestows the M.T. "Pepper" Jenkins Award to the medical student who has demonstrated exceptional clinical performance and shown enthusiasm for the specialty. The Department also recognizes a visiting student every year with the Edward R. Johnson Visiting Medical Student Award. The Richard W. Eller Anesthesiology Award is given to the fourth-year medical student at West Virginia School of Medicine who best demonstrates professionalism, academic achievement, and clinical skills during the anesthesiology rotation. Make inquiries with your Department of Anesthesiology to learn about award opportunities you may be eligible for.

Medical schools and departments of anesthesiology often have funding in the form of scholarships or grants to support student research either during the summer between the first and second year or at a later time. External awards, particularly for research, are also available. The most prestigious are national research programs sponsored by the Foundation for Anesthesia Education and Research. These are described below.

In recent years, anesthesiology has become increasingly competitive. Medical students often ask us if it's necessary to do research in the field. In the 2012 NRMP Program Director Survey, 49% cited "demonstrated involvement and interest in research" as a factor in selecting applicants to interview.[1] It's especially helpful to read the perspectives of anesthesiology residency program directors about the importance of research in the selection process. We offer you these perspectives on the next page.

Anesthesiology Research for Medical Students: Perspectives of Residency Program Directors

- "It is not critical that the student have research experience," writes the Department of Anesthesiology at Drexel University. "If the student has participated in research, it is very important that he/she be familiar enough with the research to discuss it on a residency interview."[2]

- "Do research because you are curious, because you want to learn more about the scientific method, or you are excited about a particular question or investigational project at the Medical School," writes the Department of Anesthesiology at the University of Minnesota. "In general, it is not necessary to do research as an obligatory ('merit') component of an application packet."[3]

- "Although not necessary, clinical and research experience in anesthesiology is viewed very positively and encouraged for those applying to our specialty," writes the Department of Anesthesiology at the University of Texas Houston Medical School.[4]

- As you might expect, some programs value research more than others. "Research-intensive programs, for example programs with relatively large amounts of National Institutes of Health or foundation funding, will also seek and attract applicants interested in careers as physician-scientists," writes Dr. Lee Fleisher, Chair of the Department of Anesthesiology at the University of Pennsylvania. "It is critical to acknowledge that each program has different missions, expertise, and resources, and it is critical for them to attract medical students coincident with these goals and individual strengths of the program."[5]

- Your participation in research may allow you to network with key program personnel. "If you have done research in medical school, you might also seek to participate in one of these national meetings and then you personally get the opportunity to meet the individuals with whom you will soon be interviewing," writes Dr. William McDade, Associate Professor of Anesthesiology at the University of Chicago. "It makes an enormous difference in your favor if the first time you meet someone from the program you desire to attend, it is a national meeting and you are presenting your data. When you appear for the interview, it will be as if you are speaking to a friend."[6]

Medical Student Anesthesia Research Fellowship Year-Long Program

Description: The Foundation for Anesthesia Education and Research (FAER) offers medical students the Medical Student Anesthesia Research Fellowship Year-Long Program (MSARF). This is an opportunity for students to immerse themselves in a full year of anesthesiology research. A $32,000 stipend is given to recipients. Fellows will be required to make presentations at the Association of University Anesthesiologists (AUA) and American Society of Anesthesiologists (ASA) annual meetings.

To Apply: To qualify for the MSARF program, you must be enrolled full-time in an accredited allopathic or osteopathic medical school. Eligible applicants must have completed their core clinical rotations. The application includes biographical sketch, transcript, abstract, research plan, mentor selection and mentoring plan, letters of recommendation, and IRB approval.

Deadline: The application deadline is in December. For more information, visit:

http://faer.org/programs/msarf-year-long-program/

Medical Student Anesthesia Research Fellowship Summer Program

Description: The Foundation for Anesthesia Education and Research (FAER) offers medical students the Medical Student Anesthesia Research Fellowship Summer Program (MSARF). Students who are accepted into the program receive a $400 per week stipend for eight consecutive weeks of anesthesiology research. Students work closely with a dedicated mentor, and have the opportunity to present their work at the American Society of Anesthesiologists (ASA) annual meeting. Funds are given to cover the cost of travel to the meeting.

To Apply: To qualify for the program, you must be enrolled full-time in an accredited allopathic or osteopathic medical school. The application includes CV, letter of good standing, and two reference letters. Responses to the following essay questions are also required:

- List any anesthesiology or perioperative medicine experience.
- List any past research experiences and/or peer-reviewed publications.
- In 250 words or fewer, describe, as well as possible, aspirations for professional life 10 years following medical school graduation.

Deadline: The application deadline for the MSARF program is in December. For more information, visit:

http://faer.org/programs/msarf-summer-program/

Profile of Winner

Brian Ebert, a second-year medical student at the Arizona College of Osteopathic Medicine, participated in the program during the summer of 2011. He performed his anesthesiology research at the University of Utah where he was mentored by Drs. Harriet W. Hopf and Sean Runnels. Ebert presented his abstract "Does the UU Butyrylcholinesterase genotype predict a normal clinical and biochemical response to succinylcholine? A model for personalized medicine in anesthesia" at the 2011 American Society of Anesthesiologists (ASA) annual meeting.

"Coming from a medical school that does not have its own anesthesiology residency program, my experience with MSARF was absolutely invaluable!" said Ebert. "I was able to interact with an anesthesiology program and learn things about the field that I otherwise never would have been exposed to. My summer experience with FAER has made me a more well-rounded medical student and has better prepared me for residency training. MSARF transformed my interest in anesthesiology into a desire to pursue it as a career."[7]

Rural Access to Anesthesia Care Scholarship

Description: To introduce medical students to rural anesthesia, the American Society of Anesthesiologists (ASA) has established the Rural Access to Anesthesia Care Scholarship. The award amount is up to $750 to cover the cost of travel and lodging for a rural clerkship.

To Apply: To be eligible, applicants must be in the third or fourth year of medical school and a member of ASA. A list of mentors and locations is available at the ASA website below. The application includes an essay explaining why you are interested in the program.

Deadline: There are four application cycles during the year. For more information, visit:

http://www.asahq.org/For-Students/For-Medical-Students/Rural-Access-to-Anesthesia-Care-Scholarship.aspx

References

[1]2012 NRMP Program Directors Survey. Available at:
http://www.nrmp.org/wp-content/uploads/2013/08/programresultsbyspecialty2012.pdf. Accessed June 3, 2014.

[2]Drexel University Department of Anesthesiology. Available at:
http://webcampus.drexelmed.edu/cdc/medSpecialtyAnesthesiology.asp.
Accessed January 28, 2013.

[3]University of Minnesota Department of Anesthesiology. Available at:
http://www.anesthesiology.umn.edu/residency/prospective/application/home.html. Accessed January 28, 2013.

[4]University of Texas Houston Department of Anesthesiology. Available at:
http://www.uth.tmc.edu/med/administration/student/ms4/CareerGuide.pdf.
Accessed January 28, 2013.

[5]Fleisher L, Evers A, Wiener-Kronish J, Ulatowski J. What are we looking for?
The question of resident selection. *Anesthesiology* 2012; 117 (2): 230-1.

[6]American Medical Association. Available at:
http://www.med.und.edu/fargo/documents/AMA-ResidencyInsideLook_000.pdf. Accessed January 28, 2013.

[7]Foundation for Anesthesia Education and Research. Available at:
http://faer.org/news/medical-student-program-provides-invaluable-experience/.
Accessed January 20, 2014.

Chapter 20

Dermatology Awards, Scholarships, & Grants

Dermatology is a highly competitive specialty. In the 2011 NRMP Match, approximately 370 positions were available. However, 21% of U.S. senior medical students failed to match. Almost all applicants to dermatology will have performed research and therefore if you're considering dermatology as a career, you may wish to participate in research between the first and second years of medical school.

Medical schools and departments of dermatology often have funding in the form of scholarships or grants to support student research either during the summer between the first and second year or at a later time, and this can be a valuable addition to the residency application. In a 2002 survey of 36 departments of dermatology, 21 reported at least one first- or second-year student involved in a case report or series.[1] Research experience has significant educational benefits. Beyond those benefits, research allows a student the chance to develop a relationship with their research supervisor. Establishing a mentor-mentee relationship will prove useful during the residency application process when your mentor can provide a strong letter of recommendation, based on significant personal interaction, as well as advocate on your behalf at other programs.

External awards, particularly for research, are also available. The most prestigious are national research programs sponsored by the Melanoma Research Foundation, American Skin Association, and American Dermatological Association.

Medical students who belong to minority groups underrepresented in medicine should be aware of the Diversity Medical Student Mentorship Program sponsored by the American Academy of Dermatology. A significant percentage of participants in this program have been able to successfully match into dermatology.

American Skin Association Medical Student Grants Targeting Melanoma and Skin Cancer

Description: The American Skin Association provides research grants to promote the early careers of medical students. Applications are invited from medical students working actively in the areas of melanoma and skin cancer. Up to five grants of $7,000 will be awarded each year. A second year of funding may be requested upon receipt and review of a final progress report and re-application.

To Apply: Applicants must include a title page, a letter indicating career goals and relevance of grant, CV, letter of endorsement by mentor, research proposal, and an indication of budget and past applications.

Deadline: The deadline for the application is in October, and grants are announced in January of the following year. Application forms and instructions are available at the following site:

http://www.americanskin.org

American Academy of Dermatology Diversity Medical Student Mentorship Program

Description: The American Academy of Dermatology (AAD) offers medical students who are members of underrepresented groups in medicine the opportunity to participate in the Diversity Mentorship Program. Through this program, award recipients explore the specialty under the guidance of a mentor in an academic or private practice setting. In 2013, approximately 25 students were chosen to participate in the program.

To Apply: The program is open to first- through fourth-year medical students. Applicants may choose their own mentor or select one from the AAD mentor list. The mentor must be identified prior to application submission. Mentors must be members of the AAD. The application includes CV, medical school transcript, and two letters of recommendation.

Deadline: The application deadline is in January. For more information, visit:

http://www.aad.org/members/residents-and-fellows/diversity-mentorship-program-information-for-medical-students

American Dermatological Association Medical Student Fellowship Program

Description: The American Dermatological Association sponsors the Medical Student Fellowship Program. Through this program, award recipients receive $700/month for dermatologic research.

To Apply: The program is open to U.S. and Canadian medical students. For application information, visit the website below.

Deadline: For more information, visit:

http://www.amer-derm-assn.org/MemberInfo/2013%20Medical%20Student%20Fellowship%20Application.pdf

---

Profile of a Winner

Bethaney Vincent was the recipient of the American Dermatological Association Medical Student Fellowship. The award provided funding for her summer research project investigating the role of mitochondrial DNA mutations in skin cancer. "While many medical students at Vanderbilt elect to do summer research, it is a rare accomplishment for a student to identify a project, write a proposal, and have it successfully funded during their first year," said Dr. James Sligh, her research mentor. "Bethaney is deserving of this award from the American Dermatological Society which recognizes her initiative and potential as a physician scientist."[2] Bethaney is now a dermatopathology fellow at the University of Alabama Birmingham.

Melanoma Research Foundation Grant

Description: The Melanoma Research Foundation (MRF) Grant Program provides funding to support basic and clinical research projects that explore innovative approaches to understanding melanoma and its treatment. Grant awards are $3,000 per award period. Length of award period is a minimum of three months.

To Apply: Applicants must be medical students in good academic standing at an accredited U.S. medical school or institution. Grants will not be awarded to any applicant who has previously received a MRF Grant Award.

Deadline: Applications will be accepted beginning September and ending in November. Decisions will be made and sent out via email by January. Funds will be disbursed in March. For more info, visit:

http://www.melanoma.org/research/research-grant-application-process

National Psoriasis Foundation Amgen Medical Dermatology Fellowship

Description: The National Psoriasis Foundation has established this fellowship program for medical students and residents interested in studying psoriasis and psoriatic arthritis. The goal of the program is to increase the number of scientists studying psoriatic disease. Through this program, trainees are linked with psoriatic disease researchers who serve as mentors. The award amount is $40,000 to support one year of research.

To Apply: For application information, visit the website below.

Deadline: For more information, visit:

https://www.psoriasis.org/research/our-research/grants/amgen-medical-dermatology-fellowships

Women's Dermatologic Society Medical Student Awareness Program

Description: The Women's Dermatologic Society administers the Medical Student Awareness Program. Awardees receive up to $2,000 to explore the field of dermatology by working with a leading dermatologist. According to the website, the program is not currently active but students should contact the program to see if it will be reinstituted.

To Apply: U.S. and international medical students are eligible to apply for this program. Applicants must be in the first, second or third year of medical school. Preference will be given to students attending schools without a dermatology department.

Deadline: For more information, visit:

http://www.womensderm.org/grants/medical_student.php

Did you know...

Shailee Patel, a medical student at the University of Miami, took two years off from medical school to perform dermatology research under the supervision of the Director of the Wound Healing and Regenerative Medicine Research Program. She applied for numerous research awards and programs, and was the recipient of 12 honorable distinctions. Among her honors:

- Alpha Omega Alpha Carolyn L. Kuckein Student Research Fellowship Award
- Wound Healing Society Young Investigator Award
- Medical Student Fellowship from the American Dermatological Association
- Outstanding Basic Science Oral Presentation at the Eastern-Atlantic Student Research Forum
- Dermatology Poster Award and Best Overall Poster at the 54th Annual National Student Research Forum

"Every student who spent a year doing research in our program has won one or more awards, but Shailee's success is exceptional," said Dr. Marjana Tomic-Canic, her research mentor. "In addition to her work in the laboratory, Shailee was active in collaborating with other clinical and research faculty in the department that resulted in multiple publications."[3]

References

[1]Wagner R, Ioffe B. Medical student dermatology research in the United States. *Dermatol Online J* 2005; 11(1): 8.

[2]Vanderbilt University Medical Center *Reporter*. Available at: http://www.mc.vanderbilt.edu:8080/reporter/index.html?ID=3416. Accessed June 4, 2014.

[3]University of Miami Miller School of Medicine. Available at: http://med.miami.edu/news/student-researcher-honored-with-a-dozen-accolades-in-two-years. Accessed June 3, 2014.

Chapter 21

Emergency Medicine Awards, Scholarships, & Grants

For medical students interested in receiving a scholarship, award, or grant in emergency medicine, begin by researching opportunities at your own institution. Each medical school may select a senior medical student to receive the Society for Academic Emergency Medicine (SAEM) Medical Student Excellence in Emergency Medicine Award.

External awards for community service, leadership, research, and other contributions to the field are also available. The most prestigious are awards and scholarships sponsored by the Society for Academic Emergency Medicine, Emergency Medicine Foundation, American College of Emergency Physicians, and Emergency Medicine Residents' Association.

At schools with academic emergency medicine departments, there are often opportunities to participate in research during the summer between the first and second year. If you're interested in performing EM research during this time, consider applying for the Medical Student Research Grant, which is jointly sponsored by SAEM and the Emergency Medicine Foundation. Medical students are also eligible to apply for a Research Grant from the Emergency Medicine Residents' Association.

In recent years, emergency medicine has become increasingly competitive. Medical students often ask us if it's necessary to do research in the field. In the 2012 NRMP Program Director Survey, 56% of emergency medicine residency programs cited "demonstrated involvement and interest in research" as a factor in selecting applicants to interview.[1] It's especially helpful to read the perspectives of emergency medicine residency program directors about the importance of research in the selection process. We offer you these perspectives on the next page.

Emergency Medicine Research for Medical Students: Perspectives of Residency Program Directors

- "Many applicants want to do know if they should do some research to bolster their application," writes Dr. David Overton, Professor of Emergency Medicine at the Michigan State University/Kalamazoo Center for Medical Studies. "Programs vary in how much weight they place upon research in their ranking decisions. Some give extra brownie points, others don't. Overall, however, surveys of emergency medicine program directors indicate that research is one of the least important factors in ranking candidates."[2]

- As you might expect, some programs value research more than others. "Research and leadership activities have become additional screening criteria at highly competitive programs along with board scores and/or class ranking," writes Dr. Bharath Chakravarthy, Program Director of the University of California Irvine Emergency Medicine Residency Program.[3]

- Participation in research allows the emergency medicine residency applicant to form a strong relationship with a faculty member. "This, in turn, allows the research mentor to advocate on the student's behalf," writes Dr. Shahram Lotfipour, Professor of Emergency Medicine and Associate Dean for Clinical Sciences Education at the University of California Irvine.[4]

- Starting research early in medical school can lead to publication or presentation. "The goal of the project should be presentation at a regional or national meeting in abstract/poster form, followed by submission to and publication in a peer reviewed EM journal," writes Dr. Lotfipour. "The two major national research meetings have deadlines for submissions of January (SAEM) and June (ACEP). Regional and state chapter meeting deadlines occur throughout the year. Presenting research at a national EM forum or publishing a research paper in an EM journal is viewed very favorably by many EM programs."[4]

- "Most programs are impressed with research and even more impressed with publications," writes Dr. Todd Berger, Program Director of the UT Southwestern – Austin Emergency Medicine Residency Program. "Most programs also feel the value of one month of research does not compare to four years of ongoing involvement. If you're looking to publish, a case write-up is a quick opportunity. If you see an unusual case, do a literature search. If you find minimal references, talk to your attending about submitting a case report."[5]

AAEM/RSA Medical Student Scholarship

Description: The American Academy of Emergency Medicine (AAEM) in partnership with the Resident and Student Association (RSA) awards up to two scholarships each year to students who have demonstrated dedication and passion for the specialty. The award amount is $500. Winners are recognized at the AAEM Scientific Assembly.
To Apply: Any current AAEM/RSA medical student member is eligible. Students must be nominated by an attending, fellow, or resident member of AAEM/RSA.
Deadline: Nominations are accepted from September 15 to November 15. For more information, visit:

http://www.aaemrsa.org/resources/medical-student-scholarship

American College of Emergency Physicians National Outstanding Medical Student Award

Description: The American College of Emergency Physicians (ACEP) developed this award for medical students who intend to pursue a career in emergency medicine, and who have demonstrated outstanding patient care and involvement in medical organizations or the community. A maximum of 10 students may receive awards. Winners will receive a plaque from the ACEP, a free one-year membership in ACEP, free registration to ACEP's annual meeting, and convocation at ACEP's annual meeting. Award winners will also be recognized during the ACEP awards ceremony and have their names published in ACEP News or other College publications.
To Apply: The chair of emergency medicine, emergency medicine program director or the medical student clerkship director is asked to nominate one emergency medicine bound medical student who fulfills the necessary criteria. Students are awarded for their humanism/professionalism, scholarly achievement, leadership and service to medical organizations/ACEP, community service and research/publications. See the link below for the requirements and the application form.
Deadline: The application deadline is in February. See the link for more information:

http://www.acep.org/content.aspx?id=22572

American College of Emergency Physicians Medical Student Professionalism and Service Award

Description: This award is given by the American College of Emergency Physicians (ACEP) to medical students who intend to pursue a career in emergency medicine, and who have excelled in compassionate care of patients, professional behavior, and service to the community and/or specialty. The winner will receive a certificate from the ACEP and an opportunity to attend a reception for award winners at ACEP's annual Scientific Assembly. Award recipients will also be mentioned in an ACEP publication and on the ACEP website. Monetary awards are to be decided at the local level.

To Apply: The chair of emergency medicine, emergency medicine program director or the medical student clerkship director is asked to nominate one emergency medicine bound medical student who fulfills the necessary criteria. See the link below for the requirements and the application form.

Deadline: The deadline for application submission is from October to August of the following year. Visit the link for further information:

http://www.acep.org/content.aspx?id=22570

Profile of a Winner

In 2012, Alan Johnson, a third-year medical student from The Commonwealth Medical College (TCMC), was one of the 16 recipients of the prestigious ACEP Medical Student Professionalism and Service Award. He was recognized at ACEP's annual Scientific Assembly in Denver. He received the award for this commitment to professionalism and involvement with medical organizations and the community. Mr. Johnson has also dedicated himself to the field of emergency medicine and founded the Emergency Medicine Interest Group at TCMC.[6]

American College of Emergency Physicians Best Medical Student Paper Award

Description: The American College of Emergency Physicians (ACEP) bestows the ACEP Best Medical Student Paper Award based on a review of research abstracts presented at the annual ACEP Research Forum in October.

To Apply: To be eligible, abstracts submitted by medical students must not appear in any journal prior to publication or be presented at any other scientific meeting. The student applicant must be the presenter of the abstract at the Research Forum.

Deadline: The deadline is in April. For more information, visit:

http://www.acep.org/rf/

American College of Osteopathic Emergency Medicine Case Study Poster Competition

Description: The American College of Osteopathic Emergency Medicine (ACOEP) invites students, residents, and physicians to submit their research for poster presentation. The top three presenters will be recognized during the ACOEP Spring Seminar, and will receive awards.

To Apply: For more information, visit the website below.
Deadline: The deadline is in January. For more information, visit:

http://www.acoep.org/pdf/students/2012%20Case%20Poster%20Competition.pdf

American College of Medical Toxicology Travel Scholarship for Underrepresented Minority Medical Trainees

Description: The American College of Medical Toxicology (ACMT) sponsors the Minority Student Travel Award to encourage minority medical students to attend the ACMT Annual Scientific Meeting. The award amount is $1,500.
To Apply: The application includes CV, letter of interest, and letter of support.
Deadline: For more information, visit:

http://www.acmt.net/Travel_Scholarship_for_Underrepresented_Minority_Medical_Trainees.html

Dr. Alexandra Greene Medical Student Award

Description: This award is given by the Emergency Medicine Residents' Association to a medical student who has demonstrated significant dedication to the specialty.
To Apply: Criteria for selection include compassion, professionalism, and willingness to go above and beyond for patients and colleagues. The application includes letter of support and CV. To be eligible, applicants must be medical student members of EMRA and in the third or fourth year of medical school.
Deadline: The application deadline is in February. For more information, visit:

http://www.emra.org/content.aspx?id=163

Emergency Medicine Health Equity Student Scholarship

Description: The University of Illinois at Chicago Department of Emergency Medicine provides the Emergency Medicine Health Equity Student Scholarship. Through this program, scholarship recipients gain exposure to academic emergency medicine with an exploration of the subspecialty areas of health disparities research, toxicology, ultrasound, international EM, education and simulation, resuscitation, and health policy and administration. The award amount is $1,500 and $2,000 for the 4-week and 6-week programs, respectively.
To Apply: The application includes two letters of recommendation, USMLE scores, and personal essay describing interest and/or experiences in health equity. Criteria for selection include interest and work in health equity, academic achievement, leadership, and interest in academic emergency medicine.

Deadline: For more information, visit:

http://chicago.medicine.uic.edu/UserFiles/Servers/Server_442934/Image/Emer
gency%20Medicine/Revised%20Scholarship%20Flyer%2022014.v1.pdf

Emergency Medicine Interest Group Grant

Description: The Society of Academic Emergency Medicine (SAEM) Foundation gives grants to interest groups to promote the specialty at the medical student level. The award amount is $500.

To Apply: Emergency Medicine Interest Groups at medical schools are eligible to apply. On the application, medical students should be listed as the primary applicants. A faculty member should be listed as a co-applicant. The faculty member must be a member of SAEM. Criteria for judging include educational merit, significance to emergency medicine, originality, methodology, institutional support, applicant qualifications, and appropriateness of budget.

Deadline: The deadline is in January. For more information, visit:

http://www.saem.org/saem-foundation/grants/what-we-fund/em-interest-group-
grant

Emergency Medicine Summer Clinical Externship Program for Medical Students

Description: WellSpan York Hospital invites medical students to apply for their externship program. Participants will spend the summer between the first and second year of medical school shadowing and gaining early exposure to emergency medicine. Students will shadow emergency medicine attendings and residents, participate in workshops and lectures, learn and practice procedures in the simulation center, and develop skills in medical writing and oral presentation.

To Apply: To be eligible, applicants must be completing their first year of medical school. The application includes CV and 500-word essay outlining your interest in the program.

Deadline: The application deadline is in February. For more information, visit:

http://www.yorkhospital.edu/default.aspx?program=2&type=text&content=109

EMBRS Scholarship

Description: This award is given by the Emergency Medicine Residents' Association to a medical student who has demonstrated interest in a research career and seeks to attend the EMBRS workshop. This is an 11-day, 2-session program led by seasoned research investigators.

To Apply: The application includes letter of support and CV. A cover letter indicating the reason why the applicant wishes to attend the EMBRS course, career interests, and proposed research projects is also required. To be eligible, applicants must be medical student members of EMRA. Criteria for selection include desired interest in research, dedication to investigation, and likelihood that applicant will continue research in the future.

Deadline: The application deadline is in February. For more information, visit:

http://www.emra.org/content.aspx?id=1443

EMF/SAEM Medical Student Research Grant

Description: The Emergency Medicine Foundation (EMF) and the Society for Academic Emergency Medicine (SAEM) jointly created this research grant to encourage medical students to actively participate in emergency medicine research. The grant is for a maximum of $2,400, of which at least $1,200 must be used as a student stipend. The maximum number of awards funded is determined annually. Applicants may reapply each academic year for a second term of support.

To Apply: An application form may be submitted by either a specific medical student or by an Emergency Medicine residency program wishing to sponsor a medical student research project. Please see the link below for the application form and requirements.

Deadline: The application deadline is in January, and award recipients are notified by the following May. Visit the following link for more information:

http://www.saem.org/saem-foundation/grants/what-we-fund/medical-student-research-grant

---

Profile of a Winner

In 2012 – 2013, the Emergency Medicine Foundation and Society for Academic Emergency Medicine funded two highly qualified and motivated medical students to help them pursue their strong interest in emergency medicine research.

Paul Pukurdpol, a medical student at the University of Colorado Denver, used his award to fund the *National Study of Primary Care-Treatable Emergency Department Visits as Indicators of Limited Access to Care*.

The second grant winner was Erin Conrad from the University of Michigan Medical School. She studied *Spatial Biochemical Dynamics of Central Venous Catheter Infections*.[7]

EMRA Research Grant

Description: This award is given by the Emergency Medicine Residents' Association to medical students interested in completing emergency medicine research projects during medical school. The award amount is $1,000.

To Apply: The application includes cover letter, grant proposal, and CV. Criteria for selection include perceived importance and possible impact of the research project. To be eligible, applicants must be EMRA members.
Deadline: The application deadline is in February. For more information, visit:

http://www.emra.org/content.aspx?id=167

EMRA Travel Scholarship to ACEP Leadership & Advocacy Conference

Description: This award is given by the Emergency Medicine Residents' Association to medical students planning to attend the American College of Emergency Physicians (ACEP) Leadership & Advocacy Conference. Attendees are able to refine leadership skills, stay informed of important issues, and meet with members of Congress. The award amount of $800 is provided to cover the cost of attendance. Up to three recipients are chosen.
To Apply: To be eligible, applicants must be EMRA members. Of note, international members may also apply for the scholarship. The application includes letter of intent explaining need and purpose of attendance, letter of recommendation, and CV.
Deadline: The application deadline is in February. For more information, visit:

http://www.emra.org/content.aspx?id=168

EMRA Travel Scholarship to SAEM

Description: This award is given by the Emergency Medicine Residents' Association to medical students planning to attend the Society for Academic Emergency Medicine (SAEM) Conference. The award amount is $600. Up to six winners will be chosen.
To Apply: Applicants must be EMRA members. Of note, international members may also apply for the scholarship. The application includes letter of intent explaining need and purpose of attendance, reference letter, and CV.
Deadline: The application deadline is in February. For more information, visit:

http://www.emra.org/content.aspx?id=169

EMRA Travel Scholarship to AEM Gender Consensus Conference

Description: This award is given by the Emergency Medicine Residents' Association to medical students planning to attend the AEM Gender Consensus Conference. The award amount is $500. Up to three winners will be chosen. The conference is held the day before the Society for Academic Emergency Medicine (SAEM) annual meeting.
To Apply: To be eligible, applicants must be EMRA members. Of note, international members may also apply for the scholarship. The application includes letter of intent explaining need and purpose of attendance, letter of recommendation, and CV.

Deadline: The application deadline is in February. For more information, visit:

http://www.emra.org/content.aspx?id=2058

EMRA Local Action Grants

Description: This award is given by the Emergency Medicine Residents' Association to medical students interested in community service and other activities that support the field of emergency medicine. The award amount is $1,000.

To Apply: To be eligible, applicants must be EMRA members. The application includes cover letter, grant proposal, and CV. Projects that are consistent with the mission of EMRA will be considered for funding, and examples are provided at the EMRA website.

Deadline: There are two application cycles with deadlines in February and July. For more information, visit:

http://www.emra.org/content.aspx?id=177

EMRA Be the Change Challenge

Description: This award is given by the Emergency Medicine Residents' Association to medical students interested in creating or pursuing a project of major significance to the specialty of emergency medicine. Project focus may be on education, research, practice, or policy. The award amount is $5,000.

To Apply: To be eligible, applicants must be EMRA members. The application includes project proposal form and reference letter. Criteria for selection include quality, feasibility, and novelty of the project.

Deadline: The application deadline is in July. For more information, visit:

http://www.emra.org/content.aspx?id=1652

EMRA Travel Scholarship to Scientific Assembly

Description: This award is given by the Emergency Medicine Residents' Association to medical students planning to attend the American College of Emergency Physicians Scientific Assembly. The award amount is $500. Up to six winners will be chosen.

To Apply: To be eligible, applicants must be EMRA members. Of note, international members may also apply for the scholarship. The application includes letter of intent explaining need and purpose of attendance, letter of recommendation, and CV.

Deadline: The application deadline is in July. For more information, visit:

http://www.emra.org/content.aspx?id=170

SAEM Medical Student Excellence in Emergency Medicine Award

Description: Each medical school is permitted to select a senior medical student to receive this award. Winners will receive complimentary membership in the Society for Academic Emergency Medicine (SAEM) and subscriptions to *Academic Emergency Medicine* and the SAEM Newsletter.

To Apply: Only one student at each medical school can receive this award.

Deadline: For more information, visit:

http://www.saem.org/meetings/saem-awards/medical-student-excellence-award

---

Did you know...

There are opportunities to win awards at local and regional EM meetings. Nathaniel Hunt, a medical student at Wayne State University, won the Best Medical Student Presentation award at the Society of Academic Emergency Medicine Regional Conference in Akron, Ohio. Hunt researched patient care outcomes following delays in obtaining adequate vascular access in septic shock patients. "Not every medical student gets to present research at a regional or national conference, and very few will win this type of award during their medical school career," said Dr. James Paxton, his research mentor. "I am sure that the judges saw some merit in the subject matter, but I suspect that his public speaking talent, coolness under pressure – a trait that I'm sure he perfected while working as a nurse in the emergency department – and familiarity with the study data are what really earned this award for him."[8]

References

[1]2012 NRMP Program Directors Survey. Available at:
http://www.nrmp.org/wp-content/uploads/2013/08/programresultsbyspecialty2012.pdf. Accessed June 3, 2014.

[2]Department of Emergency Medicine at Michigan State University/Kalamazoo Center for Medical Studies. Available at: http://med.wmich.edu/node/103. Michigan State University/Kalamazoo Center for Medical Studies

[3]University of California Irvine Department of Emergency Medicine. Available at:
http://www.meded.uci.edu/education/residencyselection/emergencymed.html. Accessed January 30, 2013.

[4]Lotfipour S, Luu R, Hayden S, Vaca F, Hoonpongsimanont W, Langdorf. Becoming an emergency medicine resident: a practical guide for medical students. *J Emerg Med* 2008; 35 (3): 339-44.

[5]UT Southwestern – Austin Emergency Medicine Residency Program. Available at: http://www.austingme.com/residency-programs/emergency-medicine/how-to-apply/application-advice. Accessed January 30, 2013.

[6]Times Leader. Available at:
http://www.timesleader.com/apps/pbcs.dll/article?avis=TL&date=20121021&category=news&lopenr=310219711&Ref=AR. Accessed January 20, 2014.

[7]Emergency Medicine Foundation. Available at:
http://www.emfoundation.org/EMF.aspx?id=394. Accessed January 20, 2014.

[8]Wayne State University School of Medicine *Prognosis*. Available at: http://prognosis.med.wayne.edu/article/wsus-nathaniel-hunt-wins-top-student-presentation-award-at-emergency-medicine-conference. Accessed June 4, 2014.

Chapter 22

Family Medicine Awards, Scholarships, & Grants

For medical students interested in receiving a scholarship, award, or grant in family medicine, begin by researching opportunities at your own institution. The Department of Family Medicine at Michigan State University College of Human Medicine offers the Blake W.H. Smith, PhD, Scholarship to a medical student, resident, or faculty member "engaged in furthering the goals of primary health care, or community-oriented medical education with an emphasis on international settings or underserved areas and populations in the United States."[1] The Clerkship Professionalism Award is given to one student each year by the Department of Family Medicine at the University of Washington. The award is given for exemplary professional behavior during the third year clerkship. The Department of Family Medicine at the University of Wisconsin honors a first-year medical student with the Compassion in Action Award for desire to provide "good work" in an underserved community.

External awards for community service, leadership, research, and other contributions to the field are also available. The most prestigious are awards and scholarships awarded by the American Academy of Family Practice and the Pisacano Scholars Leadership Foundation. These are described below.

Medical students may also apply for local, regional, and state awards. At the Georgia Academy of Family Physicians Meeting, three Mercer University School of Medicine students received an award for a poster presentation.

AAFP Community Outreach Award

Description: The American Academy of Family Physicians grants this award to medical students who have served in a key leadership role in a community service or advocacy project. Each awardee will receive $600 to attend the National Conference of Family Medicine Residents and Medical Students.
To Apply: To be eligible, medical student applicants must complete an application, submit a letter of support, and describe the project.
Deadline: The deadline is in May. For more information, visit:

http://www.aafp.org/about/awards-scholarships/student/nc.html

AAFP Family Medicine Interest Group Leadership Scholarship Program

Description: The American Academy of Family Physicians grants scholarships to students who have made outstanding contributions to their school's Family Medicine Interest Group and wish to travel to the National Conference of Family Medicine Residents and Medical Students. The award amount is $600.
To Apply: To be eligible, medical student applicants must complete an application and write a personal essay.
Deadline: The deadline is in May. For more information, visit:

http://www.aafp.org/about/awards-scholarships/student/nc.html

AAFP Minority Scholarships Program for Residents and Medical Students

Description: The American Academy of Family Physicians grants scholarships to AAFP student minority members. Each awardee will receive $600 to attend the National Conference of Family Medicine Residents and Medical Students.
To Apply: To be eligible, medical student applicants must complete an application and write a personal essay.
Deadline: The deadline is in May. For more information, visit:

http://www.aafp.org/about/awards-scholarships/student/nc.html

AAFP National Conference First-Time Student Attendee Award

Description: The American Academy of Family Physicians grants scholarships to students wishing to attend the National Conference of Family Medicine Residents and Medical Students. The award amount is $600.
To Apply: To be eligible, medical student applicants must complete an application and write a personal essay.
Deadline: The deadline is in May. For more information, visit:

http://www.aafp.org/about/awards-scholarships/student/nc.html

AAFP Tomorrow's Leader Award

Description: The American Academy of Family Physicians grants this award to medical students for demonstration of leadership ability. Each awardee will receive $600 to attend the National Conference of Family Medicine Residents and Medical Students.
To Apply: To be eligible, medical student applicants must complete an application and submit CV, letters of recommendation, and personal essay.
Deadline: The deadline is in May. For more information, visit:

http://www.aafp.org/about/awards-scholarships/student/nc.html

American College of Osteopathic Family Physicians Poster Presentation Competition

Description: The American College of Osteopathic Family Physicians (ACOFP) invites osteopathic medical students, family practice residents, and faculty members to present their research during the Annual Convention & Scientific Seminars in March. A certificate of participation will be given to all presenters. Three prizes will be given for Original Research for Students and Residents. In a second category of Case Reports, one student and one resident will receive awards.
To Apply: For more information, visit the website below.
Deadline: The deadline is in January. For more information, visit:

http://www.acofp.org/Journal_and_Clinical_Resources/Call_for_Poster_Presen tations/

Dr. Andrew David Bagby Scholarship

Description: This scholarship provides support for a medical student to spend four weeks in Latrobe, Pennsylvania with the family practice residency program at Latrobe Area Hospital.
To Apply: To be eligible, the applicant must have interest in becoming a family physician. The applicant must be in the second year of medical school in an allopathic or osteopathic school in the U.S. or Canada. The application includes written statement of interest in the field and letter of reference.
Deadline: The deadline is in April. For more information, visit:

http://zone.medschool.pitt.edu/sites/FMIG/Lists/Announcements/Attachments/ 5/bagbyscholarship.pdf

James G. Jones, MD, Student Scholarship Program

Description: The James G. Jones, MD, Student Scholarship provides support for one medical student to attend the Family Medicine Congressional Conference. Jointly sponsored by the American Academy of Family Physicians and the Council of Academic Family Medicine, the meeting allows student attendees to be informed of health policy issues at the Congressional level. Attendees also learn how to advocate for the specialty.
To Apply: For application information and instructions, visit the website below.
Deadline: For more information, visit:

http://www.aafpfoundation.org/online/foundation/home/programs/education/jo nesscholar.html

Joseph Collins Foundation Scholarship (See Chapter 18)

NAPCRG Student Family Medicine/Primary Care Research Award

Description: The North American Primary Care Research Group (NAPCRG) has established this award to recognize medical student research in family medicine and primary care.
To Apply: One award may be made by each department of family medicine. Contact your school's department for more information.
Deadline: For more information, visit:

http://www.napcrg.org/AboutUs/Awards/StudentResearchAward

National Conference Poster Competition

Description: Medical students and residents are invited to present their research during the National Conference for Family Medicine Residents and Medical Students sponsored by the American Academy of Family Practice. Applicants can submit research in one of four categories – Research, Clinical Inquiry, Community Project, and Educational Program. Outstanding poster presentations will be recognized during the conference with ribbons. One resident and one student will be awarded a trip to the AAFP Scientific Assembly to present their posters in October.
To Apply: The applicant must be enrolled in an ACGME/AOA accredited residency program or LCME/COCA accredited medical school and a member in good standing of the AAFP. Presenters must be able to attend the National Conference held in Kansas City in July/August. Criteria for judging include appropriateness and relevance to family medicine, originality of project, clarity of presentation, and validity of conclusions.
Deadline: The deadline is in April. For more information, visit:

http://www.aafp.org/dam/AAFP/documents/events/nc/NC-poster-factsheet.pdf

One Medical Group Scholarship

Description: This scholarship is open to medical students committed to pursuing a career in the primary care field (family medicine or internal medicine). The award amount is $10,000.
To Apply: The applicant must be in the third year of medical school with an interest in pursuing a career in primary care. The application includes two reference letters and essays. The essays should address the following questions:

- Describe how technology will change patients' experience of primary care.
- How has your extracurricular involvement aligned with your personal values of pursuing primary care?

Deadline: The deadline is in March. For more information, visit:

http://www.onemedical.com/lp/scholarship

Pisacano Scholars Leadership Foundation

Description: The Pisacano Scholars Leadership Program is a competitive program that provides career development opportunities and scholarship funding to medical students identified as future leaders of family medicine. Up to five awards are granted annually. The maximum amount of the award is $28,000.

To Apply: This award is open to third-year medical students. Criteria for selection include strong commitment to the specialty, strong leadership skills, superior academic achievement, character and integrity, and notable contributions to community service.

Deadline: The deadline is in March. For more information, visit:

http://www.fpleaders.org

STFM Medical Student Education Student Scholarship

Description: The Society of Teachers of Family Medicine (STFM) offers this award to medical students. Award winners are invited to present their work to educators and student colleagues at the Conference on Medical Student Education. Monetary support to cover the cost of conference registration and travel is provided.

To Apply: Applicants must first be nominated by medical student educators. Leadership, commitment to family medicine, and adherence to the organization's core values of integrity, openness, nurturing, learning, and excellence are the criteria educators use in the nomination process. Once nominated, students apply for the award.

Deadline: For more information, visit:

http://stfm.org/

Did you know...

Brian Laing, a medical student at UCSF, built quite a record during medical school, and this helped him become a Pisacano Scholar. His involvement outside the classroom included:

- Student Homeless Clinic Volunteer
- Mission Neighborhood Health Center Volunteer (care for Latino immigrants)
- Student Chair of UCSF Family Medicine Interest Group
- Coordinator for social activism elective and health policy elective
- Founder of UCSF Health Disparities Working Group
- Co-President of UCSF AMSA Chapter
- Student Coordinator for Physicians for a Democratic Majority
- Reviewer for Primary Care E-Letter[2]

Profile of a Winner

In 2013, Anastasia Coutinho, a fourth-year medical student at the University of Vermont College of Medicine, was named a Pisacano Scholar. After graduating from McGill University in Montreal, she completed her Master in Health Sciences in International Health at the Bloomberg School of Public Health at Johns Hopkins.

While at Hopkins, Anastasia completed her thesis in Bangladesh. She conducted interviews with ethnic minorities in rural parts of the country to learn about pregnancy-related care, including malaria prevention and treatment.

Anastasia has continued to perform at a high level as a medical student. During her second year, she developed a student-faculty collaborative clinic for the care of underserved patients. She has also made contributions as a co-leader of the Health Policy Interest Group and President of the UVM AMWA Chapter.

Recently, her focus has centered on the evaluation of a child health program in West Africa. She has been working with the Johns Hopkins University Institute of International Programs on this large-scale project.[3]

Profile of a Winner

Chandra Campbell is a fourth-year student at Loyola University Chicago Stritch School of Medicine. She was a recent recipient of this scholarship, and this allowed her to attend the STFM Annual Conference.

Before medical school, Chandra found her experiences as a health educator and group fitness instructor very fulfilling. In the future, she plans to use the skills that she has developed along with her medical expertise to make an impact through preventive medicine.

"So much of primary care is about education and working toward prevention, not just putting a Band-Aid on existing problems," said Chandra. "I'm inspired by new approaches to addressing chronic disease and patient education."

Chandra has certainly made a mark in service as a medical student. After long days in medical school, she works tirelessly as a resident manager at the Ronald McDonald House. She also developed a health education program at Loyola's clinic to fill an important need for Chicago's underserved population.

"She stands out as an exceptional student physician who has left a permanent legacy on our school that will benefit patients, students and faculty for years to come," said Dr. Aaron Michelfelder, Vice-Chair of the Department of Family Medicine at the Loyola University Chicago Stritch School of Medicine."[4]

Less well appreciated by medical students is the availability of scholarships and awards bestowed by state chapters of the American Academy of Family Physicians. Examples of these awards are shown in the following table, and you are encouraged to make inquiries with your state academy.

Awards Given by State Chapters of the American Academy of Family Physicians	
Organization	**Award/Scholarship**
Minnesota Academy of Family Physicians	The Medical Student Award for Contributions to Family Medicine is awarded to one fourth-year student for family medicine activities on a local, community, state or national level.
Nebraska Academy of Family Physicians	A number of awards are available, including the Haiti Mission Trip Scholarship, Medical Mission Trip Educational Grant, Michael Haller Scholarship, and Fay Smith Scholarship.
North Carolina Academy of Family Practice	Third- and fourth-year students considering careers as family physicians can receive scholarships ranging from $2,000 to $5,000.
California Academy of Family Physicians	Through the Student Research Grant Program, students have opportunities to perform research under the supervision of a practicing or academic family physician.
Ohio Academy of Family Physicians	Scholarships are available for students to attend the Family Medicine Education Consortium Northeast Region Meeting.

References

[1] Department of Family Medicine at the Michigan State University College of Human Medicine. Available at: http://chmfamilymedicine.msu.edu/academic-programs/student-awards/blake-smith-scholarship. Accessed June 4, 2014.
[2] UCSF School of Medicine. Available at: http://www.ucsf.edu/news/2007/08/7589/fourth-year-medical-student-wins-pisacano-scholarship. Accessed July 2, 2014.
[3] Annals of Family Medicine. Available at: http://www.annfammed.org/content/12/1/81.full. Accessed April 4, 2014.
[4] Loyola University Chicago Stritch School of Medicine. Available at: http://www.stritch.luc.edu/newswire/news/stritch-student-receives-national-family-medicine-award. Accessed January 20, 2014.

Chapter 23

General Surgery Awards, Scholarships, & Grants

For medical students interested in receiving a scholarship, award, or grant in general surgery or one of its subspecialties, begin by researching opportunities at your own institution. The Department of Surgery at North Carolina recognizes one fourth-year medical student with the George F. Sheldon, MD Leadership Award. The award is given to the student who has "demonstrated outstanding academic and clinical achievement, and who possesses personal characteristics that promise a future leadership role in surgery."[1] One student at the UT San Antonio Health Sciences Center receives the Basil A. Pruitt Jr., MD Award for outstanding research achievement during his/her medical school career. At the University of Illinois College of Medicine at Peoria, students are selected by the Chair and Clerkship Director of the Department of Surgery to receive the UICOMP Surgery Travel Award. This is a monetary award that helps to cover the cost of travel to either the American College of Surgeons Clinical Congress or Association for Surgical Education Annual Meeting. Make inquiries with your Department of Surgery to learn about award opportunities you may be eligible for.

External awards for leadership, research, and other contributions to the field are also available. These awards, scholarships, and grants are presented in this chapter.

General surgery is a very competitive specialty. Medical students often ask us if it's necessary to do research in the field. In the 2012 NRMP Program Director Survey, 56% of general surgery residency programs cited "demonstrated involvement and interest in research" as a factor in selecting applicants to interview.[2] It's especially helpful to read the perspectives of general surgery residency program directors about the importance of research in the selection process. We offer you these perspectives on the next page.

General Surgery Research for Medical Students: Perspectives of Residency Program Directors

- In a survey of general surgery residency program directors, researchers in the Department of Surgery at Stony Brook University sought to determine the importance of research in the residency selection process. A total of 134 program directors responded. The largest group of respondents were program directors of university-based programs (45.5%) followed by directors of community-based programs with university affiliations (42.5%) and community-based programs without university affiliation (11.9%). The study found that basic science or clinical research was almost always or always considered in the evaluation of general surgery residency applicants.[3]

- In the study performed by Stony Brook University researchers, basic science and clinical research were given equal importance by 54.5% of PDs.[3]

- Although most program directors value research involvement, 29.9% of program directors rarely or never placed value on research that was not published as an abstract or paper.[3]

- When asked to rank the importance of research on a scale of 1 to 5 (5 = most important), 8.2% gave basic science and clinical research a score of 5. Clearly, there is a small group of program directors who highly value research in the selection process. However, most program directors gave research a score of 3.[3]

- In discussing the survey's findings, the authors wrote "that basic science and clinical research were favorable traits in an application for general surgery residency. The student's participation in research demonstrated considerable interest in the surgical field, which is a selection factor at the top of most PDs' lists."[3]

- Since published research is most highly valued, strive to begin research early in medical school. The summer between the first and second years of medical school is an excellent time to begin such work. Follow-through during the remaining years of medical school will increase the likelihood that the work will be published prior to submission of the residency application. "Those who recognize its importance and benefits early adopt a positive attitude, are persistent, determined, and follow through," writes Dr. Adil Haider, Co-Director of the Center for Surgery Trials and Outcomes Research at Johns Hopkins School of Medicine. "They are generally more productive earlier as a result."[4]

- Even research started later in medical school can lead to publication, depending on the type of article. Case reports, letters to the editor, and review articles are examples of articles that have shorter timelines. Productivity in a short time period is "highly dependent on the supervisor, availability of research opportunities, and new 'ideas,' and the student researcher's drive, commitment, and resourcefulness."[4]

American Association for the Surgery of Trauma Research and Education Foundation Medical Student Scholarship

Description: The American Association for the Surgery of Trauma (AAST) provides medical students with monetary support to attend the AAST Annual Meeting and Clinical Congress of Acute Care Surgery.
To Apply: To be eligible, the student must be sponsored by an AAST member. The application includes cover letter, CV, and letter of sponsorship.
Deadline: The deadline is in June. For more information, visit:

http://www.aast.org/foundation/scholarships.aspx

American Society of Colon and Rectal Surgeons Medical Student Research Initiation Grant

Description: The American Society of Colon and Rectal Surgeons provides the Medical Student Research Initiation Grant for students interested in performing clinical or laboratory-based research. The award amount is $4,000. Up to 10 awards are given annually.
To Apply: U.S. and Canadian medical students are eligible to apply. The application includes research proposal, letter from research mentor, and biographical sketch. Preference is given to applicants who plan to pursue a career in Colon and Rectal Surgery.
Deadline: The application deadline is in March. For more information, visit:

http://www.fascrs.org/research_foundation/grants/

Annual Starr Poster Contest for Medical Students and Residents

Description: The Annual Starr Poster Contest for Medical Students and Residents is offered by the Association of Women Surgeons (AWS). Research posters are presented at the AWS Annual Conference which takes place during the American College of Surgeons Clinical Congress. Each year, ten medical students are invited to present their research posters. The top three medical student posters will be recognized, and these students will receive a monetary prize. The top student poster winner will also be invited to attend the AWS Awards Dinner.
To Apply: Students are eligible to apply if they are members of AWS. Written abstracts of 400 words or less should be submitted. Topics should be surgical in nature, and may reflect work in basic science, clinical outcomes, epidemiology, and health policy. Abstracts should include title, author, introduction, methodology, and results. Applicants may submit work previously sent to other conferences. No case reports will be accepted.
Deadline: The application deadline is in August. For more information and application deadline, visit:

https://www.womensurgeons.org/AWS_Foundation/Awards.asp#sthash.7o5cYYgq.dpuf

Profile of a Winner

Avianne Bunnell is a senior medical student at the University of Central Florida College of Medicine. She was the first place winner in the 7th Annual Starr Poster Contest for Medical Students and Residents for her research on abdominal compartment syndrome. She received the award at the AWS meeting which took place at the annual American College of Surgeons Clinical Congress.

UCF medical students participate in a two-year research project as part of the Focused Inquiry and Research Experience (FIRE) module. Her research project was an extension of this work under the guidance of Dr. Michael Cheatham, Director of Surgical ICU at the Orlando Regional Medical Center.

Before starting medical school, she studied physiology at the University of Arizona. "That was where I first became interested in research that allowed me to explore the body's physiology while discovering clinically applicable data," said Avianne. "I have kept that interest in becoming a physician scientist throughout medical school, and given the opportunities I received here at UCF I have been able to develop those interests through several different research projects."[5]

Association for Academic Surgery Student Research Award

Description: The Association for Academic Surgery (AAS) grants awards to those medical students who are distinguished in research efforts in the surgical field and have an interest in pursuing a career in academic surgery. From the pool of projects submitted, six awards are granted: 3 in the basic sciences and 3 in clinical research. Winners receive an invite to the Academic Surgical Congress, complementary registration for the event, and a $500 travel stipend for costs encumbered during the trip. Recipients will be presented with an award certificate and have their name published on the AAS website and newsletter.
To Apply: The applicant must be a graduating medical student. Candidates must submit the application with a 250-word summary of their project and a letter from their research mentor, stating the applicant's contributions in the project as well as the qualifications of the applicant and the mentor.
Deadline: The deadline for this award is in September. The information and application for the award is updated per annum and can be found at

http://www.aasurg.org/awards/student_award.php

Profile of a Winner

Nirmish Singla, M.D. is a recent recipient of the AAS Student Research Award. Attending medical school at the University of Michigan, Nirmish decided early on that he was interested in pursuing a surgical field, considering both neurosurgery and urology. In his 4th year, Nirmish decided to apply for the award with a project in the neurosciences under the guidance of a faculty member in the Department of Neurosurgery.

"I looked at MRI's of patients with Parkinson's Disease (PD) to see if there's a predictive correlation between white matter hyperintensities (markers of cerebrovascular pathology) on pre-operative imaging and cognitive decline following deep brain stimulation (DBS) surgery. In this way, we could determine if there is a role for pre-operative imaging in guiding surgical candidacy for this last-resort treatment of PD. Having a background in biomedical engineering and an interest in neurosurgery, I wanted to partake in a project at the intersection of the two fields, and one that would be directly applicable to clinical practice."

Though Nirmish's interests in neurosurgery were well-established, he chose to pursue urology as his career based on his exposure through additional research, international rotations, and the mentorship of his father, who is also an urologist. He is currently a urology resident at the University of Texas Southwestern, and plans to further subspecialize, "perhaps in the field of urologic oncology," after his residency training.

Source: Personal Interview

James Ewing Foundation Summer Fellowships in Oncology

Description: This fellowship supports medical student summer research in surgical oncology. The award amount is $2,000 for 2-3 months.
To Apply: Medical students in the first three years of medical school may apply.
Deadline: The deadline is in February. For more information, contact:

800 East Northwest Highway Suite 1080
Palatine, IL 60067
(708) 359-4605

Massachusetts General Hospital Division of Thoracic Surgery Summer Scholars Program

Description: The Division of Thoracic Surgery at Massachusetts General Hospital provides this opportunity for medical students interested in exploring thoracic surgery as a career. Scholars will be involved in patient care, participate in rounds, observe surgeries, and work on a clinical research project.

To Apply: To be eligible, students must be in their first or second years of medical school. The application includes CV and letter of intent.

Deadline: The deadline is in December. For more information, visit:

http://www.massgeneral.org/education/internship.aspx?id=27

Patricia Numann Medical Student Award

Description: Patricia Numann was the founder of the Association of Women Surgeons (AWS), and this award bearing her name was established to support female medical students interested in a surgical career. The award recipient will receive an Award Certificate at the AWS Awards Dinner during the AWS Fall Conference. The awardee will also be reimbursed up to $1,000 for the cost associated with conference attendance, and receive one year complimentary AWS membership.

To Apply: Applicants must be in their clinical years of medical school. Recipients are selected for their interest in surgery and potential leadership qualities or research contributions to the specialty. The application includes a CV, letter of recommendation, and personal statement. The letter of recommendation must be from a surgeon, and should address the student's future potential as a surgeon/leader and contributions to the field. In the personal statement, applicants are encouraged to write about their interest in the specialty, mentors who have shaped their interests, and a description of a situation in which leadership skills were demonstrated.

Deadline: The application deadline is in July. For more information, visit:

https://www.womensurgeons.org/AWS_Foundation/Awards.asp#

Ross Student Research Fellowship

Description: Through this 10-week program at the Carolinas HealthCare System, medical students gain exposure to surgery, trauma, and research. Participants observe patient care on the floors, ICU, and operating room. Research training includes education on research design, biostatistics, data collection, and Institutional Review Board. Participants will receive co-authorship for all work presented or published.

To Apply: For application information and instructions, contact the fellowship program.

Deadline: For more information, contact
diane.winters@carolinashealthcare.org.

Scanlan/Women in Thoracic Surgery Traveling Mentorship Program

Description: The Scanlan/Women in Thoracic Surgery (WTS) Scholarship provides funding for medical students to gain exposure to the field of cardiothoracic surgery. Award recipients are mentored by female cardiothoracic surgeons for an elective period. The award amount is $2,500.
To Apply: Female medical students are encouraged to apply. The application includes CV, letter of support, and letter of commitment from the WTS mentor.
Deadline: For more information, visit:

http://wtsnet.org/scholarship/scanlan/

Society of American Gastrointestinal and Endoscopic Surgeons Medical Student Scholarship Award

Description: The Society of American Gastrointestinal and Endoscopic Surgeons (SAGES) offer the Medical Student Scholarship Award for students to attend SAGES Surgical Spring Week. Three winners will be selected, and matched with mentors. The award amount is $2,000, and recipients will be recognized during the meeting.
To Apply: To be eligible, students must attend medical school in the U.S. or Canada. The application includes a personal essay explaining the reasons why the applicant would like to attend the meeting.
Deadline: The deadline is in February. For more information, visit:

http://www.sages2014.org/sages-2014-medical-student-scholarship-award/

Society of Vascular Surgery Minority Medical Student Travel Scholarship

Description: The Minority Medical Student Travel Scholarship, established by the Society of Vascular Surgery Diversity and Inclusion Committee, provides students with the opportunity to attend the Vascular Annual Meeting. Award recipients will work one-on-one with a mentor. During the meeting, students will attend sessions, network with leaders, participate in open and endovascular simulation training, and participate in a residency fair. The award amount is $450.
To Apply: Minority medical students in the U.S. and Canada with a strong interest in vascular surgery are encouraged to apply. The application includes demographic information and personal statement explaining the reasons for their interest in the specialty and attending the Vascular Annual Meeting.
Deadline: For more information, visit:

https://www.vascularweb.org/educationandmeetings/2013-Vascular-Annual-Meeting/Pages/Minority-Medical-Student-Travel-Scholarship.aspx

Society of Vascular Surgery Student Research Fellowship

Description: The Student Research Fellowship, established by the Society of Vascular Surgery Foundation, supports laboratory and clinical vascular research by undergraduate college students and medical school students registered at universities in the United States and Canada. Each award consists of a $3,000 student stipend and a two-year complimentary subscription to the *Journal of Vascular Surgery*. In addition, the student will receive a travel scholarship in the amount of $450 to attend the Vascular Annual Meeting.

To Apply: The award is designed for students to spend a meaningful period of time on a project either in a block of several months or spread out over a longer period of time, not to exceed 12 months.

Deadline: Applications are annually due in March. For more information, visit:

http://www.vascularweb.org/about/SVSFoundation/Pages/student-research-fellowship.aspx

Summer Internship Scholarship in Cardiothoracic Surgery

Description: The American Association for Thoracic Surgery (AATS) established the Summer Internship Scholarship in Cardiothoracic Surgery to provide students with early exposure to the field. Award recipients have the opportunity to spend eight weeks working with AATS members in a cardiothoracic surgery department. The award amount is $2,500, and winners also receive complimentary registration to the AATS Annual Meeting.

To Apply: First- and second-year medical students enrolled in North American medical schools are eligible to apply. The application includes letter of support by host sponsor and one-page outline of what the candidate hopes to accomplish during the scholarship period. Award recipients must submit a summary report following the summer experience.

Deadline: For more information, visit:

http://aats.org/research/Grants/Summer-Intern-Scholarship.cgi

Southern Thoracic Surgical Association James W. Brooks Medical Student Scholarship

Description: The Southern Thoracic Surgical Association (STSA) provides a scholarship to cover the cost of attending the STSA Annual Meeting. The award recipient will be assigned to a STSA mentor.

To Apply: To be eligible, students must be a rising second-, third-, or fourth-year medical student in an allopathic medical school. The school must be located in the STSA region. Criteria for selection include academic excellence, dedication to the field of cardiothoracic surgery, and demonstrated commitment through community service, education, and leadership.

Deadline: The deadline is in July. For more information, visit:

http://stsa.org/brooksscholarship/

Profile of a Winner

Jade Porter is a first-year medical student at the UC Davis School of Medicine. She is a recent recipient of a $2,500 scholarship from the American Association of Thoracic Surgery (AATS). This monetary award will provide support while she conducts summer research at the UC Davis Division of Cardiothoracic Surgery.

Porter plans to compare survival in patients with non-small cell lung cancer undergoing operative treatment versus those who receive nonsurgical therapy. "This summer, I will get a lot of observation time in the operating room to get a first-hand look into what goes on," said Porter in an interview with UC Health. "I will also write manuscripts and do posters on my research. Hopefully it will open some doors for me."[6]

According to the AATS, there were 87 applicants from 42 medical schools throughout North America. Awards were given to 30 students.

William J. von Liebig Summer Research Fellowship

Description: Four research fellowships are available to students who are interested in performing vascular surgery research. Funding will support research training for a period of 10-12 weeks at a Harvard-affiliated institution. The award amount is $3,500, and recipients will receive appointment at Harvard Medical School as a Research Fellow in Surgery.
To Apply: To be eligible, students must be enrolled in an LCME-accredited medical school. The application includes personal statement, CV, and letters of recommendation
Deadline: For more information, visit:

http://portal.mah.harvard.edu/templatesnew/departments/BID/vonliebig/upload ed_documents/vonliebig.htm

Women in Thoracic Surgery Scholarship Program

Description: The Women in Thoracic Surgery Scholarship covers the cost of registration, travel, and lodging for medical students to attend the Society of Thoracic Surgery Annual Meeting.
To Apply: To be eligible, students must be interested in a career in cardiothoracic surgery. The application includes a questionnaire and personal essay.
Deadline: For more information, visit:

http://wtsnet.org/mentoring-program/scholarship-information/

References

[1]University of North Carolina Department of Surgery. Available at:
http://www.med.unc.edu/surgery/aboutus/awards/sheldon_leadership.
Accessed June 3, 2014.

[2]2012 NRMP Program Directors Survey. Available at:
http://www.nrmp.org/wp-
content/uploads/2013/08/programresultsbyspecialty2012.pdf. Accessed June 3,
2014.

[3]Melendez M, Xiaoti X, Sexton T, Shapiro M, Mohan E. The importance
of basic science and clinical research as a selection criterion for general
surgery residency programs. *J Surg Educ* 2008; 65 (2): 151-4.

[4]Leow J, Mackay S, Grigg M, Haider A. Surgical research elective in the
United States: an Australian medical student's experience. *J Surg Educ*
2011; 68 (6): 562 – 7.

[5]University of Central Florida College of Medicine. Available at:
https://today.ucf.edu/college-of-medicine-student-wins-national-research-
competition/. Accessed January 20, 2014.

[6]UC Health. Available at:
http://health.universityofcalifornia.edu/2011/03/23/med-student-wins-national-
surgery-scholarship/. Accessed July 2, 2014.

Chapter 24

Internal Medicine Awards, Scholarships, & Grants

For medical students interested in receiving a scholarship, award, or grant in internal medicine or one of its subspecialties, begin by researching opportunities at your own institution. At the University of Alabama – Birmingham School of Medicine, the Department of Medicine bestows the Medical Student Research Excellence Award to three students with an interest in medical or health-related summer research. The Department of Medicine at Northwestern University honors a medical student with the American College of Physician's Award for outstanding performance in the junior medicine clerkship. External awards are also available. These are described below.

Abstract Travel Grant

Description: Medical students who have performed original research in gastroenterology or hepatology may apply for a travel grant. The award amount is up to $1,000 to cover the costs of travel to an annual meeting.
To Apply: For application information and instructions, visit the website below.
Deadline: For more information, visit:

American Digestive Health Foundation
7910 Woodmont Ave., 7th Floor
Bethesda, MD 20814-3015
Website: www.gastro.org

ACP National Abstract Competition

Description: The American College of Physicians (ACP) invites medical students to participate in the ACP National Abstract Competition. Winners will present their work in an oral or poster presentation at the national conference.
To Apply: Medical student applicants must be ACP members and listed as first author of the abstract. The abstract must be original – abstracts presented elsewhere will not be considered. Abstracts can be submitted in the categories of basic research, clinical research, quality improvement – patient safety, high value cost conscious care, and clinical vignette. Abstract competitions may also be available at the local or chapter levels.

Deadline: The deadline is in December. For more information, visit:

http://www.acponline.org/education_recertification/education/program_director
s/abstracts/#definitions

Did you know...

The American College of Physicians has local and state chapters throughout the country. These chapters may also offer clinical vignette competitions open to medical students. At the 2012 American College of Physicians Northern Illinois Associates Day Meeting, Joshua Williams, a fourth-year student at the University of Chicago, won the First Place Medical Student Oral Clinical Vignette Award for his presentation, "Eat Your Heart Out: An Atypical Presentation of Endocarditis."

American College of Osteopathic Internists Research Abstract Poster Contest

Description: The American College of Osteopathic Internists (ACOI) invites students, residents, and fellows to participate in the Research Abstract Poster Contest. This contest takes place during the Annual Convention in October. Case awards of $1,500, $1,000, and $500 will be given to the 1st, 2nd, and 3rd place poster winners, respectively. Winners will also receive reimbursement of their travel costs. Also available is a competition for interesting cases with separate cash awards of $500, $250, and $100.
To Apply: Abstracts must be related to internal medicine and its subspecialties.
Deadline: The application deadline is in July. For more information, visit:

https://www.acoi.org/ResPosterContest.html

American Gastroenterological Association Investing in the Future Student Research Fellowship

Description: Ten awards will be given to underrepresented minority undergraduate and medical students to participate in eight to ten weeks of gastroenterology research. The award amount is $5,000. Fellows are encouraged to submit an abstract for presentation at Digestive Disease Week.
To Apply: Underrepresented minority students (African American, Hispanic/Latino American, American Indian, Alaska Natives, and Natives of the U.S. Pacific Islands) are eligible to apply. For application information and instructions, visit the website below.
Deadline: The application deadline is in February. For more information, visit:

http://www.gastro.org/aga-foundation/grants/aga-investing-in-the-future-iitf-
student-research-fellowship

American Gastroenterological Association Student Research Fellowship Award/AGA-Eli and Edythe Broad Student Research Fellowship

Description: Through this fellowship, medical students receive $2,500 stipends to perform research in digestive diseases or nutrition. A minimum of ten weeks of summer research is required. Fellows are encouraged to submit an abstract for presentation at Digestive Disease Week.

To Apply: Criteria for judging includes novelty, feasibility, and significant of the proposal, attributes of the candidate, and record of the preceptor.

Deadline: The application deadline is in February. For more information, visit:

http://www.gastro.org/aga-foundation/grants/student-awards/student-research-fellowship-awards

American Gastroenterological Association Student Abstract Prizes

Description: The American Gastroenterological Association will provide eight travel awards to students who will be presenting abstracts during Digestive Disease Week. The award amount is $500. The three best abstracts submitted will receive $1,000.

To Apply: Applicants must be the designated presenter or first author of the abstract. A letter of recommendation from the faculty sponsor is required.

Deadline: The application deadline is in February. For more information, visit:

http://www.gastro.org/aga-foundation/grants/student-awards/aga-student-abstract-prizes

American Heart Association Student Scholarships in Cardiovascular Disease

Description: The American Heart Association (AHA) offers the Student Scholarships in Cardiovascular Disease to medical students interested in performing cardiovascular disease research. The award amount is $2,000. The recipient designated as the top recipient of this scholarship will be named the Howard S. Silverman Scholar, and will receive an additional $1,000.

To Apply: Medical students and mentors must be members of the AHA at the time of application. The application includes student scholar statement, preceptor statement, student/preceptor CV, and letters of recommendation.

Deadline: The application deadline is in March. For more information, visit:

http://my.americanheart.org/professional/Councils/AwardsandLectures/Scholarship/Student-Scholarships-in-Cardiovascular-Disease-and-Stroke_UCM_322561_Article.jsp

American Society of Nephrology Student Scholar Grant

Description: The American Society of Nephrology (ASN) Foundation enables medical students with an interest in either basic or clinical research to spend time (10 - 52 weeks) engaged in work full-time on a kidney research project.

The student must work with a mentor who is an ASN member. Recipients receive $500 per week. Additionally, up to $1,500 will be reimbursed to the student for travel-related expenses to attend the ASN Annual Meeting.

To Apply: To apply, a candidate must be enrolled as a medical student in good standing at a U.S. or Canadian medical school. The applicant will have to perform full-time research in a nephrology lab with a mentor who is a current ASN member.

Deadline: There are two cycles for applications with deadlines in March and September. For more information, visit:

http://www.asn-online.org/grants/students/

Profile of a Winner

Michelle Kim, a medical student at the University of Central Florida, was awarded the 2012 Student Scholarship from the American Heart Association. Prior to medical school, Michelle attended UCLA and graduated with a Master's degree in physiological science. Michelle's work focuses on describing a protein, Nur77, which is found to be decreased in mice models of heart failure. The hope for her research, mentored by Dr. Daniel Kelly of Sanford-Burnham Medical Research Institute, is to identify the physiological function of this protein to assess the implications and roles it plays in heart failure and gene expression. Clinically speaking, Michelle hopes that "preventing metabolic dysfunction in the heart might help address cardiac complications that occur in the current epidemics of obesity and diabetes."[1]

Cardiopulmonary Research Science & Technology Student Intern Program

Description: The Cardiopulmonary Research Science & Technology Student Intern Program was developed to introduce students to the clinical research medical environment. Participants are assigned a research project, and are involved in data collection, critical thinking, analysis and a written abstract. At the end of the program, students will receive a certificate and an award amount of $2,000.

To Apply: The application includes CV, essay, transcript, and two letters of recommendation. The essay should explain what qualities/experiences would make the applicant a good intern candidate, and what the applicant hopes to gain/accomplish from this experience.

Deadline: The application deadline is in February. For more information, visit:

http://www.crsti.org/index.php?page=internship

Case Western Reserve University Heart, Lung and Blood Summer Research Program (See Chapter 13)

Conquer Cancer Foundation of the American Society of Clinical Oncology Medical Student Rotation (See Chapter 13)

Crohn's & Colitis Foundation Student Research Fellowship Award

Description: The Crohn's & Colitis Foundation of America (CCFA) created this award to stimulate research interest in the area of inflammatory bowel disease (IBD). The program will financially support students to spend a minimum of 10 weeks in IBD-related research. Up to 16 awards are usually available. Each recipient will receive a one-time payment of $2,500.
To Apply: Applicants must be undergraduate, medical, or graduate students currently enrolled in an accredited institution in the United States.
Deadline: Applications are due in March, and reviewed from April through May. The start date for selected projects is in June. Visit the following link for more information:

http://www.ccfa.org/science-and-professionals/research/grants-fellowships/student-research-awards.html

Endocrine Society Summer Research Fellowship

Description: The Endocrine Society offers Summer Research Fellowships to encourage promising undergraduate students, medical students and first-year graduate school students to pursue careers in endocrinology. The Society provides a stipend to each student award recipient to participate in research projects under the guidance of a Society member for 10 to 12 weeks during the summer.
To Apply: Medical students who are beyond their first year of schooling are eligible to apply. The application includes summary of research project, mentor statement, personal statement, transcript, CV, and mentor biosketch.
Deadline: For more information, visit:

http://www.endo-society.org/awards/research_fellowship/summer.cfm

Gina M. Finzi Memorial Student Summer Fellowship

Description: The Gina M. Finzi Memorial Student Summer Fellowship Program provides funding for medical students to perform lupus research. The award amount is $4,000.
To Apply: Although undergraduate students may apply, preference will be given to graduate or medical students. For application information and instructions, visit the website below.
Deadline: The application deadline is in March. For more info, visit:

http://www.lupus.org/webmodules/webarticlesnet/templates/new_researchlfa.aspx?articleid=145&zoneid=31

Glenn/AFAR Scholarships for Research in the Biology of Aging

Description: The American Federation for Aging Research (AFAR) sponsors the Glenn/AFAR Scholarships for Research in the Biology of Aging. Scholarship recipients receive support to perform 3 – 6 months of research in aging. Up to 10 scholarships are granted. The award amount is $5,000.
To Apply: Students at any level in an allopathic or osteopathic U.S. medical school are eligible to apply for the award. Criteria for judging include qualifications and ability of the applicant, merit and feasibility of proposed research, and qualifications of designated mentor. The application includes research proposal, academic performance, statement of purpose, and letter of reference. For application information and instructions, visit the website below.
Deadline: The application deadline is in January. For more info, visit:

http://www.afar.org/research/funding/glenn-afar-scholarships/

Glorney-Raisbeck Medical Student Grants in Cardiovascular Research

Description: These grants are administered by the New York Academy of Medicine. Up to four recipients will receive a stipend of $3,000 to pursue a summer research project seeking better understanding of the causes, prevention, and treatment of cardiovascular disease.
To Apply: M.D. candidates attending medical school or performing research in the greater New York area (New York City, Long Island, Westchester County, or New Jersey) will be given preference. The application includes cover letter, research proposal, biographical sketch, letter of support from faculty mentor, and NIH biosketch of faculty member.
Deadline: For more information, visit:

http://www.nyam.org/grants/glorney-raisbeck-student.html

HONORS (Hematology Opportunities for the Next Generation of Research Scientists) Award

Description: Formally known as the Trainee Research Award, the American Society of Hematology (ASH) HONORS Award will contribute to the development of the next generation of hematologists by supporting talented medical students and residents to conduct hematology research. The award is intended for medical students and residents in the United States, Canada, or Mexico. It will provide the recipient with a $5,000 stipend to conduct either a short hematological research project for a minimum of three months, or a long hematological research project between three and 12 months.
To Apply: Eligible applicants must be a M.D. or D.O. medical student/resident in an LCME (or its equivalent) or ACGME-accredited institution. The

application includes trainee biosketch, mentor biosketch, mentor letter of support, personal statement, and research proposal.

Deadline: Applications are due at the end of February and award winners are notified in May. For more information please visit:

http://www.hematology.org/Awards/Next-Generation-Research-Scientists-Award/2627.aspx

---

Profile of a Winner

Amrita Krishnamurthy, a first-year medical student at the UC Davis School of Medicine, was the recipient of the 2013 HONORS Award from the American Society of Hematology. After being nominated by her faculty mentors, Mingyi Chen and Ralph Green, she submitted an application for her project "Chronic Anemia Post Gastric Bypass Surgery: Mimicking Myelodysplastic Syndrome: More than just Iron and Copper Deficiency." Award recipients receive a stipend for research support, and are eligible for travel awards to present findings at scientific meetings. Following medical school, Krishnamurthy plans to pursue fellowship training in hematology/oncology after completing an internal medicine residency. "As we gain a greater understanding of the molecular mechanisms underlying the various cancers and hematological disorders, it will be possible to develop targeted therapies and practice personalized medicine," said Krishnamurthy in an article written on the UC Davis School of Medicine website.[2]

HTVN Research and Mentorship Program Scholar Grants (See Chapter 13)

Infectious Disease Society of North America Scholar Program

Description: An important part of Infectious Disease Society of North America's (IDSA) mission is to promote the subspecialty of infectious diseases by attracting the best and brightest medical students to the field. Each scholarship recipient will receive $2,000 for work focused on pediatric or adult infectious diseases. The work may involve either clinical or research activities.

To Apply: Students at any level in an U.S. medical school are eligible to apply for the award. The application includes cover letter and letter from IDSA mentor.

Deadline: The application deadline is in February. For more info, visit:

http://www.idsociety.org/Medical_Scholars_Program/

Dr. James A Ferguson Emerging Infectious Diseases Fellowship Program

Description: This program is funded by the Centers for Disease Control and Prevention (CDC), and provides support for a nine-week summer program. The program was developed to provide opportunities for students from underrepresented minority groups interested in addressing health disparities related to infectious diseases. Fellows receive mentored research and professional development at a designated institution. A stipend of $4,000 is provided. Fellows are expected to submit an abstract to a national scientific meeting.
To Apply: Full-time students who are members of an underrepresented group are eligible to apply. The applicant must have at least a 3.0 GPA.
Deadline: The application deadline is in January. For more info, visit:

http://www.kennedykrieger.org/professional-training/professional-training-programs/rise-programs/ferguson-fellowship

Leah Menshouse Springer Summer Opportunities Program

Description: Through this program, medical students have the opportunity to perform oncology research for a period of ten weeks at the Siteman Cancer Center of Barnes-Jewish Hospital and Washington University School of Medicine. Participants will receive a stipend of $3,500.
To Apply: Medical students are eligible to apply.
Deadline: The application deadline is in March. For more information, visit:

http://www.siteman.wustl.edu/contentpage.aspx?id=254

Medical Student Research Program in Diabetes

Description: This program is sponsored by the National Institutes of Health and allows medical students to perform diabetes research under the supervision of an established scientist. The research must take place at an institution with one of the NIDDK-funded Research Centers.
To Apply: Students may participate in the program during the summer between the first and second year or second and third year of medical school.
Deadline: For more info, visit:

http://medicalstudentdiabetesresearch.org/

Medical Student Training in Aging Research

Description: The Medical Student Training in Aging Research (MSTAR) is administered by the American Federation for Aging Research and National Institute on Aging. Short-term scholarships are awarded to medical students interested in performing aging research. Funding provides support for 8 – 12 weeks of geriatrics research during the summer. Recipients will have the opportunity to present their work at the American Geriatrics Society Annual Meeting. The award amount is $1,748 per month.

To Apply: Students at any level in an allopathic or osteopathic U.S. medical school are eligible to apply for the award. For application information and instructions, visit the website below.

Deadline: The application deadline is in January. For more info, visit:

http://www.afar.org/research/funding/mstar

Memorial Sloan-Kettering Cancer Center Medical Student Summer Fellowship Research Program

Description: The Medical Student Summer Fellowship Research Program is an eight-week research program offered to first- and second-year medical students who have a career interest in the field of oncology. A stipend of $5,800 is given for eight weeks of research.

To Apply: First- or second-year medical students in good academic standing at allopathic and osteopathic U.S. medical schools are eligible to apply.

Deadline: All application materials must be received by January. For more info, visit:

http://www.mskcc.org/education/students/summer-fellowship

One Medical Group Scholarship (See Chapter 22)

Rheumatology Research Foundation Medical and Graduate Student Achievement Award

Description: The Rheumatology Research Foundation has developed the Student Achievement Award to recognize outstanding medical students for exemplary work in the field of rheumatology and to provide students with the opportunity to attend the American College of Rheumatology (ACR) / Association of Rheumatology Health Professionals (ARHP) Annual Meeting. Recipients will receive an award of $750. A $1,000 reimbursement for travel expenses to attend the ACR/ARHP Annual Meeting will also be given. Registration for the meeting will be complimentary.

To Apply: Students applying for this award should be actively enrolled in an accredited institution. Applicants must also be an author or co-author of an abstract that was submitted for the application year's ACR/ARHP Annual Scientific Meeting. The student will be evaluated on evidence of submission of an abstract, contribution of work to the abstract, merit and relevance of the applicant's research to rheumatology.

Deadline: The application deadline is in August, and applicants are notified of the results in September. See the following link for more information:

http://www.rheumatology.org/foundation/awards/medstudents.asp

Robert L. Mayock Student Research Fellowship

Description: The Robert L. Mayock Student Research Fellowship is administered by the Penn Lung Center. Fellows receive support to perform pulmonary research.
To Apply: M.D. students are eligible to apply for the fellowship. The application includes CV, letter of recommendation, and transcript.
Deadline: The application deadline is in April. For more info, visit:

http://www.pennmedicine.org/lung/academics/residencies-fellowships/summer-research-fellowship-mayock.html

Roswell Park Summer Research Experience Program in Oncology

Description: The Roswell Park Summer Research Experience Program in Oncology provides support to medical students interested in gaining research or clinical experience in oncology. Students can choose to work in a variety of cancer research areas. The award amount is $3,200.
To Apply: Allopathic and osteopathic medical students in their first year of graduate medical training are eligible to apply for the program. For application information and instructions, visit the website below.
Deadline: The application deadline is in February. For more info, visit:

http://www.roswellpark.edu/education/summer-programs/medical/dental/pa-students/faq

Sarnoff Cardiovascular Research Foundation

Description: The Sarnoff Cardiovascular Research Foundation provides funding for students interested in performing cardiovascular research over a period of one year. Winners must perform the research at a medical school other than the one they attend. A $30,000 stipend will be given as will funds to cover costs associated with travel to meetings to present research.
To Apply: Second and third-year medical students may apply for funding. Fourth-year medical students who have deferred graduation are also eligible to apply. Of note, MD/PhD students are not eligible. Prior research is not a requirement. The application includes personal essays, transcript, and letters of recommendation.
Deadline: The deadline is in January. For more information, visit:

www.SarnoffFoundation.org

Sidney Kimmel Comprehensive Cancer Center – CUPID Program

Description: The Cancer in the Under-Privileged, Indigent, or Disadvantaged (CUPID) Program is a summer fellowship experience at the Johns Hopkins University School of Medicine. Fellows will have a structured, mentored research experience. Part of the time will be spent in clinical care.

To Apply: Medical students with an interest in cancer research and underserved populations are encouraged to apply. First- and second-year medical students who can commit to the full 7-week program are given preference. The application includes personal photograph, personal statement, CV, and recommendation letters.
Deadline: The application deadline is in January. For more info, visit:

http://cupid.onc.jhmi.edu/?section=application

Profile of a Winner

In 2010, Joshua Balderman and Mojdeh Kappus, medical students at the University of Buffalo School of Medicine, were two of the eleven scholarship recipients from the Sarnoff Cardiovascular Research Foundation. These two second-year medical students went through a competitive application process that led to the selection of 11 recipients out of a pool of 50 applicants.

Award recipients are chosen based on scholastic and leadership ability. Research fellows will spend a period of one year immersed in cardiovascular research. A stipend is given, and funds are made available to support student travel to scientific meetings.[3]

Society of General Internal Medicine Clinical Vignette Competition

Description: Medical students, residents, and fellows are invited to present clinical vignettes at the Society of General Internal Medicine (SGIM) Annual Meeting. Top-rated clinical vignettes are selected for oral presentation. In 2012, the organization received 567 clinical vignette submissions.
To Apply: Over 12 clinical vignette submission categories are available. For more information, visit the website below.
Deadline: For more information, visit:

http://www.sgim.org/meetings/annual-meeting/call-for-abstracts-vignettes-ime-cpi/vignette-submission-info

Society of Hospital Medicine Research, Innovations, and Clinical Vignettes Competition

Description: Medical students and residents may partner with Society of Hospital Medicine (SHM) faculty to submit clinical vignette abstracts. Selected abstracts will be presented at the Hospital Medicine meeting.
To Apply: For more information, visit the website below.
Deadline: The deadline is in December. For more information, visit:

https://shm.confex.com/shm/HM14/cfp.cgi

University of Texas MD Anderson Cancer Center Summer Research Program for Medical Students

Description: Through this program, medical students have the opportunity to engage in basic or clinical sciences research at the University of Texas MD Anderson Cancer Center. At the end of the research period, students will submit their work in journal article format. A stipend of $5,000 will be given.
To Apply: Students who have successfully completed their first year of medical school are eligible to apply. The application includes CV, letters of recommendation, personal statement, and transcript.
Deadline: For more information, visit:

http://www.mdanderson.org/education-and-research/education-and-training/schools-and-programs/summer-science-programs/medical-students-summer-research-program.html

Vanderbilt University Research Training Program

Description: The Vanderbilt University School of Medicine invites applications for the summer Medical Student Research Training Program (SRTP) in Diabetes and Obesity, Kidney Disease, and Digestive Disease. Each student receives a stipend of approximately $400 per week.
To Apply: Each student chooses an established Vanderbilt investigator in the field of diabetes, hypertension, kidney disease, or obesity. Program staff will assist students in selecting a preceptor.
Deadline: The application deadline is in February. For more info, visit:

http://www.mc.vanderbilt.edu/diabetes/srtp/program-description.php

References

[1]University of Central Florida College of Medicine. Available at: http://med.ucf.edu/news/2012/10/med-student-wins-american-heart-association-scholarship/. Accessed June 2, 2014.
[2]University of California Davis School of Medicine. Available at: http://www.ucdmc.ucdavis.edu/publish/news/newsroom/7875. Accessed June 16, 2014.
[3]University of Buffalo School of Medicine. Available at: http://www.buffalo.edu/news/releases/2010/05/11396.html. Accessed April 4, 2014.

Chapter 25

Neurology Awards, Scholarships, & Grants

For medical students interested in receiving a scholarship, award, or grant in neurology, begin by researching opportunities at your own institution. At the Wayne State University School of Medicine, the Department of Neurology offers the McHenry Award in Neurology. To be considered, fourth-year students who received honors in the neurology clerkship must submit an essay in clinical neurology, experimental neurology, or historical aspects of neurology. Winners will be chosen based on the quality of essay. Make inquiries with your Department of Neurology to learn about award opportunities you may be eligible for.

There are often opportunities to participate in research during the summer between the first and second year. You may be able to secure funding through your school. External awards are also available so support research in the field. These are described in this chapter.

Medical students often ask us if it's necessary to do research in the field of neurology to enhance their chances of matching. In the 2012 NRMP Program Director Survey, 62% of neurology residency programs cited "demonstrated involvement and interest in research" as a factor in selecting applicants to interview.[1] It's especially helpful to read the perspectives of neurology program directors and faculty about the importance of research in the selection process. We offer you these perspectives on the next page.

Neurology Research for Medical Students: Perspectives of Neurology Residency Program Directors

- "Many variables are considered, including grades in medical school, board scores, academic achievements (**research, publications**, awards, etc), letters of recommendation and many others," writes the Department of Neurology at the University of Michigan.[2]

- "Published articles share information and ideas across fields and are a tangible form of currency in academia," writes Dr. Michael Perloff, Assistant Professor of Neurology at Boston University. "Thus, one obvious motive to publish is to facilitate career advancement. Publications can be a topic of discussion at residency and fellowship interviews and may be quite literally counted and reviewed when hiring faculty."[3]

- "Another great resource is faculty or neurology residents at your school - approach them about any available opportunities," writes the American Academy of Neurology. "They may have a project that would be appropriate for medical student involvement. Be sure to set clear expectations with any research mentor regarding the time and energy you are able to devote to extra-curricular work."[4]

- Participating in original research, and following it through to publication can take considerable time. For applicants who are closer to the residency application process, writing and publishing a case report is one option for strengthening credentials. The time required to publish case reports is generally much shorter.

- Some attending physicians keep a list of interesting cases, and are just waiting for an enterprising medical student to seize one of these many opportunities. "In my daily private practice I keep a list of interesting and reportable cases that I have seen in the office and the hospital," writes Dr. Richard Rison, Clinical Assistant Professor of Neurology at the University of Southern California Keck School of Medicine.[5]

- Although not all journals will publish case reports, there are many options available. "One can argue that it has never been easier to publish a case report," writes Dr. Rison. "The growth of electronic medical journals on the Internet, which are less constrained with respect to space, provide additional opportunities for the publication of case reports. Journal of Medical Case Reports is a peer-reviewed journal committed only to case reports. It is open access and remains at the forefront of clinical knowledge determination via case reporting by publishing high quality manuscripts."[5]

American Academy of Neurology Medical Student Prize for Excellence

Description: The American Academy of Neurology's (AAN) Undergraduate Education Subcommittee developed this award to recognize graduating medical students for excellence in clinical neurology. This $200 award is given to one graduating medical student from each medical school and will be presented during the institution's graduation/award ceremony.

To Apply: It is the responsibility of the neurology clerkship director, department chair, and neurology residents to evaluate the performance of all graduating medical students in the clinical neurology clerkship and to nominate one student from each medical school as the recipient of the award. To receive this award, the student must have outstanding evaluations and recommendations from faculty and residents and must show the most promise for a career in neurology. Excellent performance on the neurology shelf exam or equivalent examination may be used as supporting criteria for the nominee.

Deadline: The nomination letter deadline is in March. See the following link for more information:

http://www.aan.com

American Academy of Neurology Medical Student Scholarship to the Annual Meeting

Description: The American Academy of Neurology (AAN) and the Association of University Professors of Neurology (AUPN) have created this scholarship to cover the costs associated with travel to the AAN Annual Meeting. The award is open to students who are Student Interest Group in Neurology (SIGN) chapter members. The AAN and AUPN hope that this scholarship will help stimulate student interest in neurology. Approximately forty $1,000 scholarships are awarded to SIGN chapter members to attend the meeting. SIGN chapter presidents or designated SIGN representatives are given preference.

To Apply: Applicants must be active SIGN members and a member of the AAN. AAN membership is free for medical students. Application materials include CV, letter of interest outlining SIGN leadership and activities, and letter of support from SIGN faculty advisor or other faculty member. An online application must also be completed. Follow the link below for further information.

Deadline: Applications are due in October, and winners are notified in November. See the following link for more information:

http://www.aan.com

Profile of a Winner

James Andry, a medical student at UT Southwestern Medical School, was a recent winner of the American Academy of Neurology Medical Student Prize for Excellence. He solidified his interest in neurology during a rotation in his third-year of medical school. "I always had an intellectual interest in neurology, but I wasn't sure if the clinical day-to-day work would really capture me," said Dr. Andry in an article published by the UT Southwestern Medical Center. "But once I experienced it, that's when I knew this is what I wanted to do."

"He is a very bright student who will, without a doubt, be a leader in neurology," stated Dr. Mark Agostini, Associate Professor of Neurology and Neurotherapeutics at UT Southwestern Medical School. Dr. Andry is currently a neurology resident at Vanderbilt University Medical Center in Nashville, Tennessee.[6]

American Academy of Neurology Medical Student Summer Research Scholarship

Description: The Medical Student Summer Research Scholarship program offers members of the American Academy of Neurology's (AAN) Student Interest Group in Neurology (SIGN) a summer stipend to conduct a neuroscience-based project in either an institutional, clinical or laboratory setting where there are ongoing programs of research, service or training, or a private practice. The scholarship will be given to first- or second-year medical students who have a supporting preceptor and a project with clearly defined goals. The project should be conducted at a U.S. or Canadian institution of the student's choice and jointly designed by the student and sponsoring institution. Scholarship recipients receive a $3,000 stipend. Up to 20 first- and second-year medical students receive this award per cycle.
To Apply: Only one student will be selected from an institution. Applicants must be current AAN members and SIGN chapter members. Previous scholarship recipients are not eligible. Preference is given to first-time researchers. Students are required to submit a project proposal, CV, and two letters of recommendation. See the link below for further information.
Deadline: Preliminary materials are due for submission in February. After completion of the project, students are required to submit secondary materials by the following September. See the link for more information:

http://www.aan.com

Profile of a Winner

In 2010, David Balser, a medical student at New York University School of Medicine, was one of 20 recipients of the Summer Research Scholarship. He was awarded the scholarship for his research project on pig cortical brain injury. Mr. Balser has shown a strong dedication to the field of neurology. He has also received the American Heart Association (AHA) Stroke Medical Student Summer Research Fellowship in 2012 and won a travel award to present at the International Stroke Meeting of the AHA in 2013.[7-8]

American Academy of Neurology Medical Student Essay Award – Extended Neuroscience Award (See Chapter 15)

American Academy of Neurology Medical Student Essay Award – G. Milton Shy Award (See Chapter 15)

American Academy of Neurology Medical Student Essay Award – Roland P. Mackay Award (See Chapter 15)

American Academy of Neurology Medical Student Essay Award – Saul R. Korey Award (See Chapter 15)

American Academy of Neurology Minority Scholars Program

Description: The Minority Scholars Program was created by the American Academy of Neurology (AAN) to promote diversity in the field of neurology and to provide medical students with an opportunity to learn more about careers in neurology and neuroscience. Students are chosen based on their interest in neurology as a career, their academic achievements and community involvement, as well as their plans to maximize the AAN Annual Meeting opportunity. The recipient will receive airfare and lodging for up to four nights to attend the AAN Annual Meeting. They will also be able to register for educational programs and participate in the Medical Student rush line.
To Apply: Racial minority medical students from underrepresented and underserved populations are eligible to apply for this program. The student must be in good standing at a U.S. medical school. Preference is given to second- and third-year students. Application requirements include a one-page essay, a letter of recommendation, and CV. Visit the link below for more information.
Deadline: The deadline for application is in October. See the following link for more information:

http://www.aan.com

Profile of a Winner

In 2012, Gabriel Moreno, a third-year medical student at Wayne State University School of Medicine, was one of the eight members of AAN's Minority Scholars Program. His interest in medicine began during his childhood when concern for his father's Parkinson's disease was coupled with fascination of his mother's clinical experiences as a registered nurse.

"Gabriel is very active in his Hispanic community," said Dr. Maher Fakhouri, Assistant Professor of Neurology at Wayne State University, in his nomination letter. "He identified that our medical school has minimal representation from the Hispanic and Latino communities and formed the Latin American and Native American Medical Student Association, the first medical student association at Wayne State University committed to raising awareness of the health issues of Hispanic and Latino Americans and to increasing opportunities in medicine for Hispanic and Latinos in the Detroit area."[9]

American Brain Tumor Association Medical Student Summer Fellowship

Description: The American Brain Tumor Association provides the Medical Student Summer Fellowship to students interested in performing brain tumor research. The award amount is $3,000. The fellowship may take place in laboratories in the U.S. or Canada.

To Apply: The award is open to first-, second-, and third-year medical students. The application includes CV, letter from sponsor, letter of reference, and description of research.

Deadline: The deadline is in January. For more information, visit:

http://www.abta.org/brain-tumor-research/research-grants/

American Heart Association Student Scholarships in Cerebrovascular Disease and Stroke

Description: The American Heart Association (AHA) offers the Student Scholarships in Stroke to medical students interested in performing stroke research. The award amount is $2,000. Recipients will also receive a travel stipend to present their research at the AHA International Stroke Conference.

To Apply: Medical students and mentors must be members of the AHA at the time of application. The application includes student scholar statement, preceptor statement, student/preceptor CV, and letters of recommendation.

Deadline: The application deadline is in March. For more information, visit:

http://my.americanheart.org/professional/Councils/AwardsandLectures/Scholar ship/Student-Scholarships-in-Cardiovascular-Disease-and-Stroke_UCM_322561_Article.jsp

Consortium of Multiple Sclerosis Centers Research Scholarship

Description: The Consortium of Multiple Sclerosis Centers (CMSC) offers medical students the opportunity to participate in a research scholarship at a member institution. By working with a mentor in the field, students gain exposure to multiple sclerosis research and clinical care. Research results may be presented at the CMSC Annual Meeting.

To Apply: Prior to submitting the application, the medical school applicant must arrange a proposed research program with a CMSC mentor. The project plan must be described in the application.

Deadline: The deadline is in May. For more information, visit:

http://cmscfoundation.org/initiatives2/ms-workforce-of-the-future/fcmsc-research-scholars

Epilepsy Foundation Student Fellowships

Description: The Epilepsy Foundation supports a series of grants and fellowships to advance the understanding of epilepsy that will lead to better treatment, more effective prevention, and ultimately to a cure. The award amount is $3,000. The Behavioral Sciences Student Fellowship is available to both undergraduate and graduate students who are studying a field relevant to epilepsy research or clinical care. The Health Sciences Student Fellowship is geared toward individuals who are enrolled in medical school, a doctoral program, or other graduate program.

To Apply: For application information, visit the website below.

Deadline: All applications are due by March for funding to begin in July. A complete application must be submitted via the proposalCentral system. For more information, visit:

http://www.epilepsyfoundation.org/research/grant-and-fellowship-opportunities.cfm

Huntington Medical Research Institute Summer Student Program

Description: Through this 10-week summer research program, students have the opportunity to conduct research under the supervision of accomplished mentors. Students will attend lectures and present the results of their research.

To Apply: The application includes personal essay and official transcript. The essay should describe your motivation for doing biomedical research in the selected laboratory.

Deadline: The application deadline is in April. For more information, visit:

http://www.hmri.org/education/summer-student-program/

Joseph Collins Foundation Scholarship (See Chapter 18)

National Institute of Neurological Disorders and Stroke Summer Program in the Neurological Sciences

Description: Through this summer research program, medical students have the opportunity to conduct neuroscience research under the supervision of leading scientists in the department. At the end of the experience, participants are able to present their research.
To Apply: For application information and instructions, visit the website below.
Deadline: For more information, visit:

http://www.ninds.nih.gov/jobs_and_training/summer/

Parkinson's Disease Foundation Summer Fellowship Program

Description: The Parkinson's Disease Foundation Summer Fellowship Program supports students interested in performing Parkinson's-related summer research. For 10 weeks of clinical or laboratory research, the awardee will receive $4,000.
To Apply: The award is open to national and international medical students. The application includes research plan, academic transcript, personal statement, and letters of support.
Deadline: For more information, visit:

http://www.pdf.org/en/grant_funding_fellow#summer

Parkinson's Disease Foundation Student Travel Award

Description: The Parkinson's Disease Foundation Student Travel Award supports students intending to attend and present data at scientific conferences. Up to $1,000 will be available to cover registration, transportation, and hotel accommodations.
To Apply: The award is open to medical students who have conducted Parkinson's disease research. Applicants must show proof of an accepted abstract. The application includes copy of abstract, confirmation of abstract acceptance, personal statement, and letter of support.
Deadline: For more information, visit:

http://www.pdf.org/en/grant_funding_fellow#summer

Robinson Neurological Foundation Scholarship

Description: This scholarship is open to medical or graduate students interested in performing neurological research. The award amount is $2,500.
To Apply: The application includes CV, summary of intended project, and letter of recommendation from research mentor.
Deadline: The deadline is in July. For more information, contact:

Jenny H. Crowley
1401 Centerville Road, Suite 300
Tallahassee, FL 32308
(850) 877-5115

Swaiman Medical Scholarship

Description: The Child Neurology Foundation administers the Swaiman Medical Scholarship. Up to ten awardees will receive $3,500 to perform summer research under the supervision of a child neurologist.
To Apply: First and second-year medical students in the U.S. or Canada are eligible. The application includes cover letter, description of research project, and letter of reference from child neurology mentor.
Deadline: The deadline is in March. For more information, visit:

http://www.childneurologyfoundation.org/swaiman-scholarships/

References

[1] 2012 NRMP Program Directors Survey. Available at:
http://www.nrmp.org/wp-content/uploads/2013/08/programresultsbyspecialty2012.pdf. Accessed June 3, 2014.
[2] University of Michigan Department of Neurology. Available at:
http://www.med.umich.edu/neurology/edu/application.htm. Accessed March 3, 2013.
[3] Perloff M, Zuzuárregui J, Frank S. Writing From the Wards: Advice for Residents. *The Neurologist* 2012; 18(2): 96-8.
[4] American Academy of Neurology. Available at:
http://www.aan.com/globals/axon/assets/9784.pdf. Accessed March 7, 2013.
[5] Rison R. Neurology case reporting: a call for all. *Journal of Medical Case Reports* 2011; 5: 113.
[6] UT Southwestern Medical School. Available at:
http://www.utsouthwestern.edu/newsroom/center-times/year-2012/june/andry-neurology-prize.html. Accessed January 20, 2014.
[7] American Academy of Neurology. Available at:
http://www.aan.com/globals/axon/assets/7246.pdf. Accessed January 20, 2014.
[8] Department of Neurosurgery at New York University School of Medicine. Available at: http://neurosurgery.med.nyu.edu/education-training/medical-student-training/medical-student-research-opportunities. Accessed January 22, 2014.
[9] American Academy of Neurology. Available at:
http://prognosis.med.wayne.edu/article/som-student-one-of-eight-nationwide-selected-for-aan-foundations-minority-scholars-program. Accessed January 20, 2014.

Chapter 26

Neurosurgery Awards, Scholarships, & Grants

For medical students interested in receiving a scholarship, award, or grant in neurosurgery, begin by researching opportunities at your own institution. At Johns Hopkins University, the Department of Neurosurgery presents the Harvey Cushing Medical Student Hunterian Research Award to a medical student who has shown dedication and achievement in neurosurgical research. Make inquiries with your Department of Neurological Surgery to learn about award opportunities you may be eligible for.

External awards are also available. The most prestigious are awards and scholarships sponsored by the American Association of Neurological Surgeons, Council of State Neurosurgical Societies, Neurosurgery Research and Education Foundation, Campagna Scholarship, and the Pauletta and Denzel Washington Family Gifted Scholars Program. These are described below.

Medical students often ask us if it's necessary to do research in the field of neurosurgery to enhance their chances of matching. In the 2012 NRMP Program Director Survey, 86% of neurosurgery residency programs cited "demonstrated involvement and interest in research" as a factor in selecting applicants to interview.[1] It's especially helpful to read the perspectives of neurosurgery program directors and faculty about the importance of research in the selection process. We offer you these perspectives on the next page.

Neurosurgery Research for Medical Students: Perspectives of Neurosurgery Residency Program Directors

- Dr. Mitchel Berger is the Chairman of the Department of Neurosurgery at UCSF. He describes the importance of research in the specialty. "Pressures to publish begin during medical school. Evidence of scholarship has become a prerequisite for a residency in academic neurological surgery, and residents must produce a substantial body of published work during training if they plan to seek a faculty appointment."[2]

- "While research is not technically required, it can be a huge help and is recommended especially if it is in the neurosciences," writes Dr. Ben Roitberg, Program Director of the Neurosurgery Residency Program at the University of Chicago.[3]

- The Department of Neurosurgery at Drexel University provides some insight as to how research experience is viewed in the selection process. "Since this is such a highly competitive specialty, students invited for interview have similar academic records. Thus anything that can be done to differentiate you is highly recommended. Research is one of those methods."[4]

- Neurosurgery is "highly competitive," writes Dr. Mark Linskey, Program Director of the Neurosurgery Residency Program at the University of California Irvine. "However, other factors are considered to be as important. These include personal characteristics of sound judgment, integrity, and capacity for hard work. **Some research experience is also advantageous.**"[5]

- "Research opportunities allow students to work with neurosurgeons at the end of their first year and potentially throughout their medical school experience," writes Dr. Chikezie Eseonu, a neurosurgical resident at Johns Hopkins University. "Through this opportunity a student is allowed to explore interests in neurosurgery as well as to establish a mentoring relationship with a neurosurgeon that can be continued throughout medical school. The summer after the student's first year is an optimal time for medical students to participate in research conducted by neurosurgeons and residents."[6]

American Association of Neurological Surgeons Young Neurosurgeons Committee Medical Student in Organized Neurosurgery Fellowship

Description: The American Association of Neurological Surgeons Young Neurosurgeons Committee sponsors the Medical Student in Organized Neurosurgery Fellowship. This is a two-year fellowship which provides a medical student with the opportunity to participate on subcommittees. The award amount is $1,000.

To Apply: Medical student applicants must submit a research topic addressing a system/practice issue. The award recipient will present the project as an abstract upon completion of the fellowship. Criteria for selection include CV and personal essay.

Deadline: The deadline is in September. For more information, visit:

http://www.aans.org/en/Young%20Neurosurgeons/Medical%20Students/Research%20Opportunities.aspx

Campagna Scholarship

Description: The Campagna Scholarship provides support for a 10-week summer research experience in neurosurgery. One scholar will be selected annually. The scholar will perform research under the supervision of a neurosurgical mentor at Oregon Health & Science University. The scholar will receive $5,000. An additional $2,500 will be made available to support travel to a national neurosurgical meeting to present research results.

To Apply: U.S. medical students in their first or second year of medical school are eligible to apply. The application includes personal essay, CV, letters of recommendation, Dean's letter, and scholarship application form.

Deadline: The deadline is in February. For more information, visit:

http://www.ohsu.edu/xd/education/schools/school-of-medicine/departments/clinical-departments/neurosurgery/news-events/campagna-scholarship.cfm

Council of State Neurosurgical Societies Medical Student Summer Fellowship in Socioeconomic Research

Description: The Council of State Neurological Societies and Congress of Neurological Surgeons sponsor the Medical Student Summer Fellowship in Socioeconomic Research. This scholarship provides $2,500 to support medical student research on a socioeconomic issue affecting neurosurgery. The funding is for 8 – 10 weeks of supervised research.

To Apply: Medical student from the U.S. and Canada are eligible. The application includes two reference letters, CVs of applicant and mentors, and photo. Criteria for selection include originality of proposed project, significance, feasibility of project completion, and applicant qualifications.

Deadline: The deadline is in January. For more information, visit:

http://w3.cns.org/education/fellowshipDescr.asp?ID=15

Neurosurgery Research and Education Foundation Medical Student Summer Research Fellowship

Description: The Neurosurgery Research and Education Foundation offers the Medical Student Summer Research Fellowship program to medical students interested in spending the summer performing neurosurgical research. Up to twenty fellowships will be awarded annually in the amount of $2,500. Fellows will be mentored by a neurosurgical investigator who is a member of the Association

To Apply: U.S. and Canadian medical students who have completed one, two, or three years of medical school are eligible to apply. The application includes sponsor statement and letters of recommendation.

Deadline: For more information, visit:

http://www.nref.org/MSSRF.aspx

Pauletta and Denzel Washington Family Gifted Scholars Program in Neuroscience

Description: The Pauletta and Denzel Washington Family Gifted Scholars Program is administered by the Cedars Sinai Medical Center. This award supports the education of medical students with an interest in neuroscience. The awardee will perform research in the Department of Neurosurgery at Cedars Sinai under the supervision of Dr. Keith Black. The position provides funding for a period of one year. Funding will also cover the expense to attend a national neuroscience meeting if the awardee's abstract is accepted.

To Apply: Medical student applicants must be citizens or permanent residents of the United States. The application includes letters of reference and personal essay.

Deadline: The deadline is in March. For more information, visit:

http://www.cedars-sinai.edu/Patients/Programs-and-
Services/Neurosurgery/Training-Program/Documents-and-
Images/WashingtonApplication-2013-EXTENDED.pdf

Texas Brain & Spine Institute Medical Student Research Program

Description: The Texas Brain & Spine Institute offers a summer research program for medical students. Up to five students are selected. Students perform research four days of the week. One day is set aside every week to observe neurosurgical procedures.

To Apply: The application includes summer project goals and research background.

Deadline: For more information, visit:

http://www.txbsi.com/education/student-research-program

Did you know...

Look for opportunities to present your research at scientific meetings where you may be eligible for awards. Garrett Banks, a medical student at Columbia University's College of Physicians and Surgeons, won the Top Neurosurgery Form Poster in Neurotrauma and Critical Care at a recent meeting of the Congress of Neurological Surgeons.

Banks was recognized for his stroke research. He investigated the integrity of the white matter pathways following hemorrhagic stroke, and compared the findings to levels of consciousness.[7]

References

[1] 2012 NRMP Program Directors Survey. Available at: http://www.nrmp.org/wp-content/uploads/2013/08/programresultsbyspecialty2012.pdf. Accessed June 3, 2014.

[2] Eastwood S, Derish P, Berger M. Biomedical publication for neurosurgery. Neurosurgery 2000; 47 (3): 739-48.

[3] University of Chicago Pritzker School of Medicine. Available at: http://pritzker.uchicago.edu/current/students/ResidencyProcessGuide.pdf. Accessed March 3, 2013.

[4] Drexel University Department of Neurosurgery. Available at: http://webcampus.drexelmed.edu/cdc/medSpecialtyNeurologicalSurgery.asp. Accessed March 3, 2013.

[5] University of California Irvine Department of Neurosurgery. Available at: http://www.meded.uci.edu/education/residencyselection/neuosurgery.html. Accessed March 3, 2013.

[6] Attracting top medical students to neurosurgery. Available at: http://www.aansneurosurgeon.org/NS-v19n3-1118-finaltoweb.pdf. Accessed March 3, 2013.

[7] Columbia University Medical Center. Available at: http://www.columbianeurosurgery.org/2013/11/columbia-med-student-wins-best-neuro-trauma-paper-national-neurosurgery-meeting/. Accessed July 22, 2014.

Chapter 27

Obstetrics & Gynecology Awards, Scholarships, & Grants

For medical students interested in receiving a scholarship, award, or grant in obstetrics and gynecology, begin by researching opportunities at your own institution. At the University of Wisconsin School of Medicine and Public Health, the Department of Obstetrics and Gynecology presents the T.A. Leonard Award to medical students for exemplary performance during the third year core clerkship. The Department of Obstetrics, Gynecology and Reproductive Sciences at the University of Texas Medical School at Houston offers the Drs. Emil and Anna Steinberger Endowed Research Award in Reproductive Biology. This award is available to medical students who pursue summer research in reproductive biology. Make inquiries with your Department of Obstetrics & Gynecology to learn about award opportunities you may be eligible for. External awards are also available. These are described below.

Medical students often ask us if it's necessary to do research in the field of obstetrics and gynecology to enhance their chances of matching. In the 2012 NRMP Program Director Survey, 54% of obstetrics and gynecology residency programs cited "demonstrated involvement and interest in research" as a factor in selecting applicants to interview.[1] It's especially helpful to read the perspectives of obstetrics and gynecology program directors and faculty about the importance of research in the selection process. We offer you these perspectives on the next page.

American Congress of Obstetricians and Gynecologists John Gibbons Medical Student Awards

Description: The American Congress of Obstetricians and Gynecologists (ACOG) provide these awards to students interested in the specialty. The monetary support covers the costs associated with travel to ACOG meetings.
To Apply: Applicants must apply through their ACOG district. Each district has its own application process.
Deadline: For more information, visit:

https://www.acog.org/About_ACOG/ACOG_Departments/Medical_Students

Obstetrics and Gynecology Research for Medical Students: Perspectives of Residency Program Directors

- "I would agree that published research does not rank as high as many other criteria," writes Dr. Eugene Toy, Program Director of The Methodist Hospital Obstetrics and Gynecology Residency Program. "For instance, clinical performance on medical school rotations, commitment to the specialty, attitude and ability to work with people, performance on the standardized tests, and work ethic are more important. Nevertheless, if two students are equally qualified in these areas, and one has research, then that student would be ranked higher."[2]

- "Many research projects are long term and therefore, getting started on a project in the first or second year of medical school is advantageous," writes Dr. Carol Major, Program Director of the Obstetrics and Gynecology Residency Program at the University of California Irvine.[3]

- Production is valued more than participation by many programs when it comes to evaluating an applicant's involvement in research. "Research will improve the chances of obtaining a residency if it is published or presented at a meeting," writes Dr. Carol Major.[3]

Profile of a Winner

Lori Homa was the 2011 recipient of the John Gibbons Medical Student Award. Her involvement in ACOG began during her first year of medical school when she attended the ACOG Annual Meeting. Following this, Lori showed great initiative in starting a forum for students interested in pursuing obstetrics and gynecology as a career. The forum was so well received that it was developed into a full day medical student workshop at the Annual Clinical Meeting. The award has allowed Lori the opportunity to attend ACOG meetings, and her involvement has allowed her to assume a leadership role in the organization.

Center for Reproductive Medicine Summer Internship

Description: The Center for Reproductive Medicine is a research program of the Cleveland Clinic Glickman Urological & Kidney Institute and the Ob/Gyn & Women's Health Institute. The Center provides opportunities for students to conduct research in human fertility and reproductive biology under the supervision of scientists and faculty. Participants will be involved in the writing of research articles, reviews, and/or book chapters in the field.
To Apply: For application information and instructions, visit the website below.
Deadline: For more information, visit:

http://www.clevelandclinic.org/ReproductiveResearchCenter/info/traininfo_int 5.html

CREOG / APGO Student/Resident Award for Excellence in Educational Research

Description: The Council on Resident Education in Obstetrics and Gynecology (CREOG) and the Association of Professors of Gynecology and Obstetrics (APGO) invites medical students, residents, fellows, and faculty to submit abstracts to be considered as oral or poster presentations at the Annual Meeting. A $500 award is presented in the student/resident category. In 2014, a $500 award was also available for Exxcellence in Life-Long Learning or Pearls of Exxcellence, and funded by the Foundation for Exxcellence in Women's Health Care.
To Apply: For application information and instructions, visit the website below.
Deadline: For more information, visit:

https://www.apgo.org/bulletin/613-2014-creog-a-apgo-annual-meeting-call-for-abstracts.html

References

[1]2012 NRMP Program Directors Survey. Available at:
http://www.nrmp.org/wp-content/uploads/2013/08/programresultsbyspecialty2012.pdf. Accessed June 3, 2014.
[2]The Successful Match: Getting into Obstetrics and Gynecology. Available at:
http://studentdoctor.net/2010/05/the-successful-match-getting-into-obstetrics-and-gynecology/. Accessed February 10, 2013.
[3]University of California Irvine Department of Obstetrics and Gynecology.
Available at:
http://www.meded.uci.edu/education/residencyselection/obgyn.html. Accessed February 10, 2013.

Chapter 28

Ophthalmology Awards, Scholarships, & Grants

For medical students interested in receiving a scholarship, award, or grant in ophthalmology, begin by researching opportunities at your own institution. At the University of Pennsylvania Perelman School of Medicine, the Department of Ophthalmology gives the Jeffrey W. Berger Medical Student Research in Ophthalmology Award to support medical student research in the field over a period of three months. The Washington University Department of Ophthalmology and Visual Sciences has several awards for outstanding medical student research. Make inquiries with your Department of Ophthalmology to learn about award opportunities you may be eligible for.

External awards for research are also available. The most prestigious are awards and scholarships sponsored by the Fight for Sight and Research to Prevent Blindness. These are described in this chapter.

Medical students often ask us if it's necessary to do research in the field of ophthalmology to enhance their chances of matching. It's especially helpful to read the perspectives of ophthalmology residency program directors and faculty about the importance of research in the selection process. We offer you these perspectives on the next page.

Fight for Sight Summer Student Scholarship

Description: Fight for Sight funds basic or clinical research in ophthalmology, vision or related sciences for individuals with limited or no other research funding. Summer Student Fellowship stipends are made payable to the institution and forwarded to the sponsor in June. Applicants must be matriculated at the institution where the research is conducted during the precise time the Fight for Sight grants are awarded.
To Apply: Grant applicants are eligible to apply regardless of citizenship, but should be affiliated with a North American institution for their research. The grants program is administered by the scientific review committee.
Deadline: All applications, including Post-Docs, Grants-In-Aid, and Summer Student Fellowships must be completed and submitted online by February. For more information, visit:

http://www.fightforsight.org/Grants/Guidelines/

Ophthalmology Research for Medical Students: Perspectives of Residency Program Directors

- "Research in ophthalmology is not the be-all, end-all to getting an interview, but it certainly helps," writes the Department of Ophthalmology at Loyola University in Chicago. "It helps you to get more experience in a field you are passionate about and it helps to align yourself with someone in the department."[1]

- Research, particularly work that leads to publication, is highly valued by programs. "Yes, Research can sometimes separate applicants who are academically similar otherwise," writes Dr. Jeremiah Tao, Program Director of the Ophthalmology Residency Program at the University of California Irvine. "Having publications demonstrates work ethic, intellectual curiosity, and commitment to the field (if paper is related to ophthalmology). Peer reviewed publications within ophthalmology are the gold standard."[2]

- Students may have the opportunity to perform laboratory or clinical research. For applicants who wish to be published sooner rather than later, a clinical project may be preferable. Dr. Simmons Lessell, Director of Medical Student Education at Massachusetts Eye and Ear, writes that "a well-designed [clinical] project performed under the direct supervision of a faculty member and with advanced planning that permits the student to 'hit the ground running' can be accomplished in a month."[3]

- When choosing among research electives, an important consideration is the degree of contact you will have with a faculty member. According to Dr. Lessell, you should "choose an elective in which there will be direct supervision by a faculty member since, should the student decide to apply for residency, it will be important to obtain a recommendation from an ophthalmologist who has directly observed the student's performance."[3]

- For applicants who develop a late interest in ophthalmology, it may not be possible to participate in research before submitting the application. However, all is not lost. "It is important to have research experience," writes Dr. Susan Ksiazek, Program Director of the Ophthalmology Residency Program at the University of Chicago. "However, this research can be done in any field as long as students are able to discuss it during their interviews and they can speak to the experience with some authority."[4]

- If you are considering performing a year of ophthalmology research during or after medical school, you will be interested in the results of a recent survey of ophthalmology residency program directors. Sixty-four percent believed that a year of research was helpful in moving a borderline applicant into the matched pool. Twenty-five percent indicated that a year of research would transform a good application into a great one. Not all program directors valued long-term research. Thirty percent believed that such research was of little value in improving the odds of matching.[5]

North American Neuro-Ophthalmology Society Best Abstract Award

Description: The North American Neuro-Ophthalmology Society offers the Best Abstract Award. This award recognizes the best poster or platform presentation.
To Apply: For application information and instructions, visit the website below.
Deadline: For more information, visit:

http://www.nanosweb.org/i4a/pages/index.cfm?pageid=3365

Rabb-Venable Research Award

Description: Drs. Maurice Rabb, Jr. and H. Phillip Venable were two prominent African American ophthalmologists who made significant contributions to the field through research. This award bearing their name is open to medical students involved in ophthalmology research. Awardees have the opportunity to present research at the National Medical Association Annual Convention and meet with a representative of the National Eye Institute.
To Apply: Three Rabb-Venable Awards for Outstanding Research will be given. Criteria used to judge include importance of research question, potential impact, quality of study data, data analysis, background knowledge of subject, and knowledge/discussion of study limitations.
Deadline: The application deadline is in March. For more information, visit:

http://ophthalmology.nmanet.org/index.php/rabb-venable-reseach-program

Research to Prevent Blindness Medical Student Fellowship

Description: The Research to Prevent Blindness Medical Student Fellowship allows medical students to spend one year fully immersed in research. Funding in the amount of $30,000 will be made available to fellows.
To Apply: The fellowship must take place prior to the third or fourth year of medical school. For application instructions and information, visit the website below.
Deadline: The deadline for the application is in February. For more information, visit:

https://www.rpbusa.org/rpb/grants/grants/medical_student_fellowships/

Sigma Xi Scientific Research Society Grants-in-Aid of Research Program (See Chapter 10)

Sjogren's Syndrome Foundation Student Fellowship

Description: The Sjogren's Syndrome Foundation has established this fellowship program to support medical students interested in performing research in the area. Three fellowships are available.
To Apply: The research must take place at a U.S. institution. See the website below for more information.
Deadline: The deadline for the application is in February. For more information, visit:

https://www.sjogrens.org/home/research-programs/student-fellowships

Sjogren's Syndrome Foundation Student Fellowship – Contact Lens Association of Ophthalmologists Education and Research Foundation

Description: The Sjogren's Syndrome Foundation provides this fellowship to medical students interested in performing research in dry eye and ocular surface disease.
To Apply: See the website below for more information.
Deadline: The deadline for the application is in November. For more information, visit:

http://www.sjogrens.org/home/research-programs/student-fellowships/clao-erf

References

[1]Loyola University Chicago's Ophthalmology Look Book. Available at: www.meddean.luc.edu/.../LUHS_Ophthalmology_Look_Book.pdf. Accessed May 20, 2012.
[2]University of California Irvine Department of Ophthalmology. Available at: http://www.meded.uci.edu/education/residencyselection/ophtho.html. Accessed May 22, 2012.
[3]Lessel S. Advising medical students about ophthalmology electives and residencies. *Journal of Academic Ophthalmology* 2009; 2 (1): 19 – 22.
[4]University of Chicago Pritzker School of Medicine Residency Process 2012. Available at: pritzker.uchicago.edu/current/students/ResidencyProcessGuide.pdf. Accessed May 19, 2012.
[5]Nallasamy S, Uhler T, Nallasamy N, Tapino P, Volpe N. Ophthalmology resident selection: current trends in selection criteria and improving the process. *Ophthalmology* 2010; 117 (5): 1041-7.

Chapter 29

Orthopaedic Surgery Awards, Scholarships, & Grants

For medical students interested in receiving a scholarship, award, or grant in orthopaedic surgery, begin by researching opportunities at your own institution. At the Wayne State University School of Medicine, the Palmer Award is given to two senior medical students pursuing a career in orthopaedic surgery. These are scholarships to offset medical school expenses. Make inquiries with your Department of Orthopaedic Surgery to learn about award opportunities you may be eligible for. External awards for research are also available. These are described below.

Medical students often ask us if it's necessary to do research in the field of orthopaedic surgery to enhance their chances of matching. In the 2012 NRMP Program Director Survey, 71% of orthopaedic surgery residency programs cited "demonstrated involvement and interest in research" as a factor in selecting applicants to interview.[1]

Benjamin Fox Orthopaedic Research Scholar Award

Description: The Benjamin Fox Orthopedic Research Scholar Award allows medical students to perform clinical orthopaedic research at The Children's Hospital of Philadelphia. This "year-out" program can be done before the third or fourth year of medical school. Opportunities to present and publish research are available. Completion of the program provides participants with a significant edge in the orthopaedic surgery residency selection process. Recipients will receive a $20,000 stipend.

To Apply: Most applicants will be completing their third year of medical school. In some cases, highly qualified students finishing their second year will be considered. To be eligible, applicants must have completed the USMLE Step 1 exam. The application includes letter of recommendation, personal essay, and CV.

Deadline: The deadline for the application is in February. For more information, visit:

http://www.chop.edu/service/orthopaedic-surgery/resources-for-professionals/education-fellowships/ben-fox-ortho-research-scholar.html

Hospital for Special Surgery Medical Student Summer Research Fellowship

Description: This fellowship offered by the Hospital for Special Surgery is a mentored research program designed to introduce students who have completed their first year of medical school to research opportunities in orthopaedic basic science, translational science, and clinical research in orthopaedics. The 8-week program runs from mid-June to mid-August and includes a $2,400 stipend. Up to 15 fellowship awards will be granted.

To Apply: To apply for the program, eligible students should first contact an orthopaedic surgeon or scientist who is offering a research project that is of interest. Once the student has been accepted by the surgeon or scientist, the student and mentor may apply for the fellowship together.

Deadline: The deadline is in March. Students and mentors will be notified in May. For more information, visit:

http://www.hss.edu/medical-student-summer-research-fellowship.asp

John Cuckler Senior Orthopaedic Visiting Medical Student Scholarship

Description: This scholarship is offered by the Division of Orthopaedic Surgery at the University of Alabama at Birmingham to increase diversity in the specialty. Four students receive the scholarship each year. Award winners receive on-campus housing during the rotation along with a $500 travel stipend.

To Apply: To be considered, applicants must be a member of an underrepresented minority (African-American, Latino, or Native American) group. Women applicants as well as those who can bring "a unique dimension to our residency program" are also invited to apply. This is a merit-based award, and criteria for judging include academic performance, board scores, volunteer activities, research experience, and personal statement.

Deadline: The deadline is in March. For more information, visit:

http://www.uab.edu/medicine/surgery/orthopaedics/education-training/john-cuckler-senior-orthopaedic-visiting-medical-student-scholarship

New England Baptist Hospital Aufranc Summer Research Scholars Program

Description: The New England Baptist Hospital offers the Otto E. Aufranc Fellowship in Adult Reconstructive Surgery. Fellows are able to conduct novel orthopaedic research and observe surgery during the course of a summer. Fellows receive a stipend of $4,000.

To Apply: The application includes CV and personal statement.

Deadline: The deadline is in March. For more information, visit:

https://www.med.upenn.edu/mdresearchopps/documents/AufrancResearchFellowship2013.pdf

Nth Dimensions Educational Solutions Orthopaedic Summer Internship Program

Description: Twenty medical students will have the opportunity to participate in this eight-week clinical and research internship under the supervision of orthopaedic surgeons across the U.S. Mentors continue to support students after the internship, and facilitate relationship building with other orthopaedic surgeons.

To Apply: The program is open to first-year medical students. The application includes transcripts, MCAT scores, AMCAS application, personal statement, letters of recommendation, and CV.

Deadline: The deadline is in January. For more information, visit:

http://www.nthdimensions.org/Site/program_details.aspx?id=13

Nth Dimensions Educational Solutions Orthopaedic Interview Grants

Description: Grants are available to cover the costs of travel and lodging associated with orthopaedic surgery residency interviews.

To Apply: The program is open to fourth-year medical students. The application includes CV, list of interviews, and hotel/travel receipts.

Deadline: For more information, visit:

http://www.nthdimensions.org/Site/program_details.aspx?id=10

Nth Dimensions Educational Solutions Orthopaedic Book Scholarships

Description: Scholarships are available for the purchase of orthopaedic surgery textbooks.

To Apply: The program is open to fourth-year medical students who have matched in the specialty. Scholarships are given out on a first come first serve basis.

Deadline: For more information, visit:

http://www.nthdimensions.org/Site/program_details.aspx?id=9

RJOS Medical Student Achievement Awards

Description: To stimulate interest in the specialty of orthopaedic surgery, the Ruth Jackson Orthopaedic Society (RJOS) offers the Medical Student Achievement Award. Up to $1,500 is provided for recipients to attend the American Academy of Orthopaedic Surgeons (AAOS) Annual Meeting. Winners are recognized at the RJOS Breakfast Meeting, and are registered for the Student/Resident Workshop.

To Apply: Applicants must be current female medical students. Awardees are chosen based on achievements in community service/volunteerism, research, leadership, mentoring, and athletics. The applicants must be or become a member of the Ruth Jackson Orthopaedic Society. The application includes CV and letter of recommendation from a medical school faculty member. Applicants are asked to answer the following questions:

- "Describe, in 400 words or less, why you are interested in orthopaedic surgery, and how you hope to promote women in orthopaedic surgery and/or improve women's musculoskeletal health.
- Briefly describe the achievement of which you are most proud, and why."[2]

Deadline: The application deadline is in November. For more information, visit:

http://www.rjos.org/web/awards/Student%20Awards.html

RJOS Resident & Medical Student Workshop Scholarship

Description: The Ruth Jackson Orthopaedic Society (RJOS) has made available scholarships to offset the cost of travel to the RJOS Annual Meeting.
To Apply: Medical students and residents are eligible to apply. Applicants must submit a CV, and provide a brief answer to the question, "What do you hope to gain from attending the 2014 RJOS Meeting?"
Deadline: The application deadline is in November. For more information, visit:

http://www.rjos.org/web/awards/index.htm

Profile of a Winner

Casey deDeugd is a fourth-year medical student at the University of Central Florida College of Medicine, and a recent recipient of the Ruth Jackson Orthopaedic Society award. As a charter member of the Alpha Omega Alpha Honor Society, Casey has performed at a high level academically.

She has made important service contributions by organizing the event "Joining Forces." This event allowed veterans and V.A. healthcare providers to meet and discuss important health issues encountered by veterans after completing military service. She is also actively involved in the medical school's "Adopt a Senior" program. In this program, students are paired with senior citizens in the community.

"Your accomplishments thus far are very impressive!" wrote Gloria Gogola, M.D. chair of the society's scientific committee, in notifying deDeugd of her award. "We look forward…to welcoming you to our field of orthopaedic surgery."[3]

References

[1]2012 NRMP Program Directors Survey. Available at:
http://www.nrmp.org/wp-content/uploads/2013/08/programresultsbyspecialty2012.pdf. Accessed June 3, 2014.
[2]Ruth Jackson Orthopaedic Society. Available at:
http://www.rjos.org/web/awards/Student%20Awards.html. Accessed January 20, 2014.
[3]University of Central Florida College of Medicine. Available at:
http://today.ucf.edu/ucf-medical-student-wins-national-orthopaedic-award/. Accessed February 1, 2014.

Chapter 30

Otolaryngology Awards, Scholarships, & Grants

For medical students interested in receiving a scholarship, award, or grant in otolaryngology, begin by researching opportunities at your own institution. At the Oregon Health Science University, the Ed Everts Medical Student Summer Research Award is available to fund one basic science summer research fellow. The Department of Otolaryngology at the University of Michigan Medical School bestows the Albert C. Furstenberg Award to a medical student for outstanding performance in Otolaryngology. The recipient is chosen based on scholastic achievement, clinical work, research efforts, and interest in the specialty. Make inquiries with your Department of Otolaryngology to learn about award opportunities you may be eligible for. External awards are also available. These are described below.

Medical students often ask us if it's necessary to do research in the field of otolaryngology to enhance their chances of matching. In the 2012 NRMP Program Director Survey, 82% of otolaryngology residency programs cited "demonstrated involvement and interest in research" as a factor in selecting applicants to interview.[1] It's especially helpful to read the perspectives of otolaryngology residency program directors and faculty about the importance of research in the selection process. We offer you these perspectives on the next page.

Association for Research in Otolaryngology Medical Student Travel Award

Description: The Association for Research in Otolaryngology (ARO) provides these awards to cover the cost of travel and lodging incurred by medical students attending the ARO MidWinter Meeting.
To Apply: The application includes cover letter, CV, submitted abstract for presentation at conference, and letter of recommendation.
Deadline: The deadline for the application is in October. For more information, visit:

http://www.aro.org/mwm/documents/Resident_MedicalStudentApplication.pdf

---

Otolaryngology Research for Medical Students: Perspectives of Residency Program Directors

- "A publishable project in the field is desirable and most programs highly value a commitment to research," writes the Department of Otolaryngology at UCSF.[2]

- "Research experience is extremely helpful when applying for Otolaryngology residency," writes the Department of Otolaryngology at Oregon Health Sciences University.[3]

- "Research experience, including presentations and publications are looked upon very favorably," writes Dr. Alan Micco, ENT Career Advising Coordinator at Northwestern University. "Otolaryngology research is ideal, but any research is good. Start as early as possible."[4]

- Presenting your work at scientific meetings not only offers an opportunity to strengthen your credentials but you also may meet and interact with key personnel from other residency programs. "Posters also allow more dialogue and interaction," writes Dr. Michael Stewart, Professor in the Department of Otolaryngology at Weill Cornell Medical College. "Most meetings have meet-the-author receptions for presenters to discuss their work, and at many meetings blocks of time are dedicated to poster viewing and discussion."[5]

- "It is not essential to do a research project, but it may be helpful," writes the Department of Otolaryngology at the University of Mississippi. "A publication or research project is one of many factors considered in granting you an interview. If you have significant research exposure in any area in the past that may well be adequate. If you have no exposure, you may want to consider doing a project with us either as a separate block or during your rotation. The residency directors are simply looking to find the most motivated and curious students. Research work is one marker for this. By no means does the lack of a research project exclude you as we have successfully matched a number of students without any research background. There are only a handful of programs in the country that would deny you an interview on this basis alone. However, the topic comes up frequently during interviews, and you may feel more comfortable if you have done some type of project."[6]

Johns Hopkins Department of Otolaryngology – Head and Neck Surgery Clership Program for Underrepresented Minority Students

Description: The Department of Otolaryngology at Johns Hopkins University offers this clerkship program to members of underrepresented minority groups interested in pursuing careers in otolaryngology – head and neck surgery. Program participants will be mentored by Hopkins faculty. Two types of clerkships are available:

- Clinical Clerkship (one month)
- Research Clerkship (three months)

A $500/month stipend will be given. Students who have taken part in this program have been able to publish their research, and match at competitive otolaryngology residency programs.

To Apply: To be eligible, medical student applicants must be a member of an underrepresented minority group as designated by the AAMC. U.S. and Canadian medical students are eligible to apply after at least one year of medical school education.

Deadline: Application materials must be submitted 3-6 months prior to the desired elective. For more information, visit:

http://www.hopkinsmedicine.org/otolaryngology/education/medical_school_clerkship.html

---

Profile of a Winner

Vishal Dhandha took a year off from medical school to perform research in the Department of Otolaryngology at the University of North Carolina-Chapel Hill School of Medicine. His poster, "Effects of Maxillary Antrostomy Configuration and Size on Nasal Spray Deposition in the Maxillary Sinus: A Virtual Surgery Study Using Computational Fluid Dynamics, won first place in the Allergy/Rhinology category at the Triological Society Annual Meeting.

"My advice to future poster authors is to keep the audience and readers in mind when designing the poster," said Dhandha in an interview with *ENT Today*. "There are usually many posters to look at over the course of a short poster session, so displaying a concise, efficient poster allows observers to broadly understand your topic. More specific questions and information can be addressed during a meet-the-author/Q & A session."[7]

References

[1] 2012 NRMP Program Directors Survey. Available at:
http://www.nrmp.org/wp-content/uploads/2013/08/programresultsbyspecialty2012.pdf. Accessed June 3, 2014.

[2] UCSF Department of Otolaryngology. Available at:
http://meded.ucsf.edu/ume/career-information-otolaryngology. Accessed March 29, 2013.

[3] Oregon Health Sciences University Department of Otolaryngology. Available at: http://www.ohsu.edu/xd/health/services/ent/training/medical-student-education/career_guide.cfm. Accessed March 29, 2013.

[4] Northwestern University Department of Otolaryngology. Available at: http://www.feinberg.northwestern.edu/education/current-students/career-development-residency/career-development-program/career-advising-specialties/otolaryngology.html. Accessed March 27, 2013.

[5] Stewart M, Chandra R, Chiu A, Hanna E, Kennedy D, Kraus D, Gleeson M, Levine P, Niparko J, O'Malley B, Rosenfeld R, Ruben R, Sataloff R, Smith R, Weber P. The value of resident presentations at scientific meetings. *I Head Neck Surg* 2013; 139 (1): 100.

[6] University of Mississippi Department of Otolaryngology. Available at: http://www.umc.edu/Education/Schools/Medicine/Clinical_Science/Otolaryngology___Communicative_Sciences/Academics(Otolaryngology___Communicative_Science)/Residency_FAQ.aspx. Accessed March 30, 2013.

[7] ENT Today. Available at:
http://www.enttoday.org/details/article/2464831/COSM_2012_TRIO_Poster_Winners_Discuss_their_Projects.html. Accessed June 3, 2014.

Chapter 31

Pathology Awards, Scholarships, & Grants

For medical students interested in receiving a scholarship, award, or grant in pathology, begin by researching opportunities at your own institution. At the University of California San Diego, up to four medical students will receive travel awards to cover the costs associated with attending a scientific meeting. Students are eligible if they have performed a project in the Department of Pathology. At the University of Oklahoma College of Medicine, the Department of Pathology presents the Robert M. O'Neal Award to the sophomore medical student who has performed at an outstanding level in the course, "Introduction to Human Illness." The Department of Laboratory Medicine and Pathology at the University of Minnesota School of Medicine awards the Dr. Kenneth F. Ernst Award for superior research in pathology.

External awards for research are also available. The most prestigious are awards and scholarships sponsored by the American Society for Clinical Pathology and American Society for Investigative Pathology. These are described below.

Academic Excellence and Achievement Award in Pathology

Description: The American Society for Clinical Pathology (ASCP) annually offers the Academic Excellence and Achievement Award for exemplary medical students who demonstrate excellence in pathology and laboratory medicine. This award honors medical students who have achieved "academic excellence, leadership ability, and a strong interest in the pathology profession."[1] Ten medical students will be awarded each year. Of the ten, one student will receive the prestigious Gold Award.
To Apply: Only students from medical schools within the United States, Canada and Puerto Rico are eligible for this award. See the ASCP nomination form in the link below.
Deadline: The ASCP usually accepts nominations starting in March and ending in May. See the link below for further information:

http://www.ascp.org/Functional-Nav/Medical-Students/Awards#tabs-0

American Society for Investigative Pathology Summer Research Opportunity Program in Pathology

Description: The American Society for Investigative Pathology (ASIP) and Intersociety Council for Pathology Information (ICPI) offer this opportunity for underrepresented minority students. Program participants will visit, learn, and engage in research at the University of Pittsburgh over the summer. The award amount is $3,000.

To Apply: For application instructions and information, visit the website below.

Deadline: The deadline is in April. For more information, visit:

https://www.asip.org/awards/sropp.cfm

Profile of a Winner

Chao Ying Xu, a medical student at Yale University School of Medicine, was the 2012 Gold Award (Academic Excellence and Achievement Award in Pathology) recipient. Her interest in pathology stemmed from her studies during her high school and undergraduate years when she was involved in various microscopy projects and attended related courses at the University of Toronto.

"I really enjoy the critical reasoning and investigative aspect of pathology," said Ms. Xu in the ASCP article. In his nomination letter for Ms. Xu, Dr. Marcus Bosenberg, Associate Professor of Dermatology and Pathology at Yale University School of Medicine, wrote, "I can honestly say that during my years as a faculty member at Yale, Harvard, and the University of Vermont, I have never met another first-year medical student with Sarah's enthusiasm and talent for the field of pathology."[2]

Another award winner, Alexander Gallan, a Boston University School of Medicine student, has been actively involved in researching techniques for lung cancer diagnosis. Dr. Daniel G. Remick, Chair and Professor of Pathology at Boston University School of Medicine, wrote in his nomination letter, "Alex Gallan is the type of medical student representing the future of our field."[2]

ICPI Trainee Travel Award

Description: The Intersociety Council for Pathology Information (ICPI) provides these travel awards to support trainee participation in scientific pathology meetings. There are two types of travel awards:

- Awards for trainees who do not submit an abstract ($500)
- Awards for trainees who do submit an abstract ($750)

To Apply: To be eligible, medical student applicants must be a member of one of the designated ICPI pathology organizations. The application includes cover letter, letter of recommendation, and proof of membership in pathology organization.

Deadline: The deadline for the application is at least 30 days prior to the meeting. For more information, visit:

http://www.pathologytraining.org/awards_grants/documents/Travel%20Award.pdf

References

[1]American Society of Clinical Pathology. Available at:
http://www.ascp.org/Functional-Nav/Medical-Students/Awards#tabs-0. Accessed July 2, 2014.
[2]American Society of Clinical Pathology. Available at:
From http://www.ascp.org/Newsroom/ASCP-Recognizes-Stellar-Medical-Students-with-Promising-Futures-in-Pathology.html. Accessed January 14, 2014.

Chapter 32

Pediatrics Awards, Scholarships, & Grants

For medical students interested in receiving a scholarship, award, or grant in pediatrics, begin by researching opportunities at your own institution. At the West Virginia University School of Medicine, the Ruth Phillips-Trotter Award is given to a single female medical student from the Morgantown campus by the Department of Pediatrics. The award recognizes outstanding performance in the field, leadership qualities, and compassion. The Division of General Pediatrics at the Mt. Sinai School of Medicine bestows the Golden Family Community Pediatric Award to a medical student interested in participating in a mentored service or research project in community pediatrics.

External awards for research are also available. Well-known awards and scholarships include those sponsored by the American Academy of Pediatrics, American Pediatric Association, American Pediatric Society, and Society for Pediatric Research. These are described below.

Alex's Lemonade Stand Foundation Oncology Student Training Program

Description: Alex's Lemonade Stand Foundation sponsors the Oncology Student Training Program to support medical students interested in performing pediatric oncology research. A maximum of $6,000 will be provided for 8 to 10 weeks of summer research.
To Apply: Incoming and current medical students are eligible to apply. Students must have a research mentor prior to application submission. For application information and instructions, visit the website below.
Deadline: The application is due in February. For more information, visit:

http://www.alexslemonade.org/grants/post

American Academy of Pediatrics Clinical Case Competition

Description: The American Academy of Pediatrics (AAP) Section on Medical Students, Residents, and Fellowship Trainees sponsors the annual "Clinical Case Competition." Abstracts of interesting cases are submitted by medical students, and ten authors are selected to present their cases in poster format at the AAP National Conference and Exhibition. The first place winner will be announced at the poster presentation, and the case will be published in *Pediatrics in Review*.

To Apply: For more information, visit the website below.

Deadline: The deadline is in April. For more information, visit:

http://www2.aap.org/sections/ypn/r/funding_awards/clinical_case_pres.html

American Pediatric Association Student Research Award

Description: The American Pediatric Association honors student research in the fields of general pediatrics (including public health, epidemiology, health policy, and underserved populations), health services research, education, adolescent medicine, child abuse, developmental/behavioral pediatrics, emergency medicine, and hospitalist medicine. Award recipients will be chosen based on the quality of the submitted abstract.

To Apply: Medical students are eligible to apply but must present the abstract before graduating. The applicant must be the first author of the abstract, and the abstract must be accepted for publication at the Pediatric Academic Societies (PAS) Annual Meeting. The application must include a letter from the research mentor indicating that the research was performed by the applicant, and reasons why the study is worthy of a national award.

Deadline: For more information, visit:

http://www.pas-meeting.org/2013dc/awards.asp#APA Student

American Pediatric Society Student Research Program

Description: The American Pediatric Society and Society for Pediatric Research offers this program to stimulate interest in pediatric research among medical students. Program participants will have the opportunity to perform research at institutions other than their own medical school. The award amount is up to $5,508 for a 2-3 month period.

To Apply: Applicants must be enrolled in a U.S. or Canadian medical school. The application includes personal data form, dean's letter, and faculty recommendation forms.

Deadline: The deadline is in January. For more information, visit:

https://www.aps-spr.org/get-involved/student-research/

American Society of Pediatric Nephrology Trainee Research Award

Description: The American Society of Pediatric Nephrology Trainee Research Award will be given to medical students, residents, or fellows performing research in pediatric nephrology. One award is available for the best abstract on patient-oriented research. Another award will be given for the best basic science abstract. Winners will receive a monetary prize, complimentary conference registration, and funding to offset the cost of travel to the conference.

To Apply: The applicant must be planning a career as a pediatric nephrologist. Only applicants who are named as first author on abstracts submitted to the Annual Meeting will be considered.

Deadline: For more information, visit:

http://www.pas-meeting.org/2013dc/awards.asp#APA Student

Children's Hospital of Pittsburgh Student Research Training Program

Description: The Student Research Training Program provides medical students with the opportunity to conduct research under the direct supervision of faculty at the Children's Hospital of Pittsburgh. Students may perform research in a wide variety of areas, including molecular genetics, rheumatology, infectious diseases, surgery, gastroenterology, pulmonary, and neonatology. At the end of this eight-week summer research experience, participants will present their research in the form of a poster presentation.

To Apply: Medical school applicants must have completed two semesters of coursework. The application includes personal statement of interest in pediatric biomedical research and career goals, CV, and transcript.

Deadline: The application deadline is in February. For more information, visit:

http://www.chp.edu/CHP/student+research+training+program

Cystic Fibrosis Foundation Student Traineeships

Description: The Cystic Fibrosis Foundation Student Traineeship was established to introduce students to research related to cystic fibrosis and develop and maintain an interest in this area of biomedicine. The stipend is $1,500 and is paid directly to the sponsoring institution. Up to $300 of this stipend may be requested for project-related research supplies. Students receiving traineeships from the Cystic Fibrosis Foundation may reapply for support in a subsequent year.

To Apply: Applicants must be students in or about to enter a doctoral program (M.D., Ph.D., or M.D./Ph.D.). Senior-level undergraduates planning to pursue graduate training may also apply.

Deadline: Applications are accepted on an on-going basis. For more information, visit:

http://www.cff.org/research/ForResearchers/FundingOpportunities/TrainingGrants/#Student_Traineeships

JACK's Summer Scholars Program

Description: Through this program, scholars have the opportunity to explore neonatology and pediatric subspecialties through clinical mentoring and research at Virginia Commonwealth University.
To Apply: The application includes several essay questions. Applicants are asked to describe their interest in the program, future plans, previous research experience, and past teamwork experiences.
Deadline: The application deadline is in March. For more information, visit:

http://www.pediatrics.vcu.edu/pediatric_specialties/neonatal/jacks.html

Los Angeles Children's Hospital Summer Oncology Fellowship

Description: The Los Angeles Children's Hospital/ USC School of Medicine Summer Oncology Fellowship is intended to provide the highest quality experience for first-year medical school students pursuing interests in oncology research. The students are paid a weekly stipend of $300 for a minimum of six weeks or maximum of ten weeks. A limited amount of funds are available as reimbursement for travel and housing on a case-by-case basis for those students from outside the greater Los Angeles area.
To Apply: While the program has traditionally been designed for students who have completed their first year of medical school, highly qualified undergraduates majoring in health science fields may be considered.
Deadline: Each year, the program's executive committee reviews and selects approximately 20 applicants by early March. Prospective fellows are asked to download, complete and submit the application form by late January. For more info, visit:

http://www.chla.org/site/c.ipINKTOAJsG/b.4434829/k.8F5A/Summer_Oncolo gy_Fellowship.htm#.UaOhgxjIyXM

NASPGHAN Foundation Summer Student Mentor Program

Description: Through this program, medical students can participate in a 10-week research experience under the mentorship of basic or clinical scientists with a research focus in pediatric gastroenterology, hepatology, or nutrition. Stipends of $4000 for at least a 10 week experience will be provided to each student. NASPGHAN Foundation will support up to 3 students this year through this program.
To Apply: Students in good standing at accredited medical schools in the U.S. and Canada who have completed their first year of medical training may apply.
Deadline: The deadline for application is in March. For more info, visit:

http://www.naspghan.org/wmspage.cfm?parm1=4#lib2

St. Baldrick's Summer Fellowship Award

Description: The St. Baldrick's Summer Fellowship Award provides medical students with the opportunity to perform pediatric oncology research. The award amount is $2,500.
To Apply: The mentor and research plan have to be established before the application is submitted. For more information, visit the website below.
Deadline: The deadline is in April. For more information, visit:

http://www.stbaldricks.org/grant-types/

St. Jude Children's Research Hospital Pediatric Oncology Education Program

Description: Through this program, students can gain biomedical and oncology research experience. Students can perform laboratory or clinical research in a variety of departments, including anesthesiology, biochemistry, chemical biology & therapeutics, developmental neurobiology, diagnostic imaging, epidemiology and cancer control, oncology, immunology, infectious diseases, neuro-oncology, pathology, pharmaceutical sciences, radiation oncology, and structural biology. The program awards nearly 20 medical student positions. Students are expected to devote 9 weeks during the summer.
To Apply: To be eligible, medical students must meet minimum GPA requirements. Prior research experience and letter of recommendation from a research mentor are other components of the application. Only applicants from U.S. medical schools will be considered.
Deadline: The deadline is in February. For more information, visit:

http://www.stjude.org/poe

Society for Pediatric Research Student Research Award

Description: The Society for Pediatric Research honors medical students with the Student Research Award. Winners are chosen based on the quality of the submitted research abstract. The award amount is $1,000. Three to six awards are given annually.
To Apply: Medical students are eligible to apply but must present the abstract before graduating. The applicant must be the first author of the abstract, and the abstract must be accepted for publication at the Pediatric Academic Societies (PAS) Annual Meeting. The application must include a letter from the research mentor indicating that the research was performed by the applicant, and reasons why the study is worthy of a national award.
Deadline: For more information, visit:

http://www.pas-meeting.org/2013dc/awards.asp#Student_Research

Strong Children's Research Center Summer Training Program

Description: Strong Children's Research Center in Rochester, New York, sponsors a 10-week summer research program for medical students. Students can engage in basic or clinical research. A $3,000 stipend is given to program participants.
To Apply: Incoming and current medical students are eligible to apply. The completed application includes CV, recommendation letters, and transcript.
Deadline: The application is due in February. For more information, visit:

http://www.urmc.rochester.edu/pediatrics/research/Summer-Training-Program.aspx

Summer Medical Student Respiratory Research Fellowship

Description: Through the Summer Medical Student Respiratory Research Fellowship, medical students have the opportunity to conduct pediatric pulmonary-related basic science and clinical research in the Department of Pediatrics at the University of Cincinnati College of Medicine. This is a nine-week program where students will work with established scientists in such areas as asthma, cystic fibrosis, sleep disorders, lung remodeling, and acute lung injury. Participants will receive a stipend of $5,390.
To Apply: Visit the website below.
Deadline: For more information, visit:

http://www.cincinnatichildrens.org/education/research/respiratory-research-fellowship/default/

Did you know...

State chapters of the American Academy of Pediatrics often have scientific poster competitions. Medical students and residents are eligible to participate, and there may be opportunities to win awards. Check with your state chapter for more information.

Chapter 33

Physical Medicine & Rehabilitation Awards, Scholarships, & Grants

For medical students interested in receiving a scholarship, award, or grant in physical medicine & rehabilitation, begin by researching opportunities at your own institution. At the University of North Carolina School of Medicine, the Department of Physical Medicine & Rehabilitation bestows the Best Student Physiatrist Award to the medical student who "best demonstrates caring and compassion for persons with physical disabilities and exemplifies an interdisciplinary treatment philosophy to improve quality of life and function."[1]

External awards for research are also available. The most prestigious are awards and scholarships sponsored by the American Academy of Physical Medicine and Rehabilitation, Association of Academic Physiatrists, and Rehabilitation Institute of Chicago. These are described below.

American Academy of Physical Medicine and Rehabilitation Medical Student Mentor Program

Description: Through this program, students considering physical medicine and rehabilitation as a career have opportunities to identify a mentor.
To Apply: For more information, visit the website below.
Deadline: For more information, visit:

https://www.aapmr.org/members/activities/mentors/Pages/default.aspx

Association of Academic Physiatrists The Electrode Store Best Paper Competition

Description: The Association of Academic Physiatrists (AAP) administers an annual best paper competition. Medical students are eligible for this award. Winners receive complimentary registration to the AAP Annual Meeting, a monetary award, and the opportunity to present their work at the meeting.
To Apply: For more information, visit the website below.
Deadline: For more information, visit:

http://www.physiatry.org/?page=training_students

Association of Academic Physiatrists Best Paper by an Author 'In Training"

Description: The best paper published annually in the *American Journal of Physical Medicine and Rehabilitation* by a medical student, resident, or fellow will be recognized at the Association of Academic Physiatrists annual meeting. The winner will also receive a plaque and monetary award.
To Apply: To be eligible, the medical student must be first author. For more information, visit the website below.
Deadline: For more information, visit:

http://www.physiatry.org/?page=Awards_research

Association of Academic Physiatrists Medical Student Summer Clinical Externship Program

Description: The Association of Academic Physiatrists (AAP) offers the Medical Student Summer Clinical Externship Program to medical students interested in a clinical experience in the specialty. This is an 8-week summer program which provides students with inpatient and outpatient experiences.
To Apply: To be eligible, applicants must be enrolled in an accredited allopathic or osteopathic U.S. medical school. The application includes grades, MCAT scores, letter of recommendation, and essay.
Deadline: For more information, visit:

http://www.physiatry.org/?page=programs_MSSCE

Myofascial Trigger Points Research Scholarship

Description: The Myofascial Trigger Points Research Scholarship provides support to medical students interested in conducting research to advance the understanding and treatment of myofascial trigger points. The award amount is up to $500. Up to three awards will be granted annually.
To Apply: For application information and instructions, visit the website below.
Deadline: For more information, visit:

http://lifeafterpain.com/info/myofascial-trigger-point-reasearch-scholarship/

National Institute of Arthritis and Musculoskeletal and Skin Diseases Summer Institute Program in Biomedical Research

Description: Through this 8-week summer program, medical students have the opportunity to work closely with experts in the field. Participants receive training in cutting-edge basic and clinical research, are mentored by leading investigators, attend lectures, network with members of the NIH scientific community, and bolster credentials.

To Apply: For application information, visit the website below.
Deadline: For more information, visit:

http://www.niams.nih.gov/research/Ongoing_Research/Branch_Lab/Career_De
velopment_Outreach/summer.asp

National Student Injury Research Training Program

Description: Since 2005, more than 70 students have participated in research training during the summer at the Center for Injury Research and Policy (CIRP), each completing at least one scientific article based on their findings. The goal of this program is to provide research training to future physician-investigators while introducing them to the field of injury research and prevention. Four selected participants will receive a $3,000 stipend. This program gives medical students the opportunity to conduct their own research under the supervision and guidance of CIRP faculty and researchers.

To Apply: In collaboration with a faculty mentor, each participant will choose an injury topic, perform a literature review, develop a research hypothesis, analyze data to evaluate the topic and test the hypothesis, interpret and summarize findings in a manuscript for which he/she will serve as first author, and submit the paper to a peer-reviewed scientific journal for publication.

Deadline: The deadline for applications is in February. Accepted applicants will be notified by March. For more information, visit:

http://www.nationwidechildrens.org/cirp-national-student-injury-research-
training-program

Rehabilitation Research Experience for Medical Students Program Award

Description: The Rehabilitation Research Experience for Medical Students Program Award is offered by the Association of Academic Physiatrists (AAP). The program offers medical students the opportunity to perform research under the guidance of accomplished PM&R specialists. Recipients will receive a $4,000 stipend, and participate in an eight-week summer externship following the first year of medical school. Additional funds will be given to cover travel to the AAP Annual Meeting.

To Apply: To be eligible, applicants must be enrolled in an accredited U.S. medical school. The program is open to medical students at any level. The Association may give preference to certain research topics. Students are expected to identify mentors from an approved list available on the AAP website. AAP encourages applicants to choose mentors outside of their own institution. The experience can take place in the United States or Canada. Applicants should send a proposal, personal statement, and CV. Although letters of recommendation are not required, letters will be accepted. The research mentor must submit an NIH Bio-sketch.

Deadline: The application deadline is in March. For more information, visit:

http://www.physiatry.org/?page=RREMS_students

Rehabilitation Institute of Chicago Summer Research Experience

Description: This is an eight-week physical medicine and rehabilitation externship at the Rehabilitation Institute of Chicago. Students will have opportunities to participate in patient care and research.
To Apply: Students from all medical schools are eligible to apply. For more information, visit the website below.
Deadline: For more information, visit:

http://www.ric.org/professionals/medical-student-education/#.UzMs2oUb3d4

Profile of a Winner

Christopher Jackson is a Wayne State University medical student, and recent winner of the Rehabilitation Research Experience for Medical Students Award. He developed an interest in athletic rehabilitation because of injuries he suffered and the experiences he had as an athletic trainer. This led him to pursue research in the Department of Physical Medicine and Rehabilitation at Wayne State University.

"My interest in spinal cord research came from working as an athletic trainer prior to coming to medical school," said Jackson. "As an athletic trainer I unfortunately had to provide emergency care for two high school athletes who had suffered cervical spine injuries, one of which required extensive medical treatment and rehabilitation. Seeing one of the athletes that I cared for struggle through his rehabilitation made me realize that I wanted to be involved in research in order to improve the care that he and other patients can receive."

With the help of dedicated faculty mentors, Christopher won the award for his project, "The Role of Rehabilitation in Potentiating the Effects of Human Neural Progenitor Cells in Severe Spinal Cord Injury." His work was presented at the AAP annual meeting.[2]

Spaulding Rehabilitation Network Research Fellowship

Description: The Spaulding Rehabilitation Network offers the Research Fellowship for medical students interested in performing research. At the end of the project, the fellow receives a fellowship certificate from Harvard Medical School. The research experience is for a minimum of six months. No salary support is offered.
To Apply: Eligible applicants include international medical students, residents, fellows, or physicians. The application includes CV and cover letter.

Deadline: For more information, visit:

http://www.spauldingrehab.org/education-and-training/research-fellowship

References

[1]University of North Carolina School of Medicine. Available at:
http://www.med.unc.edu/phyrehab/news/lunsford-named-best-physiatrist.
Accessed July 2, 2014.
[2]Wayne State University School of Medicine. Available at:
http://prognosis.med.wayne.edu/article/wsu-student-wins-rehabilitation-
research-experience-for-medical-students-award. Accessed January 20, 2014.

Chapter 34

Plastic Surgery Awards, Scholarships, & Grants

For medical students interested in receiving a scholarship, award, or grant in plastic surgery, begin by researching opportunities at your own institution. At the University of Virginia School of Medicine, the Larry S. Nichter Award for Plastic Surgical Research is given to a medical student for exemplary research in the field. External awards for research are also available. These are described below.

American Society for Reconstructive Microsurgery Medical Student Travel Grant

Description: The American Society for Reconstructive Microsurgery (ASRM) provides scholarships to medical students interested in attending the ASRM Annual Meeting. The award provides funds to cover the costs associated with travel and accommodations.

To Apply: Eligible applicants must be medical students at the time of the meeting and not be presenting during the meeting. A letter of support from the applicant's program director is required.

Deadline: The application deadline is in September. For more information, visit:

http://www.microsurg.org/grants/annual-meeting-medical/

Bitar Cosmetic Surgery Institute Internship Program

Description: The Bitar Cosmetic Institute Internship Program provides an opportunity for medical students to spend the summer at the institute. Participants will observe the high quality of care given to patients, learn about administrative aspects of practice, and perform research. No financial compensation is offered during the internship.

To Apply: Medical students are eligible to apply. The application includes CV, letter of intent, and reference letter.

Deadline: For more information, visit:

http://www.bitarinstitute.com/internship-program/

Texas Society of Plastic Surgeons Medical Student Poster Competition Award

Description: The Texas Society of Plastic Surgeons invites medical students to enter the medical student poster competition. This competition takes place during the 2014 Annual Meeting in September. The best overall poster will receive a plaque.
To Apply: For more information, visit the website below.
Deadline: The application deadline is in July. For more information, visit:

http://www.tsps.net/

Women's Microsurgery Group Travel Scholarship

Description: The Women's Microsurgery Group provides travel scholarships to stimulate interest in reconstructive microsurgery among women medical students. The scholarship helps to defray the cost of travel and accommodations to the American Society for Reconstructive Microsurgery Annual Meeting.
To Apply: Eligible applicants must be female medical students interesting in pursuing a career in reconstructive microsurgery. Applicants who will be presenting an abstract during the Annual Meeting will not be considered for the scholarship. The application includes personal statement, CV, and letter of recommendation. The letter should address the following:

- Explaining that the applicant has demonstrated true interest in reconstructive microsurgery.
- Why the applicant is deserving of the fellowship
- Verify that the applicant is a medical student in good standing in an American or Canadian program.

Deadline: The application deadline is in October. For more information, visit:

http://www.microsurg.org/grants/womens-microsurgery-group-scholarship/

Chapter 35

Psychiatry Awards, Scholarships, & Grants

For medical students interested in receiving a scholarship, award, or grant in psychiatry, begin by researching opportunities at your own institution. At the Indiana University School of Medicine, third-year medical students are eligible to win two awards offered by the Department of Psychiatry. The Arthur B. Richter Award in Clinical and Adolescent Psychiatry is a monetary award for a student interested in the field. The Arthur B. Richter Scholarship in Research in Child and Adolescent Psychiatry is given to a medical student for research in the field. At the University of Kansas School of Medicine, medical students are eligible for several awards bestowed by the Department of Psychiatry, including the Award for Best Psychiatric Paper, Award for Psychiatry Elective Performance, and Award for Psychiatry Clerkship Performance.

External awards for research are also available. The most prestigious are awards and scholarships sponsored by the American Academy of Child and Adolescent Psychiatry and American Psychiatric Association. These are described below.

Advanced Medical Student Fellowship in Alcohol and Other Drug Dependency

Description: Through funding provided by the Scaife Family Foundation, the Institute for Research, Education, and Training in Addictions (IRETA) offers this program to medical students interested in gaining training in addiction treatment and recovery. The program includes lectures, patient contact, group sessions with clients, and rounds with resident physicians. Fellows will receive $150 per week for the three-week program. For those living outside the Pittsburgh area, an additional $200 will be given for travel. Eight students are selected as fellows per session. There are two sessions held in the summer.

To Apply: Students attending medical school in the U.S. are eligible to apply.

Deadline: For more information, visit:

http://ireta.org/scaifestudentprogram

Ascona Prize for Students (See Chapter 15)

American Academy of Addiction Psychiatry Medical Student Travel Award

Description: The American Academy of Addiction Psychiatry (AAAP) offers travel awards to students interested in attending the AAAP Annual Meeting.
To Apply: Candidates are assessed on their interest and potential for contributions to the specialty. The application includes CV, reference letter, and personal essay about interest and achievements in the field.
Deadline: The application deadline is in August. For more information, visit:

http://www2.aaap.org/meetings-and-events/annual-meeting/travel-awards

American Academy of Child and Adolescent Psychiatry Summer Medical Student Fellowship

Description: The American Academy of Child and Adolescent Psychiatry (AACAP) has established this fellowship program to provide medical students with opportunities to explore a career in the specialty. Through this program, fellows are able to meet leaders in the field. The award amount is $3,500 for 12 weeks of clinical or research training. Fellows are required to attend the AACAP Annual Meeting.
To Apply: To be eligible, the applicant must be enrolled in an accredited U.S. medical school. The application includes CV, statement of interest, and letter of support from proposed mentor.
Deadline: The deadline is in February. For more information, visit:

https://www.aacap.org/AACAP/Awards/Medical_Students_Awards/Summer_
Medical_Student_Fellowships.aspx

American Academy of Child and Adolescent Psychiatry Jeanne Spurlock Research Fellowship in Substance Abuse and Addiction

Description: The American Academy of Child and Adolescent Psychiatry (AACAP) has established this fellowship program to provide medical students with opportunities to explore a research career in substance abuse. Fellows will also be able to meet with leaders in the specialty. The award amount is up to $4,000 for 8 - 12 weeks of summer research. The research must be presented at the AACAP Annual Meeting. A travel stipend will be given to cover the costs associated with attending the meeting.
To Apply: The applicant must be enrolled in an accredited U.S. medical school. Students must be members of one of the following underrepresented groups: African-American, Native American, Alaskan Native, Mexican American, Hispanic, Asian, and Pacific Islander. The application includes CV, statement of interest, and letter of support from proposed mentor.
Deadline: The deadline is in February. For more information, visit:

https://www.aacap.org/AACAP/Awards/Medical_Students_Awards/Spurlock_
Research_Fellowship.aspx

American Academy of Child and Adolescent Psychiatry Life Members Mentorship Grants for Medical Students

Description: The American Academy of Child and Adolescent Psychiatry (AACAP) has established Life Members Mentorship Grants. Through this program, seven medical students will have the opportunity to attend the AACAP Annual Meeting where they will gain exposure to the specialty. There are considerable opportunities to meet and network with leaders in the field. The award amount is $1,000.

To Apply: To be eligible, applicants must be enrolled in accredited U.S. medical schools. The application includes CV, personal statement explaining the reasons for wanting to attend the meeting, and reference letter.

Deadline: The deadline is in July. For more information, visit:

https://www.aacap.org/AACAP/Awards/Medical_Students_Awards/Life_Members_Mentorship_Grants.aspx

American Academy of Psychosomatic Medicine Trainee Travel Award

Description: The American Academy of Psychosomatic Medicine (APM) offers trainee travel awards to cover the costs associated with attending the APM Annual Meeting.

To Apply: Eligible trainees include medical students whose abstracts have been accepted for the annual meeting. The application includes a personal essay indicating interest and future plans in psychosomatic medicine.

Deadline: The application deadline is in August. For more information, visit:

http://www.apm.org/awards/trainee-travel.shtml#how_to_apply

American Psychiatric Association Minority Medical Student Summer Mentoring Program

Description: The American Psychiatric Association (APA) has established this program to identify ethnic minority medical students with an interest in psychiatry. Through this program, students are paired with mentors in the field. The award amount is $1,500.

To Apply: To be eligible, the applicant must be enrolled in an accredited U.S. medical school and a member of one of the following ethnic minorities: American Indian, Alaska Native, Native Hawaiian, Asian American, African American, and Hispanic/Latino. The program is open to students in all four years of medical school. The application includes statement of interest and CV.

Deadline: The deadline is in March. For more information, visit:

http://www.psychiatry.org/medical-students/electives-awards

American Psychiatric Association Minority Student Summer Externship in Addiction Psychiatry

Description: The American Psychiatric Association (APA) has established this clinical shadowing program to identify ethnic minority medical students with an interest in substance abuse. Through this program, students are paired with mentors in the field and will spend one month receiving an in-depth look at how substance abuse patients are treated. The award amount is $1,500.

To Apply: To be eligible, the applicant must be enrolled in an accredited U.S. medical school and a member of one of the following ethnic minorities: American Indian, Alaska Native, Native Hawaiian, Asian American, African American, and Hispanic/Latino. The program is open to students in all four years of medical school. The application includes statement of interest and CV.

Deadline: The deadline is in March. For more information, visit:

http://www.psychiatry.org/minority-fellowship

American Psychiatric Association Resident and Medical Student Poster Competition

Description: The American Psychiatric Association (APA) invites medical students and residents to present posters at the APA Meeting. One winning poster will be selected from each of the 4 categories – Psychosocial and Biomedical, Community Service, Patient Care and Epidemiology, Curriculum Development and Education. In 2014, over 400 posters were received.

To Apply: Visit the website below for more information.

Deadline: For more information, visit:

http://www.psychiatry.org/residents/resident-poster-competition

American Psychiatric Association Travel Scholarship for Minority Medical Students

Description: The American Psychiatric Association (APA) offers travel scholarships for approximately 10 minority medical students to attend the APA Annual Meeting or Institute on Psychiatric Services (IPS) Meeting. Scholarship recipients will have opportunities to learn more about the field, attend sessions, and work with a mentor.

To Apply: Visit the website below for more application information and instructions.

Deadline: The deadline for the APA Annual Meeting is in January. The deadline for the IPS Meeting is in June. For more information, visit:

http://www.psychiatry.org/medical-students/electives-awards

Betty Ford Summer Institute for Medical Students

Description: Through this program, the Betty Ford Institute provides students with the opportunity to work closely with alcoholics and addicts in the recovery process. "SIMS is an amazing, once-in-a-lifetime, priceless experience," wrote Nataly, a medical student at Yale University. "I truly think it is going to change the way I practice medicine related to addiction."[1]
To Apply: For more information, visit the website below.
Deadline: For more information, visit:

http://www.bettyfordinstitute.org/education/summer-institute-for-medical-students.php

Geriatric Mental Health Foundation's Scholars Fund

Description: Through this fund, medical students are exposed to the field of geriatric psychiatry. The fund provides for mentorship and educational development of students. Scholars receive membership in American Association for Geriatric Psychiatry (AAGP), individual mentorship, and travel support to attend the AAGP Scholars Program.
To Apply: Medical students will be nominated for these positions by psychiatry clerkship and residency program directors. Please see the website below for application information and instructions.
Deadline: The deadline is in October. For more information, visit:

http://www.aagponline.org/index.php?src=gendocs&ref=ScholarsProgram&category=Main

Joseph Collins Foundation Scholarship (See Chapter 18)

Leah J. Dickstein, M.D. Award

Description: The Association of Women Psychiatrists (AWP) offers the Leah J. Dickstein M.D. Award. The award winner will receive the honor at the Annual Meeting of the Association of Women in Psychiatry, receive a plaque, and be invited to join the awards committee for the following year. This meeting occurs during the American Psychiatric Association Annual Meeting. The winner will receive $1,000 to cover the expense associated with attending the meeting.
To Apply: Female medical students are eligible to apply for the award. Applicants must be nominated through either the Dean's Office or the Office of Women in Medicine. The application includes a nomination letter, two additional letters of reference, an award application, and one page personal statement. Criteria for judging include superior academic achievement, creativity, and leadership.
Deadline: The application deadline is in March, and the winner is notified in April. For more information, visit:

http://www.associationofwomenpsychiatrists.com/awards.aspx

M-STREAM Program

Description: The M-STREAM Program is designed to give medical students an opportunity to explore an interest in the field of geriatric mental health through a variety of research opportunities. Student participants will have an opportunity to experience first-hand the excitement of cutting edge research. Selected trainees will spend 8-12 weeks working closely with a faculty mentor(s) on a research project in which the student will learn the basic elements of experimental design, research methodology, and interpretation of experimental data. M-STREAM gives students the opportunity to foster a relationship with a mentor in the field that will serve as a role model throughout their medical career.

To Apply: Applications are welcome from students in any year of medical school that are interested in the field of geriatric research.

Deadline: For more information, visit:

https://mstream.ucsd.edu/

Rock Sleyster, MD Memorial Scholarship

Description: The Rock Sleyster, MD Memorial Scholarship is given to medical students pursuing careers in psychiatry. The award amount is $2,500.

To Apply: Criteria for judging include academic ability, demonstrated interest in psychiatry, and financial need. The application includes three letters of reference (Dean's letter, psychiatry faculty letter), financial aid form, and transcript. The applicant must also submit a letter outlining career goals in psychiatry.

Deadline: The application deadline is in May. For more information, visit:

http://www.aie.org/scholarships/detail.cfm?id=13611

University of Pittsburgh Program in Mental Health Research

Description: The University of Pittsburgh offers the Program in Mental Health Research to medical students interested in a 12-month research experience. During the year, students will work closely with a faculty mentor, perform research, and prepare research for presentation and publication. The award amount is $21,180.

To Apply: Students may enter the program after their second or third years of medical school. Women, members of underrepresented minority groups, and individuals from disadvantaged backgrounds are encouraged to apply.

Deadline: For more information, visit:

http://www.psychiatry.pitt.edu/education/medical%20students/nimh-medical-student-fellowship

Zucker Hillside Hospital Medical Student Research Fellowship

Description: The Zucker Hillside Hospital Medical Student Research Fellowship offers medical students the opportunity to perform psychiatric research. Fellows will be paired with primary investigators based on stated interests in the specialty. An award amount of $1,250 per month will be provided for this summer fellowship.

To Apply: The fellowship is available to medical students during the summer between the first and second years. The application includes CV and a letter of interest.

Deadline: For more information, visit:

https://www.med.upenn.edu/mdresearchopps/documents/MedicalStudentResea rchFellowship.pdf

References

[1]Betty Ford Institute. Available at:
http://www.bettyfordinstitute.org/education/summer-institute-for-medical-students.php. Accessed June 3, 2014.

Chapter 36

Radiation Oncology Awards, Scholarships, & Grants

For medical students interested in receiving a scholarship, award, or grant in radiation oncology, begin by researching opportunities at your own institution. At the University of Maryland, the Department of Radiation Oncology is able to provide an annual scholarship opportunity to one medical student interested in performing radiation oncology research. To be eligible, the student must complete a research project in the department during the second, third, or fourth year of medical school. Make inquiries with your Department of Radiation Oncology to learn about award opportunities you may be eligible for.

External awards for research are also available. The most prestigious are awards and scholarships sponsored by the American Society of Radiation Oncology, Radiologic Society of North America, and Simon Kramer. These are described in this chapter.

Medical students often ask us if it's necessary to do research in the field of radiation oncology to enhance their chances of matching. In the 2012 NRMP Program Director Survey, 89% of radiation oncology residency programs cited "demonstrated involvement and interest in research" as a factor in selecting applicants to interview.[1] It's especially helpful to read the perspectives of radiation oncology residency program directors and faculty about the importance of research in the selection process. We offer you these perspectives on the next page.

Radiation Oncology Research for Medical Students: Perspectives of Residency Program Directors

- "Most successful applicants to residency programs have not only done research in the field, but either published it or presented it in at least poster form at national meetings," writes the Department of Radiation Oncology at the University of Washington.[2] How important is research experience to radiation oncology residency programs? According to Dr. Samir Sejpal, Radiation Oncology Career Advising Coordinator at Northwestern University, it is "very important and it always helps to do a research project related specifically to RO."[3] The Department of Radiation Oncology at the University of California Davis agrees with Dr. Sejpal. "Research is highly desirable; showing research interest and initiative adds to competitiveness."[4] "Coming into radiation oncology, we like people who have had a research interest," writes Dr. Barbara-Ann Millar, Program Director of the Radiation Oncology Residency Program at the University of Toronto. "If they have been able to present or publish on their work, that's great."[5]

- Pursuing research experience early in medical school is recommended. "Although it is not a 'mistake', developing an interest in radiation oncology late, particularly if one does not have a demonstrated excellent research portfolio in another medical specialty, is a challenge," writes the Department of Radiation Oncology at the University of Washington. "It is one thing for an MD/PhD student to identify rad onc as a career option at the beginning of 4th year; it is another for an otherwise strong student with no research experience to identify rad onc in September of 4th year."[2]

- Is it possible to match into radiation oncology without research experience? It is but applicants recognize the competitiveness of the specialty, and strive to strengthen their candidacy through research. "Indeed, for those medical students interested in matching into radiation oncology, because it is one of the most competitive graduate medical training programs to match into, many seek involvement in one or more research projects," writes Dr. Ariel Hirsch, Associate Professor and Director of Education in the Department of Radiation Oncology at Boston University.[6]

- "Clinical or basic science research of any kind but particularly in radiation oncology or general oncology related fields demonstrates not only interest and enthusiasm but initiative and resourcefulness" writes Dr. Jeffrey Kuo, Program Director of the Radiation Oncology Residency Program at the University of California Irvine. "Research resulting in publishable or published findings is often considered to show aptitude for an academic career. Though by no means mandatory, research experience is considered desirable."[7]

- It can take time to complete a research project, and applicants who wish to publish or present their work are urged to perform research sooner rather than later. "In general, the one-month rotation is not sufficient time to design and implement even a simple research project," writes the Department of Radiation Oncology at the University of Colorado.[8]

American Society of Radiation Oncology Minority Summer Fellowship Award

Description: The American Society of Radiation Oncology (ASTRO) offers this award to students interested in exploring the specialty. A total of $2,400 will be given to the award recipient to support basic, clinical, or translational research performed during the summer. Recipients will also receive $600 to attend the ASTRO Annual Meeting.

To Apply: Although preference is given to students in their first or second years, all medical students enrolled in U.S. medical schools are eligible to apply. The applicant must be a member of an underrepresented group in medicine. For application information and instructions, visit the website below.

Deadline: The deadline is in March. For more information, visit:

https://www.astro.org/Research/Funding-Opportunities/ASTRO-Supported-Grants/Minority-Summer-Fellowship/Index.aspx

Emory University Radiation Oncology Medical Student Scholarship

Description: The Department of Radiation Oncology at Emory University offers scholarships to medical students for mentored research by a faculty member in the department. Scholarship recipients will receive $3,500. Additional funds are available for students who submit an approved abstract for a national meeting.

To Apply: For application information, visit the website below.

Deadline: The deadline is in May. For more information, visit:

http://radiationoncology.emory.edu/news/2014/med-stdnt-schlrs-awrd-2014.html

Radiologic Society of North America Research Medical Student Grant

Description: The Radiologic Society of North America (RSNA) provides grants to medical students interested in performing medical imaging research. Award recipients are expected to engage in full time research for at least 10 weeks. This can take place during personal/vacation time or during a research elective. The award amount is $3,000. Another $3,000 will be provided by the sponsoring institution.

To Apply: To be eligible, students must be an RSNA member enrolled full time in an accredited North American medical school. The project must take place in a department of radiology, radiation oncology, or nuclear medicine. For application information and instructions, visit the website below.

Deadline: The deadline is in February. For more information, visit:

https://www.rsna.org/Research_Medical_Student_Grant.aspx

Simon Kramer Summer Externship in Radiation Oncology

Description: The Department of Radiation Oncology at Thomas Jefferson University offers the Simon Kramer Society Externship in Radiation Oncology. This externship allows students to gain exposure to the specialty. Up to two students are selected annually, and given the opportunity to spend six weeks in the department. Award recipients will participate in clinical, educational, and research activities.

To Apply: To be eligible, students must be in their first or second year of medical school in an accredited U.S. institution. For application instructions and information, visit the website below.

Deadline: The deadline is in March. For more information, visit:

http://www.jefferson.edu/university/jmc/departments/radiation_oncology/educa tion/Simon_Kramer_Externship.html

St. Jude Children's Research Hospital Pediatric Oncology Education Program

Description: Through this program, students can gain biomedical and oncology research experience. Students can perform laboratory or clinical research in a variety of departments, including anesthesiology, biochemistry, chemical biology & therapeutics, developmental neurobiology, diagnostic imaging, epidemiology and cancer control, oncology, immunology, infectious diseases, neuro-oncology, pathology, pharmaceutical sciences, radiation oncology, and structural biology. The program awards nearly 20 medical student positions. Students are expected to devote 9 weeks during the summer.

To Apply: To be eligible, medical students must meet minimum GPA requirements. Prior research experience and letter of recommendation from a research mentor are other components of the application. Only applicants from U.S. medical schools will be considered.

Deadline: The deadline is in February. For more information, visit:

http://www.stjude.org/poe

UCSF Radiation Oncology Medical Student Fellowship

Description: The Department of Radiation Oncology at UCSF offers an annual fellowship to fourth-year medical students. An award amount of $500 is given to support 8 weeks of research and clinical care in the department. A research paper may be written.

To Apply: To be eligible, you must have completed three years of medical school. The application includes CV, statement of interest, Dean's letter, transcripts, and letters of recommendation.

Deadline: The deadline is in April. For more information, visit:

http://radonc.ucsf.edu/academics_training/medical_programs/medical_student_ fellowship.html

References

[1] 2012 NRMP Program Directors Survey. Available at:
http://www.nrmp.org/wp-content/uploads/2013/08/programresultsbyspecialty2012.pdf. Accessed June 3, 2014.

[2] University of Washington Department of Radiation Oncology. Available at:
www.uwmedicine.org/.../Dept-Career-Advisors-Survey04072011.pdf.
Accessed March 4, 2013.

[3] Northwestern University Department of Radiation Oncology. Available at:
http://www.feinberg.northwestern.edu/education/current-students/career-development-residency/career-advising-specialties/radiation-oncology.html.
Accessed July 2, 2014.

[4] University of California Davis Department of Radiation Oncology. Available
at: http://www.slideshare.net/simon23/specific-residency-advice. Accessed
March 22, 2013.

[5] University of Toronto Department of Radiation Oncology. Available at:
http://cancerkn.com/interview-with-dr-barbara-ann-millar/. Accessed March
23, 2013.

[6] DeNunzio N, Parekh A, Hirsch A. Mentoring medical students in radiation
oncology. *J Am Coll Radiol* 2010; 7: 722-728.

[7] University of California Irvine Department of Radiation Oncology. Available
at: http://www.meded.uci.edu/education/residencyselection/radonc.html.
Accessed March 21, 2013.

[8] University of Colorado Department of Radiation Oncology. Available at:
http://www.ucdenver.edu/academics/colleges/medicalschool/departments/radiationoncology/Education/Documents/Medical%20student%20rotation%20objectives%2012.2009.pdf. Accessed March 23, 2013.

Chapter 37

Radiology Awards, Scholarships, & Grants

For medical students interested in receiving a scholarship, award, or grant in radiology, begin by researching opportunities at your own institution. At Stanford University, the Norman Bland Award is given to a senior medical student for Outstanding Performance in Radiology or Radiology Research. Ramin Saketkhoo was a recent recipient of this award. He received the honor because faculty members noted that he "embodies the qualities of an excellent radiologist; he is pleasant, polite, meticulous, smart, detail-oriented, and devoted to patient care. In addition, he is very productive; he completed four full-length manuscripts, wrote one book chapter and presented three abstracts in radiology."[1] Make inquiries with your Department of Radiology to learn about award opportunities you may be eligible for.

External awards for research are also available. The most prestigious are awards and scholarships sponsored by the Association of University of Radiologists, Society of Interventional Radiology, Mallinckrodt Institute, and Radiologic Society of North America. These are described in this chapter.

Medical students often ask us if it's necessary to do research in the field of radiology to enhance their chances of matching. In the 2012 NRMP Program Director Survey, 66% of radiology residency programs cited "demonstrated involvement and interest in research" as a factor in selecting applicants to interview.[2]

AMSER Henry Goldberg Medical Student Award

Description: The AMSER Henry Goldberg Medical Student Award is given annually to the student who submits an outstanding abstract for a paper, poster, or electronic exhibit for presentation at the Association of University Radiologists (AUR) Annual Meeting. The award amount is $500, and the winner will be recognized at the Annual Meeting.

To Apply: To be eligible, the applicant must be the first author or presenter of the research.

Deadline: The application deadline is in October. For more information, visit:

https://www.aur.org/Secondary.aspx?id=53

Association of University Radiologists Memorial Award

Description: The Association of University Radiologists (AUR) honors deceased members by bestowing the Memorial Award to the medical student, resident, or first-year fellow who submits an outstanding original paper in any aspect of radiology. The award amount is $1,000. The winning paper will be published in *Academic Radiology*. The winner will be asked to present the essay during the Annual Meeting.
To Apply: To be eligible, the applicant must be an AUR member. For application information and instructions, visit the website below.
Deadline: The application deadline is in October. For more information, visit:

http://www.aur.org/Secondary.aspx?id=56

Association of University Radiologists Trainee Prize

Description: The Association of University Radiologists (AUR) gives Trainee Prizes to medical students, residents, or first-year fellows for abstracts. Three prizes will be offered for the best papers, posters, or exhibits. The award amount is $750 for first place, $500 for second place, and $250 for third place. Winners will be asked to present abstracts during the Annual Meeting.
To Apply: To be eligible, the applicant must be the primary author and presenter of an accepted abstract.
Deadline: The application deadline is in October. For more information, visit:

http://www.aur.org/Secondary.aspx?id=58

Mallinckrodt Institute of Radiology Summer Research Program

Description: The Mallinckrodt Institute of Radiology offers this program to provide medical students with opportunities to perform research in the radiological sciences. Award recipients will receive $5,000 to perform research over a 10-week period during the summer.
To Apply: To be eligible, students must be enrolled in a United States medical school. Criteria for selection include academic record, coursework, essays, and recommendations. For application information and instructions, visit the website below.
Deadline: The deadline is in January. For more information, visit:

http://www.mir.wustl.edu/education/internal.asp?NavID=95

Radiologic Society of North America Research Medical Student Grant

Description: The Radiologic Society of North America (RSNA) provides grants to medical students interested in performing medical imaging research. Award recipients are expected to engage in full-time research for at least 10 weeks. This can take place during personal/vacation time or during a research elective. The award amount is $3,000. Another $3,000 will be provided by the sponsoring institution.

To Apply: To be eligible, students must be an RSNA member enrolled full time in an accredited North American medical school. The project must take place in a department of radiology, radiation oncology, or nuclear medicine. For application information and instructions, visit the website below.

Deadline: The deadline is in February. For more information, visit:

https://www.rsna.org/Research_Medical_Student_Grant.aspx

Society of Interventional Radiology Student Research Grant

Description: The Society of Interventional Radiology has created the Student Research Grant to provide funding for a summer project in an area important to the advancement of interventional radiology. Up to $4,000 will be awarded.

To Apply: To be eligible, students must be enrolled in an osteopathic or allopathic medical school in the United States or Canada. The application includes a detailed research plan, project budget, letter from Chairman of department where research will take place, and letter from designated research project advisor.

Deadline: The deadline is in February. For more information, visit:

http://www.sirfoundation.org/grants-awards/

Society of Interventional Radiology Medical Student Travel Scholarship

Description: The Society of Interventional Radiology provides medical students with complimentary meeting registration and travel stipend to attend the annual meeting. The award amount is $500.

To Apply: To be eligible, students must be enrolled in medical school. The application includes CV, letter of recommendation (optional), and answers to three essay questions:

- Besides IR, what other specialty most interests you? Please briefly compare and contrast what you perceive to be the strengths and weaknesses of that specialty with the strengths and weaknesses of IR.
- What do you hope to gain by attending the annual SIR meeting?
- Describe your exposure to the field of International Radiology at this point in your career. What is it about Interventional Radiology that has sparked your interest to explore the field in more depth?

Deadline: The deadline is in October. For more information, visit:

http://www.sirmeeting.org/index.cfm?do=cnt.page&pg=1039

References

[1]Stanford University. Available at:
http://news.stanford.edu/news/2004/june16/med-awards-616.html. Accessed
July 2, 2014.
[2]2012 NRMP Program Directors Survey. Available at:
http://www.nrmp.org/wp-
content/uploads/2013/08/programresultsbyspecialty2012.pdf. Accessed June 3,
2014.

Chapter 38

Urology Awards, Scholarships, & Grants

For medical students interested in receiving a scholarship, award, or grant in urology, begin by researching opportunities at your own institution. The Department of Urology at the University of Texas Southwestern Medical School honors one senior medical student with the John D. McConnell Award for Excellence in Urology. At the Northwestern University Feinberg School of Medicine, the top student rotating in urology receives the Urology Student Award. The C.R. Bard Urological Award is given to an Albany Medical College student who had the best performance during the clinical rotation in the Division of Urological Surgery. External awards for research are also available. The most prestigious are awards and scholarships sponsored by the American Urological Association, Urology Care Foundation, American Society of Andrology, Endourology Society, and New York Academy of Medicine. These are described below.

American Society of Andrology Outstanding Trainee Investigator Award

Description: The American Society of Andrology (ASA) offers the Outstanding Trainee Investigator Award to a trainee member who has presented the best original laboratory or clinical research report in andrology at the ASA Annual Meeting.
To Apply: Medical students are considered eligible for the award. For application information and instructions, visit the website below.
Deadline: For more information, visit:

http://andrologysociety.org/about/awards.aspx#7

American Society of Andrology Thomas S.K. Chang Trainee Travel Award

Description: The American Society of Andrology (ASA) offers the Thomas S.K. Chang Trainee Travel Award to cover the costs of travel to the ASA Annual Meeting.
To Apply: To be eligible, medical students must be first authors of accepted abstracts. Financial need is also a consideration.

Deadline: For more information, visit:

http://andrologysociety.org/about/awards.aspx#7

Arkansas Urologic Society Summer Medical Student Fellowship Program

Description: The Urologic Care Foundation and the Arkansas Urologic Society sponsor the Summer Medical Student Fellowship Program. Up to four grants will be given to medical students for summer research in the field. The fellowship may be completed at any institution but the student must return to the University of Arkansas following the fellowship.
To Apply: This program is open to medical students at the University of Arkansas.
Deadline: For more information, visit:

http://www.auanet.org/research/summer-medical-student-fellowships.cfm

CURE-UAB Travel Scholarship

Description: The Congress of Urologic Research and Education on Aging Underactive Bladder offers scholarships to cover the cost of travel to the conference. The award amount is $900.
To Apply: Ten scholarships will be given to women, minorities, and persons with disabilities. Eight scholarships will be given to junior investigators, which include medical students.
Deadline: The application deadline is in December. For more information, visit:

http://meded.beaumont.edu/cure-uab

Endourology Society Summer Student Scholarship

Description: The Endourology Society provides scholarships to medical students interested in conducting summer urologic research. Three recipients will receive the award annually. A recipient will be selected from the U.S., Asia, and Europe.
To Apply: For application information and instructions, visit the website below.
Deadline: The deadline is in January. For more information, visit:

http://www.endourology.org/about/summerscholarship.php

Ferdinand C. Valentine Medical Student Research Grant

Description: The New York Academy of Medicine has established The Ferdinand C. Valentine Medical Student Grant specifically for research in Urology. Up to three grants will be awarded with a stipend of $3,500 for students pursuing a clinical or basic science research project in the field of urology in the summer of the upcoming year. The stipend will be paid directly to the student in two equal installments (at the beginning and end of grant period).
To Apply: Competition is open to M.D. candidates attending medical school or conducting research in the greater New York area (New York City, Long Island, Westchester County, or New Jersey).
Deadline: The deadline is in May. For more information, visit:

http://www.nyam.org/grants/valentine-student.html

Herbert Brendler, MD Summer Medical Student Fellowship Program

Description: The Urology Care Foundation offers the Herbert Brendler Program to encourage medical students to join the field of urology through a summer fellowship. Up to six fellowships will be provided each year. Three fellowships will be made possible through the support of the Herbert Brendler, MD Research Fund and the Brendler Family. In addition, the Urology Care Foundation will sponsor up to three fellowships.
To Apply: The applicant must be an entering or current medical student immediately following the fellowship period. The sponsoring institution must be an accredited medical research institution or department of urology within the geographic boundaries of the American Urology Association Sections.
Deadline: The deadline is in February. For more information, visit:

http://www.urologyhealth.org/research/Brendler/intro.cfm

SMSNA Scholars in Sexuality Grants Program

Description: The Sexual Medicine Society of North America (SMSNA) awards grants to young investigators with an interest in conducting sexuality research. The amount of the award will vary depending upon the award recipient's experience, duration of research, and scope of project. The maximum award amount will be $5,000. Grant recipients must agree to present research abstracts at either the SMSNA Research Meeting or American Urological Association Annual Meeting.
To Apply: Medical students performing sexual medicine research in a variety of departments are eligible, including urology, psychology, psychiatry, gynecology, internal medicine, geriatrics, public health, physiology, genetics, molecular biology, social work, and law. The application includes a detailed description of the research question, letter of support from faculty mentor, one

page career development plan, two additional letters of support, and estimated time for project completion.

Deadline: The application deadline is in February. For more information, visit:

http://www.smsna.org/V1/index.php/grants/2014-research-grant-submission

Society for the Scientific Study of Sexuality Student Research Grants

Description: The Society for the Scientific Study of Sexuality (SSSS) awards two grants annually to students with an interest in performing human sexuality research. The award amount is $1,000. Names of award winners are announced during the SSSS Annual Meeting.

To Apply: Applicants must be SSSS members and enrolled in a degree-granting program. The application includes a 150-word abstract of the proposed research, longer abstract with bibliography, biographical sketch, and proposed budget. At the end of the research project, winners must submit a final report of their research.

Deadline: There are two application cycles with deadlines in February and June. For more information, visit:

http://www.sexscience.org/honors/student_research_grants/

Society for Male Reproduction and Urology Traveling Scholars Award

Description: The Society for Male Reproduction and Urology provides these awards to cover the costs of attending the American Society for Reproductive Medicine Annual Meeting.

To Apply: Medical students are eligible for the award. The applicant must be the presenting (first) author of an abstract. The application includes CV, letter of recommendation, and statement of career goals.

Deadline: For more information, visit:

http://www.smru.org/SMRUTravelingScholarsProgram/

Chapter 39

Medical Awards and Scholarships in Alabama

Medical students attending school in Alabama are eligible for a number of scholarships, awards, and grants. We recommend starting with your Office of Financial Aid and your school's website. Donors have provided funds to each medical school, and you may be eligible for these school-specific internal awards and scholarships. Students may also benefit from reviewing scholarship and award opportunities posted on the websites of other Alabama medical schools. Alabama residents who are attending medical school in other states may also be eligible for scholarships posted on the financial aid websites of Alabama medical schools. Below is a list of Alabama medical schools along with their websites.

Financial Aid Websites of Alabama Medical Schools	
Medical School	**Website**
University of Alabama School of Medicine	http://www.uab.edu/medicine/home/future-students/admissions/tuition-costs-and-payments/school-of-medicine-scholarships
University of South Alabama College of Medicine	http://www.southalabama.edu/finaid/com/
Alabama College of Osteopathic Medicine	http://www.acomedu.org/

State medical associations often have information about scholarships and loans available for students from the state or attending school in the state:

Medical Association of the State of Alabama
P.O. Box 1900
Montgomery, AL 36102-1900
(334) 954-2500
http://www.masalink.org/

Inquiries with your county medical society or association are recommended as well. We also encourage you to check with community foundations in the area in which you live to see if you are eligible for scholarships. Community Foundations in the State of Alabama are listed below.

Community Foundations in Alabama
Community Foundation of Baldwin County
Community Foundation of Greater Birmingham
Black Belt Community Foundation
Central Alabama Community Foundation
Community Foundation of Huntsville/Madison County
Community Foundation of Northeast Alabama
Community Foundation of Greater Decatur
Elmore County Community Foundation
Greater Huntsville Foundation
Riverbend Foundation
Community Foundation of South Alabama
Community Foundation of Southeast Alabama
Walker Area Community Foundation
Community Foundation of West Alabama

Alabama Board of Medical Scholarship Award

Description: Through this program, medical students in Alabama receive forgivable loans if they agree to practice primary care in a medically underserved community.
To Apply: For application information, visit the website below.
Deadline: For more information, visit:

http://www.bmsa.alabama.gov/

Alabama College of Osteopathic Medicine Blumberg Scholars (See Chapter 17)

Alabama Osteopathic Medical Association Scholarship (See Chapter 17)

Joanna F. Reed Memorial Scholarship

Description: Residents of Alabama and Northwest Florida who attend or have been accepted to private medical schools may apply for this award.
To Apply: Criteria for selection include academic performance, recommendations from instructors, financial need, and applicant's motivation, character, ability and promise as a practicing physician. Preference may be given to those seeking a career as general practitioners or internists.
Deadline: The application deadline is in May. For more information, visit:

http://www.athens.edu/financial/scholarships/Reed%20Medical%20Scholarship.pdf

Madison County Medical Society Scholarship

Description: These scholarships are available to medical students whose legal residence is Madison County (Alabama) at the time of medical school matriculation. The award amount is $10,000.

To Apply: Second, third, and fourth-year medical students are eligible to apply. Criteria for selection include academic performance. The completed application includes class rank and medical school transcript.

Deadline: The deadline is in July. For more information, visit:

http://www.madisoncountydoctors.org/alliance

Chapter 40

Medical Awards and Scholarships in Alaska

State medical associations often have information about scholarships and loans available for students from the state:

Alaska State Medical Assn
4107 Laurel Street
Anchorage, AK 99508
(907) 562-0304
https://www.asmadocs.org/

Inquiries with your county medical society or association are recommended as well. We also encourage you to check with community foundations in the area in which you live to see if you are eligible for scholarships. These foundations include the Alaska Community Foundation, Arctic Slope Community Foundation, and the Homer Foundation.

Arthur N. Wilson, M.D., Scholarship

Description: The American Medical Association (AMA) Foundation's Arthur N. Wilson, M.D. Scholarship was established for medical students who have graduated from a high school in Southeast Alaska. One $5,000 tuition assistance scholarship is awarded annually to a qualified medical student who is a graduate of a high school in Southeast Alaska and has consistently earned academic honors.
To Apply: Medical students who have graduated from a Southeast Alaskan high school may apply in any year of their enrollment in a U.S. accredited medical school and may apply multiple times during their medical education. Applicants must be permanent residents or citizens of the United States.
Deadline: The application deadline is usually in June. Please see the following link for further information:

http://www.ama-assn.org/ama/pub/about-ama/ama-foundation/our-programs/medical-education/arthur-n-wilson.page

Profile of a Winner

In 2012, the Arthur N. Wilson, M.D. Scholarship was awarded to Richard Stein, a second-year medical student at the University of Washington. Richard grew up in Sitka, Alaska and graduated from Sitka High School. He attended Brown University for his undergraduate studies.

"Richard has shown the initiative to pursue a diverse array of academic and cultural experiences," stated Dr. Clarence Chou, AMA Foundation Present, in an AMA article. "I am confident that whatever path he chooses, he will succeed and will impact the people of Alaska as well as patients around the world."[1]

Richard showed his dedication to the patients of Alaska when he worked with the native Alaskan youth in Southeast Alaska and volunteered with a physician in Sitka. He is also an Eagle Scout, a talented writer and the recipient of the University of Washington School of Medicine Service Award.

Northwest Osteopathic Medical Association Scholarships (See Chapter 17)

Osteopathic Foundation of Central Washington Scholarship (See Chapter 17)

Osteopathic Foundation of Yakima Scholarship (See Chapter 17)

References

[1]American Medical Association. Available at: http://www.ama-assn.org/resources/doc/ama-foundation/press-release-2012.pdf. Accessed January 14, 2014.

Chapter 41

Medical Awards and Scholarships in Arizona

Medical students attending school in Arizona are eligible for a number of scholarships, awards, and grants. We recommend starting with your Office of Financial Aid and your school's website. Donors have provided funds to each medical school, and you may be eligible for these school-specific internal awards and scholarships. Students may also benefit from reviewing scholarship and award opportunities posted on the websites of other Arizona medical schools. Arizona residents who are attending medical school in other states may also be eligible for scholarships posted on the financial aid websites of Arizona medical schools. Below is a list of Arizona medical schools along with their websites.

Financial Aid Websites of Arizona Medical Schools	
Medical School	**Website**
A.T. Still University School of Osteopathic Medicine in Arizona	http://www.atsu.edu/financial_aid/
Midwestern University Arizona College of Osteopathic Medicine	http://www.midwestern.edu/programs-and-admission/student-financial-services/loans.html
University of Arizona College of Medicine	http://financial-aid.medicine.arizona.edu/

State medical associations often have information about scholarships and loans available for students from the state or attending school in the state:

Arizona Medical Assn.
810 W. Bethany Home Rd.
Phoenix, AZ 85013 (602) 246-8901
http://www.azmed.org/

Inquiries with your county medical society or association are recommended as well. We also encourage you to check with community foundations in the area in which you live to see if you are eligible for scholarships. Community Foundations in the State of Arizona are listed on the following page.

Community Foundations in Arizona

Arizona Community Foundation
Cochise Community Foundation
FESAC Nogales
Greater Green Valley Community Foundation
Hopi Foundation
Legacy Foundation of Southeast Arizona
Oro Valley Community Foundation
Page/Lake Powell Community Foundation
Patagonia Regional Community Foundation
Scottsdale Charro Community Foundation
Sedona Community Foundation
Community Foundation for Southern Arizona
Sun Lakes Community Foundation
Tempe Community Foundation
Tuba City Community Foundation
Yavapai County Community Foundation
Yuma Community Foundation

Arizona Osteopathic Medical Association Clinical Case and Poster Forum

Description: The Arizona Osteopathic Medical Association invites students to submit entries for the Case Forum or abstracts for the poster competition. The top three entries to the Case Forum will be presented during the convention in April. All poster abstracts will be presented. $500 will be given to the winners of the Case Forum and Poster Competition.
To Apply: For more information, visit the website below.
Deadline: The deadline is in February. For more information, visit:

http://www.az-osteo.org/?page=StudentsResidents

Arizona Osteopathic Medical Association Scholarship

Description: The Arizona Osteopathic Medical Association awards two scholarships to osteopathic medical students each year. One is given to a student at the Arizona College of Osteopathic Medicine in Glendale and the other is awarded to a student at the School of Osteopathic Medicine in Mesa.
To Apply: To be eligible, the applicant must submit an essay addressing the question, "Why I Chose to Become an Osteopathic Physician."
Deadline: The deadline is in February. For more information, visit:

http://www.az-osteo.org/?page=StudentsResidents

Guinn B. Burton Medical Scholarship

Description: This scholarship provides support to undergraduate and graduate students pursuing a career in medicine.
To Apply: To be eligible, the applicant must demonstrate financial need. Preference is given to applicants from Arizona involved in community service. For application information and instructions, visit the website below.
Deadline: For more information, visit:

https://azfoundation.academicworks.com/opportunities/957

Yuma Unified Medical Associates Scholarship

Description: This scholarship provides support for a student to earn a medical degree and then return to Yuma to practice for at least one year.
To Apply: To be eligible, the applicant must be a legal resident of Yuma County, Arizona. For application information and instructions, visit the website below.
Deadline: For more information, visit:

https://azfoundation.academicworks.com/opportunities/972

Chapter 42

Medical Awards and Scholarships in Arkansas

Medical students attending school in Arkansas are eligible for a number of scholarships, awards, and grants. We recommend starting with your Office of Financial Aid and your school's website. Donors have provided funds to each medical school, and you may be eligible for these school-specific internal awards and scholarships. Arkansas residents who are attending medical school in other states may also be eligible for scholarships posted on the financial aid websites of Arkansas medical schools.

State medical associations often have information about scholarships and loans available for students from the state or attending school in the state:

Arkansas Medical Society
10 Corporate Hill Dr., Ste 300
Little Rock, AR 72205
(501) 224-8967
http://www.arkmed.org/

Inquiries with your county medical society or association are recommended as well. We also encourage you to check with community foundations in the area in which you live to see if you are eligible for scholarships. Community Foundations in the State of Arkansas are listed on the following page.

Conway Regional Health System Scholarship

Description: Ten scholarships are given annually to aid area students pursuing a career in a health-related field. Medical students are eligible to apply. The award amount is $1,000 to $2,500.
To Apply: The applicant must provide a copy of his or her class schedule and previous semester's grades. Criteria for selection include academic performance, leadership ability, references, essay, personal interview, and financial need.
Deadline: The deadline is in February. For more information, visit:

http://www.conwayregional.org/Scholarships

Community Foundations in Arkansas

Arkansas Community Foundation
Carroll County Community Foundation
Clark County Community Foundation
Cleburne County Community Foundation
Columbia County Community Foundation
Conway County Community Foundation
Craighead County Community Foundation
Endowment Foundation of Cross County
Delta Area Community Foundation
Community Foundation of Faulkner County
Fayetteville Area Community Foundation
Fort Smith Area Community Foundation
Endowment Foundation of Greene County
Hot Springs Area Community Foundation
Johnson County Community Foundation
Community Foundation of Lee County
Mississippi County Community Foundation
Monroe County Community Foundation
Endeavor Foundation
Ouachita Valley Community Foundation
Ozark Community Foundation
Phillips County Community Foundation
Pine Bluff Area Community Foundation
Pope County Community Foundation
Southeast Arkansas Community Foundation
St. Francis County Community Foundation
Texarkana Area Community Foundation
Twin Lakes Community Foundation
Union County Community Foundation
White County Community Foundation

Dr. Russell Harris Scholarship

Description: This scholarship is administered by the Arkansas Community Foundation, and is awarded to past graduates from Dumas County or Star City High School who are currently or planning to major in a medical related field. The award amount is $500.
To Apply: For application information and instructions, visit the website below.
Deadline: For more information, visit:

http://www.arcf.org/scholarships/ourscholarships/tabid/426/default.aspx

Greene and Clay Counties Medical Society and Auxiliary Scholarship

Description: This scholarship is administered by the Arkansas Community Foundation, and is awarded to pre-medical or medical students who are graduates of schools located in Greene County, Arkansas. The award amount is $1,000.
To Apply: For application information and instructions, visit the website below.
Deadline: For more information, visit:

http://www.arcf.org/scholarships/ourscholarships/tabid/426/default.aspx

L.A. Darling Company Scholarship

Description: This scholarship is administered by the Arkansas Community Foundation, and is awarded to pre-medical or medical students who are graduates of schools located in Greene County, Arkansas. The award amount is $1,000.
To Apply: For application information and instructions, visit the website below.
Deadline: For more information, visit:

http://www.arcf.org/scholarships/ourscholarships/tabid/426/default.aspx

Monroe County Medical Professionals Scholarship

Description: This scholarship is administered by the Arkansas Community Foundation, and is awarded to residents of Monroe County who are pursuing a degree in medical school, pharmacology, or nurse practitioner program. The award amount is $1,000.
To Apply: For application information and instructions, visit the website below.
Deadline: For more information, visit:

http://www.arcf.org/scholarships/ourscholarships/tabid/426/default.aspx

Chapter 43

Medical Awards and Scholarships in California

Medical students attending school in California are eligible for a number of scholarships, awards, and grants. We recommend starting with your Office of Financial Aid and your school's website. Donors have provided funds to each medical school, and you may be eligible for these school-specific internal awards and scholarships. Students may also benefit from reviewing scholarship and award opportunities posted on the websites of other California medical schools. California residents who are attending medical school in other states may also be eligible for scholarships posted on the financial aid websites of California medical schools. Below is a list of California medical schools along with their websites.

Financial Aid Websites of California Medical Schools	
Medical School	**Website**
Loma Linda	http://www.llu.edu/students/financial-aid/types-of-aid.php
Stanford	http://med.stanford.edu/md/financial_aid/
Touro University	http://studentservices.tu.edu/financialaid/
UCLA	http://www.medstudent.ucla.edu/offices/fao/current/
UC Davis	http://www.ucdmc.ucdavis.edu/financialaid/
UC Irvine	http://www.ofas.uci.edu/content/medical.aspx
UC Riverside	http://medschool.ucr.edu/admissions/financial_aid.html
UCSD	http://meded.ucsd.edu/index.cfm/asa/financial_aid/
UCSF	http://finaid.ucsf.edu/
USC	http://keck.usc.edu/en/About/Administrative_Offices/Office_of_Student_Affairs/Financial_Aid.aspx
Western University	https://www.westernu.edu/financial/financial-welcome/financial-about/

State medical associations often have information about scholarships and loans available for students from the state or attending school in the state:

California Medical Association
1201 J Street, Ste. 200
Sacramento, CA 95814
(916) 444-5532
http://www.cmanet.org/

Inquiries with your county medical society or association are recommended as well. We also encourage you to check with community foundations in the area in which you live to see if you are eligible for scholarships. Community Foundations in the State of California are listed below.

Community Foundations in California	
Amador Community Foundation	Community Foundation of Mendocino County
Anaheim Community Foundation	Community Foundation of Merced County
Avila Beach Community Foundation	Mission Viejo Community Foundation
Basin Wide Foundation	Greater Modesto Community Foundation
Bayview Hunter's Point Community Foundation	Community Foundation for Monterey County
Belvedere Community Foundation	Napa Valley Community Foundation
Berkeley Community Fund	North Valley Community Foundation
Calaveras Community Foundation	Community Foundation for Oak Park
California Community Foundation	Orange County Community Foundation
Central Valley Foundation	Palo Alto Community Fund
Claremont Community Foundation	Paradise Community Foundation
Coalinga Community Foundation	Pasadena Community Foundation
Coastal Community Foundation	Placer Community Foundation
Community Foundation Serving Riverside & San Bernadino Counties	Plumas Community Foundation
	Rancho Santa Fe Foundation
Community Foundation of San Joaquin	Richmond Community Foundation
Community Foundation of the Verdugos	Community Foundation of Richvale
Corcoran Community Foundation	River Valley Community Foundation
Corte Madera Community Foundation	Sacramento Region Community Foundation
Crockett Community Foundation	Community Foundation for San Benito County
Del Mar Foundation	San Diego Foundation
Desert Community Foundation	San Francisco Foundation
East Bay Community Foundation	Community Foundation San Luis Obispo County
El Dorado Community Foundation	
Fresno Regional Foundation	Santa Barbara Foundation
High Desert Community Foundation	Community Foundation Santa Cruz County
Community Foundation of Howard County	Valley Foundation
Humboldt Area Foundation	Saratoga Monte Sereno Community Foundation
Imperial Valley Community Foundation	Shasta Regional Community Foundation
Kern Community Foundation	Silicon Valley Community Foundation
La Palma Community Foundation	Solano Community Foundation
Lafayette Community Foundation	Community Foundation Sonoma County
Laguna Beach Community Foundation	Sonora Area Foundation
South Lake Tahoe Area Fund	Stanislaus Community Foundation
Legacy Endowment	Sutter Creek Community Benefit Foundation
Lincoln Community Foundation	Tahoe Truckee Community Foundation
Long Beach Community Foundation	Ventura County Community Foundation
Los Altos Community Foundation	Westside Community Foundation
Marin Community Foundation	Yolo Community Foundation
Martinez Community Foundation	

Aetna Foundation/NMF Healthcare Leadership Program (See Chapter 13)

Beca Foundation/Alice Newell Joslyn Medical Scholarship

Description: These scholarships are available to Latino students living in San Diego County. The award amount ranges from $500 to $2,000.
To Apply: For application information, visit the website below.
Deadline: The deadline is in March. For more information, visit:

http://www.becafoundation.org/scholarship.htm

Burbank Health Care Foundation – Medical Scholarship

Description: These scholarships are available to medical students who are from the Burbank area. The award amount is up to $10,000.
To Apply: Medical students from the Burbank area are eligible to apply. Preference is given to applicants who intend to work in Burbank following completion of residency.
Deadline: The deadline is in November. For more information, visit:

http://www.burbankhcf.org

California Academy of Family Physicians Student Research Grant Program

Description: The California Academy of Family Physicians administers the Student Research Grant Program to provide students with the opportunity to conduct research under the supervision of a practicing or academic family physician. The typical research experience takes place in the summer over a 2 – 3 month period.
To Apply: Students attending medical school in California are eligible to apply. The application includes a research proposal, CV, and letter of support from mentor.
Deadline: For more information, visit:

http://www.cafpfoundation.org/programs/research-grant-program/

California Community Service-Learning Program

Description: This program is administered by National Medical Fellowships. It provides an opportunity for medical students to make significant contributions in community service. Scholars will conduct a self-directed community health project at a site of their choice under the supervision of a mentor. The award amount is $5,000. Fourteen awards are available.
To Apply: California medical students are eligible to apply. Criteria for selection include demonstrated leadership and commitment to serving medically underserved communities. Applicants must be members of one of the following underrepresented groups: African American, Latino, or Native American.
Deadline: For more information, visit:

http://www.nmfonline.org/ccslp

California Medical Association Medical Student Community Leadership Grant

Description: The California Medical Association (CMA) Foundation offers grants to medical student organizations in California seeking support for health-related programs. The award amount is $250 to $1,000.
To Apply: Funding is available for initiatives in advocacy, community service, and other outreach efforts benefitting California communities.
Deadline: For more information, contact Leslie Barron-Smith at barron@thecmafoundation.org.

Dr. James L. Hutchinson and Evelyn Ribbs Hutchinson Scholarship

Description: This is a scholarship administered by the Silicon Valley Community Foundation. Medical school applicants must have graduated from high school in San Mateo or Santa Clara County. The award amount is $2,000.
To Apply: To be eligible, the applicant must have graduated from high school in San Mateo or Santa Clara County or have resided in that area during high school. Criteria for selection include personal motivation for excellence, academic achievement, integrity, leadership, and community involvement. The application includes personal statement, letters of reference, transcript, and financial need.
Deadline: The deadline is in May. For more information, visit:

http://www.siliconvalleycf.org

eQuality Scholarship Collaborative

Description: This scholarship is given to medical students who have demonstrated service to the lesbian/gay/bisexual/transgender community.
To Apply: Students attending medical school in California or California residents who are attending medical school out-of-state are eligible to apply.
Deadline: For more information, visit:

http://www.equalityscholarship.org/

Ethel O. Gardner Scholarship

Description: This scholarship is given by the California State Chapter of P.E.O.
To Apply: Female medical students are eligible to apply. Criteria for selection include integrity of character, scholastic ability, school/community activities, and financial need.
Deadline: The deadline is in February. For more information, visit:

http://www.peocalifornia.org/eogssc-public-page-no-menu.html

Fresno – Madera Medical Society Scholarship

Description: These scholarships are available to medical students who have been legal residents of either Fresno or Madera County for at least one year.
To Apply: For application information and instructions, visit the website below.
Deadline: The deadline is in May. For more information, visit:

http://www.fmms.org

Hellenic-American Medical & Dental Society of Southern California S. James Vamvas Scholarship (See Chapter 12)

Jayne M. Perkins Memorial Scholarship (See Chapter 18)

Jewish Vocational Service Scholarship

Description: The Jewish Vocational Service provides financial assistance to Jewish students from the Los Angeles area.
To Apply: To be eligible, the applicant must be Jewish, a U.S. citizen or permanent resident, and legal resident of Los Angeles County. Financial need is a major factor in granting awards.
Deadline: The deadline is in March. For more information, visit:

www.jvsla.org

Kaiser Permanente Medical Student Scholarship

Description: This scholarship is available to third-year medical students who demonstrate commitment and achievement in community leadership or population-based research. The amount of the award is $5,000.
To Apply: Applicants must be third-year medical students in good academic standing at an accredited U.S. medical school. Criteria for selection also include demonstrated commitment and achievement in community leadership or population-based research and two letters of support. Applicants must also have an interest in completing residency training in Northern California.
Deadline: The application deadline is in March. For more information, visit:

http://residency.kp.org/ncal/scholarships/

Kaiser Permanente Oliver Goldsmith, M.D. Scholarship

Description: Kaiser Permanente provides this scholarship to medical students who are committed to serving disadvantaged communities. Each awardee receives $5,000. Awardees are mentored by a Kaiser physician and are able to rotate at a Kaiser facility.

To Apply: This award is open to allopathic and osteopathic medical students. Scholarships are available to medical students entering their third or fourth years of medical school. Criteria for selection include demonstrated commitment to the advancement of culturally responsive care through leadership, research, or community involvement, intent to practice medicine in Southern California, and ability to participate in a rotation at a Kaiser facility. The application includes personal essay, letters of recommendation, and school transcript.

Deadline: The deadline is in February. For more information, visit:

http://residency.kp.org/scal/general_information/scholarship.html

---

Profile of a Winner

In 2010, Kevin Izquierdo and Marizabel Orellana, two medical students at the UCLA David Geffen School of Medicine, were among a group of students who received the Oliver Goldsmith, M.D., Scholarship. Scholarship winners receive a monetary award, participate in a mentoring program with Kaiser Permanente clinicians, and complete rotations at the institution.

Izquierdo was founder and director of the Street Medicine program at UC Riverside. Through this program, students work with volunteer physicians to provide care to homeless patients. "It touches people when they see that a physician has taken the time and effort to see them on their own terms," said Izquierdo.[1]

Orellana had developed the Junior Interns Program at the Renacimiento Community Center in Pomona. In this program, youth between the age of 11 and 18 years participate in leadership development activities to stimulate interest in the pursuit of higher education and careers in health care.[1]

Lakewood Medical Center Foundation Scholarships

Description: These scholarships are available to medical students who have a permanent address in certain California cities.

To Apply: To be eligible, the applicant must have a permanent address in one of the following cities: Lakewood, Bellflower, Paramount, Downey, Compton, Signal Hill, Hawaiian Gardens, Norwalk, Cypress, or Long Beach. Criteria for selection include academic achievement, financial need, and extracurricular activities.

Deadline: The deadline is in February. For more information, visit:

http://www.campusrn.com/scholarships/564/L/Lakewood_Medical_Center_Foundation_Scholarship.html

Mission Bay Hospital Auxiliary Scholarship

Description: The Mission Bay Hospital Auxiliary Scholarship is available to students pursuing a career in medicine. The average award amount is $5,000.
To Apply: To be eligible, the applicant must be a resident of San Diego County. Criteria for selection included minimum GPA and financial need.
Deadline: The deadline is in January. For more information, visit:

http://www.sdfoundation.org

Rebecca Lee, M.D. Scholarship Award (See Chapter 11)

Richard B. Irvine MD Memorial Scholarship Award

Description: Medical students who reside in or graduated high school from one of the following California cities are eligible to apply: Concord, Clayton, Antioch, Pittsburg, Benicia, Vallejo, Walnut Creek Pacheco, Pleasant Hill, Martinez, or Lafayette.
To Apply: Financial need is a consideration. The application includes proof of ties to the area (high school diploma or proof of residence) and letter of recommendation.
Deadline: For more information, contact:

Mt. Diablo Medical Center
Clinical Education Committee
2540 East Street
PO Box 4110
Concord, CA 94524-4110
(925) 674-2188.

Riverside County Medical Association Medical Student Scholarship Program

Description: This is a scholarship administered by the Riverside County Medical Association. It was developed to help students from Riverside County attend medical school.
To Apply: Allopathic and osteopathic medical students (or parents of medical students) who have been residents of California's Riverside County area for at least 5 years are eligible to apply. Financial need is a consideration. Preference is given to applicants who intend to return to the area to practice medicine.
Deadline: For more information, visit:

http://www.rcmanet.org/Physicians/INeedMedicalStudentResources.aspx

Ruth G. White Scholarship

Description: This scholarship is given by the California State Chapter of P.E.O.
To Apply: Female medical students who are residents of California are eligible to apply. Criteria for selection include integrity of character, scholastic ability, school/community activities, and financial need.
Deadline: The deadline is in February. For more information, visit:

http://www.peocalifornia.org/dlwrgw-public-page-no-menu.html

Scholarship Foundation of Santa Barbara

Description: Medical students who have graduated from high school in Santa Barbara County may apply for this scholarship. The award amount ranges from $500 to $5,000.
To Apply: To be eligible, the applicant must be a full-time medical student who graduated from high school in Santa Barbara County. The applicant must also have attended at least four of the six years between grades 7-12 at a Santa Barbara school. Following submission of the completed application, a personal interview is required.
Deadline: The deadline is in January. For more information, visit:

http://www.sbscholarship.org

Soroptomist International of Los Angeles Graduate Student Fellowship Award

Description: This scholarship is given by Soroptomist International of Los Angeles to support women in graduate study. The award amount is $3,500.
To Apply: Female medical students who are residents of California are eligible to apply. Criteria for judging include outstanding academic achievement, community service, and financial need. The application includes transcript and letters of recommendation. A personal interview is required.
Deadline: For more information, visit:

http://www.soroptimist-losangeles.com/awards.html#fellow

Southern California Lambda Medical Association Scholarship

Description: This scholarship is given by the Southern California Lambda Medical Association.
To Apply: All LGBT medical students are eligible to apply.
Deadline: For more information, visit:

http://sclma.org/directory/scholarships.php

Victor Grifols Roura Scholarship (See Chapter 13)

Washington Hospital Healthcare Foundation Scholarships

Description: This scholarship is given to two college students pursuing a career in medicine. The amount of the award is $2,500.
To Apply: Applicants must be enrolled in or have proof of admission to medical school. To be eligible, the applicant must be a resident or former resident of the Washington Township Health Care District or have significant ties to the District.
Deadline: For more information, contact the Foundation at (510) 791 – 3428.

West Los Angeles Japanese American Scholarship

Description: This scholarship honors the memory of Chiyo Hattori. The award amount is $2,500.
To Apply: Incoming and current medical students are eligible to apply. Criteria for selection include ongoing membership with JACL, WLA Chapter. For application information and instructions, visit the website below.
Deadline: For more information, contact Jean Shingematsu at (310) 207 – 3688.

Whittier Hospital Volunteer Scholarship

Description: Applicants having a permanent address in certain California cities may apply for the Whittier Hospital Volunteer Scholarship. The award amount ranges from $1,500 to $2,500.
To Apply: To be eligible, the applicant must have a permanent address in one of the following cities in the Whittier area: Whittier, La Habra, La Habra Heights, La Mirada, Santa Fe Springs, Pico Rivera, Hacienda Heights, La Puente, Rowland Heights, El Monte, and Norwalk. Criteria for selection include academic achievement, personal character, financial need, and commitment to hospital-related career.
Deadline: The deadline is in April. For more information, contact:

Muriel R. Biddinger
Chairman, Scholarship Committee
9080 Colima Road
Whittier , CA 90605
Tel: (562) 945-3561 ext. 6322

William E. Dochterman Scholarship

Description: The Sierra Sacramento Valley Medical Society administers this scholarship to medical students who completed high school in certain counties (see below).
To Apply: Medical students who completed high school in El Dorado, Sacramento, or Yolo counties may apply. Applicants must be enrolled in an accredited U.S. medical school on a full-time basis. The application includes

high school and college transcripts and three letters of reference. Criteria for selection include academic achievement and financial need.

Deadline: The application deadline is in July. For more information, visit:

http://www.ssvms.org/Programs/MedicalStudentScholarshipFund.aspx

References

[1]University of California Riverside. Available at: http://newsroom.ucr.edu/2379. Accessed April 2, 2014.

Chapter 44

Medical Awards and Scholarships in Colorado

Medical students attending school in Colorado are eligible for a number of scholarships, awards, and grants. We recommend starting with your Office of Financial Aid and your school's website. Donors have provided funds to each medical school, and you may be eligible for these school-specific internal awards and scholarships. Students may also benefit from reviewing scholarship and award opportunities posted on the websites of other Colorado medical schools. Colorado residents who are attending medical school in other states may also be eligible for scholarships posted on the financial aid websites of Colorado medical schools. Below is a list of Colorado medical schools along with their websites.

Financial Aid Websites of Colorado Medical Schools	
Medical School	**Website**
University of Colorado School of Medicine	http://www.ucdenver.edu/academics/colleges/medicalschool/education/Admissions/FinancialAid/Pages/financialaid.aspx
Rocky Vista University College of Osteopathic Medicine	http://www.rockyvistauniversity.org/financial_aid.asp

State medical associations often have information about scholarships and loans available for students from the state or attending school in the state:

Colorado Medical Society
7351 Lowry Blvd.
Denver, CO 80230
(720) 859-1001
http://www.cms.org/

Inquiries with your county medical society or association are recommended as well. We also encourage you to check with community foundations in the area in which you live to see if you are eligible for scholarships. Community Foundations in the State of Colorado are listed on the following page.

Community Foundations in Colorado

Aspen Community Foundation
Community Foundation Serving Boulder County
Broomfield Community Foundation
Community Foundation of Northern Colorado
Denver Foundation
Douglas County Community Foundation
Greater Eaton Community Foundation
Fort Lupton Community Area Fund
Grand Foundation
Community Foundation Serving Greeley & Weld County
Community Foundation of the Gunnison Valley
Longmont Community Foundation
Montrose Community Foundation
Pikes Peak Community Foundation
Rocky Mountain Community Foundation
Rose Community Foundation
Southern Colorado Community Foundation
Community Foundation Serving Southwest Colorado
Summit Foundation
Telluride Foundation
Trinidad Community Foundation
Vail Valley Foundation
Western Colorado Community Foundation
Windsor Community Foundation
Yampa Valley Community Foundation

Clinical Emergency Medicine & Research for the Underserved – Scholarship and Externship

Description: This scholarship is sponsored by the Committee for Diversity Awareness of the Denver Health Emergency Medicine Residency. Scholars have the opportunity to participate in patient care and research. Six scholarships are available. The award amount is $1,500 for the 4-week rotation.

To Apply: The program is open to fourth-year students at any U.S. medical school except the University of Colorado Denver. The application includes CV, letter of recommendation, USMLE Step 1 score, and transcript.

Deadline: For more information, visit:

http://denverem.org/index.php?option=com_content&view=article&id=272&Itemid=126

Colorado Society of Osteopathic Medicine Scholarship

Description: The Colorado Society of Osteopathic Medicine awards scholarships to upcoming second- and third-year osteopathic students. To be eligible, the applicant must be either a Colorado resident or a graduate of a Colorado high school, college or university. The applicant must intend to practice within the State of Colorado.

To Apply: For application information and instructions, contact the organization below.

Deadline: For more information, contact the organization at (303) 322 – 1722 or (800) 527 – 4578.

Colorado Springs Osteopathic Foundation Scholarships

Description: The Colorado Springs Osteopathic Foundation awards up to five $10,000 scholarships to osteopathic medical students. Also available is the Walter S. Strode, D.O. Memorial Scholarship, a $1,000 scholarship given to one of the winners for fees, books, supplies, and equipment.

To Apply: To be eligible, applicants must be U.S. citizens and residents of Colorado with preference given to those from Southern Colorado. Applicants must be entering their third year of medical school at an accredited osteopathic institution. Awards may be renewed for an additional year if recipients remain in good standing. Criteria for selection include merit, motivation and service to the community, and financial need. The application includes class rank, transcript, GPA for first three semesters, MCAT scores, extracurricular activities, community service, personal essay, and CV.

Deadline: The deadline is in February. For more information, visit:

http://csof.org/scholarships.html

C.W. Smith Healthcare Scholarship

Description: The Parkview Foundation provides a healthcare scholarship to a Pueblo County resident enrolled in a healthcare program in Colorado. The award amount is $2,500.

To Apply: To be eligible, applicants must be a Pueblo County resident. Minimum GPA of 3.0 is required. Two letters of recommendation and an official transcript must be submitted.

Deadline: The deadline is in May. For more information, visit:

http://www.parkviewmc.com/ways-to-give/foundation-scholarship-program/

Denver Osteopathic Foundation Scholarship

Description: The Denver Osteopathic Foundation awards scholarships to osteopathic students who plan to practice in Colorado.

To Apply: To be eligible, applicants must either be residents of Colorado or have lived, worked, or attended college in Colorado. Only third- and fourth-year medical students can apply. The expectation is that scholarship winners will practice in Colorado following completion of training. Criteria for selection include academic performance, class standing, commitment to the osteopathic profession, references, extracurricular activities, volunteerism, intent to practice in Colorado, and financial need. The application includes letters of recommendation, medical school transcript, class rank, GPA, CV, statement of intent to practice in Colorado, personal statement, and copy of the most recent year's federal tax return.

Deadline: The deadline is in March. For more information, visit:

http://www.dofound.org/medicalenrichment/scholarship.html

La Plata Medical Society Scholarship

Description: The La Plata Medical Society awards scholarships to medical students with an interest in primary care. The award amount is $1,500.

To Apply: To be eligible, applicants should be third- or fourth-year medical students from Southwest Colorado. Preference will be given to those from La Plata, Montezuma, and Archuleta counties.

Deadline: The deadline is in August. For more information, visit:

http://laplatamedicalsociety.org/scholarships/

Medical Staff Healthcare Scholarship

Description: The Parkview Foundation provides a healthcare scholarship to a Pueblo County resident enrolled in a healthcare program in Colorado. The award amount is $5,000.

To Apply: To be eligible, applicants must be a Pueblo County resident. Minimum GPA of 3.0 is required. Two letters of recommendation and an official transcript must be submitted.

Deadline: The deadline is in May. For more information, visit:

http://www.parkviewmc.com/ways-to-give/foundation-scholarship-program/

Saccomanno Higher Education Foundation Scholarship

Description: Medical students who are residents of Mesa County in Colorado or Carbon County in Utah are eligible for this scholarship. Criteria for selection include financial need, strength of character, and sincerity in pursuing higher education to improve the lives of others.

To Apply: For application information and instructions, contact the organization below.

Deadline: The deadline is in April. For more information, contact Saccomanno Higher Education Foundation, Attention: Joanne Cornell or Marsha Harbert, P.O. Box 3788, Grand Junction, CO 81502-3788 or call (877) 808-7878.

Chapter 45

Medical Awards and Scholarships in Connecticut

Medical students attending school in Connecticut are eligible for a number of scholarships, awards, and grants. We recommend starting with your Office of Financial Aid and your school's website. Donors have provided funds to each medical school, and you may be eligible for these school-specific internal awards and scholarships. Students may also benefit from reviewing scholarship and award opportunities posted on the websites of other Connecticut medical schools. Connecticut residents who are attending medical school in other states may also be eligible for scholarships posted on the financial aid websites of Connecticut medical schools. Below is a list of Connecticut medical schools along with their websites.

Financial Aid Websites of Connecticut Medical Schools	
Medical School	**Website**
University of Connecticut School of Medicine	http://studentservices.uchc.edu/financial/
Yale University School of Medicine	http://medicine.yale.edu/education/finaid/index.aspx
Frank H. Netter School of Medicine at Quinnipiac University	http://www.quinnipiac.edu/academics/colleges-schools-and-departments/school-of-medicine/financial-aid/

State medical associations often have information about scholarships and loans available for students from the state or attending school in the state:

Connecticut State Medical Society
160 St. Ronan Street
New Haven, CT 06511
(203) 865-0587
http://csms.org/

Inquiries with your county medical society or association are recommended as well. We also encourage you to check with community foundations in the area in which you live to see if you are eligible for scholarships. Community Foundations in the State of Connecticut are listed on the following page.

Community Foundations in Connecticut

Branford Community Foundation
Jewish Foundation of Greater New Haven
Community Foundation of Northwest Connecticut
Connecticut Community Foundation
Community Foundation of Central Connecticut
Essex Community Fund
Fairfield County Community Foundation
Guilford Foundation
Hartford Foundation for Public Giving
Madison Foundation
Main Street Community Foundation
Meriden Foundation
Community Foundation of Middlesex County
Community Foundation of Greater New Britain
New Canaan Community Foundation
Community Foundation for Greater New Haven
Orange Foundation
Community Foundation of Eastern Connecticut
Valley Community Foundation

Aetna Foundation/NMF Healthcare Leadership Program (See Chapter 13)

Community Foundation of Eastern Connecticut Scholarship

Description: The Community Foundation of Eastern Connecticut offers scholarships to medical students.
To Apply: For application information and instructions, visit the website below.
Deadline: For more information, visit:

http://www.cfect.org/Scholarships/HowtoApplyforaScholarship/tabid/211/Default.aspx

Dr. Frank and Florence Marino Scholarship

Description: The Hartford Foundation for Public Giving provides this scholarship to medical students who have attended Connecticut public/parochial schools for at least eight years.
To Apply: To be eligible, the applicant must have attended public/parochial schools in Connecticut for at least eight years. Only applicants who have graduated from Connecticut high schools will be considered. Applicants should be in their second, third, or fourth year of medical school. Criteria for selection include academic achievement and financial need.

Deadline: The deadline is in May. For more information, contact Sarah Carlson at scarlson@hfpg.org or (860) 548 – 1888.

Hellenic Medical Society of New York Scholarship (See Chapter 12)

Henry I. Russek Travel Awards for FITs and Medical Students

Nolan Scholarship

Description: This is a scholarship administered by the Connecticut Academy of Family Physicians. Medical students from Middlesex County in Connecticut may apply.
To Apply: To be eligible, the applicant must be from Middlesex County in Connecticut.
Deadline: The deadline is in June. For more information, visit:

http://www.ctafp.org/scholarships

Orazio DiMauro Foundation Scholarship

Description: This is a scholarship administered by the Orazio DiMauro Foundation. This program is open to medical students who are residents of Bridgeport, Connecticut or surrounding areas.
To Apply: To be eligible, the applicant must be from Bridgeport or surrounding areas in Connecticut. Only allopathic medical students are eligible. The application includes honors, extracurricular activities, and personal statement.
Deadline: The deadline is in April. For more information, visit:

http://oraziodimauro.org/

Roberta and Joseph Czarsty Endowment Fund Scholarship Loan Program

Description: Through this program, non-interest scholarship loans are provided to medical students. Loans are forgiven for applicants who complete a residency in family practice.
To Apply: Preference is given to medical students from Connecticut who have demonstrated commitment to family practice. Students from other states with a commitment to the specialty will also be considered. Only applicants who have completed at least one year of medical school may apply.
Deadline: The deadline is in June. For more information, contact Craig Czarsty, M.D., Connecticut Academy of Family Physicians, P.O. Box 30 Bloomfield, CT 06002 or (800) 600-CAFP.

Rocco D. LaPenta Scholarship

Description: This scholarship provides assistance for tuition incurred by medical students. Only medical students who have attended secondary schools for at least three years in the states of Connecticut, New Hampshire, and Massachusetts are eligible. Applicants from New Hampshire are given preference.
To Apply: Criteria for selection include academic aptitude, achievement, and willingness to contribute to others or the community.
Deadline: For more information, visit:

http://www.citizensbank.com/scholarships/

Ryu Family Foundation Scholarship (See Chapter 12)

Swiss Benevolent Society Scholarship (See Chapter 12)

Wellsford and Mildred Clark Medical Memorial Scholarship

Description: This scholarship is administered by the Waterbury Medical Association. Third-year medical students who are residents of Connecticut may apply.
To Apply: Applicants must be residents of Connecticut for at least five years. Applicants must be enrolled in a not-for-profit medical school accredited by the AMA and/or the World Health Organization. The application includes transcript, board scores, extracurricular activities, community service, two letters of recommendation, Dean's letter, and personal statement describing the applicant's plan for his or her medical career. Financial need is also a consideration.
Deadline: The application deadline is in April. For more information, visit:

http://www.waterburymedicalassociation.org/Scholarship.html

Windham County Medical Association Scholarship

Description: This scholarship is available to medical students who are permanent residents of Windham County.
To Apply: Applicants must be enrolled in a U.S. or Canadian medical school. Proof of permanent residence in Windham County is required. The application includes a personal statement describing the reasons for submitting an award application and the motivations for pursuing a career in medicine.
Deadline: The application deadline is in May. For more information, contact:

Windham County Medical Association
Scholarship Committee
One Regency Drive, P.O. Box 30
Bloomfield , CT 06002-0030
Tel: (860) 243-3977
Tel: (800) 223-WCMA

Chapter 46

Medical Awards and Scholarships in Delaware

State medical associations often have information about scholarships and loans available for students from the state:

Medical Society of Delaware
131 Continental Dr., Ste. 405
Newark, DE 19713
(302) 658-7596
http://www.medsocdel.org/

Inquiries with your county medical society or association are recommended as well. We also encourage you to check with community foundations in the area in which you live to see if you are eligible for scholarships. These foundations include the Delaware Community Foundation and Greater Lewes Foundation.

Delaware Postsecondary Scholarship

Description: The state of Delaware administers this scholarship program for students who are residents of the state. The award amount is up to $2,200.
To Apply: Criteria for selection include financial need and merit.
Deadline: The application deadline is in April. For more information, contact:

Delaware Postsecondary Educational Commission
Carvel State Office Building
820 North French Street
Wilmington, DE 19801
(302) 571-3240

Dr. David & Ethel Platt Summer Fellowship

Description: Through the Dr. David & Ethel Platt Summer Fellowship, medical students are able to work closely with family physicians over a four-week period in Delaware. The mission of the fellowship is to excite medical students about the specialty of family medicine. The award amount is $2,500. Four fellowships are offered each year.

To Apply: The application includes two letters of recommendation.
Deadline: The application deadline is in April. For more information, visit:

http://www.delfamdoc.org/awards.php

Elsie B. Moore Scholarship

Description: Medical students who are legal residents of Delaware may apply.
To Apply: For application information and instructions, contact the organization below.
Deadline: For more information, contact Robbie.Testa@pncadvisors.com.

H. Fletcher Brown Scholarship

Description: Medical students who were born in Delaware and are residents of the state may apply for this scholarship.
To Apply: Osteopathic and allopathic medical students are eligible to apply.
Deadline: For more information, contact Robbie.Testa@pncadvisors.com.

Henry H. Stroud, MD Scholarship

Description: Medical students who are legal residents of Delaware may apply. The scholarship is administered by the Delaware Community Foundation.
To Apply: For application information and instructions, contact the organization below.
Deadline: For more information, contact SRP-CSR@ets.org

Ida Foreman Fleisher Fund (See Chapter 12)

Mark B. Holzman Scholarship

Description: Medical students who are residents of Delaware may apply for the Mark B. Holzman Scholarship. The award amount is up to $2,000.
To Apply: Criteria for selection include academic achievement and financial need. For application information and instructions, contact the scholarship trust.
Deadline: For more information, contact

Mark B. Holzman Scholarship Trust
c/o Wilmington Trust Company
Att: Personal Trust and Private Banking
3 South DuPont Highway
Georgetown, DE 19947-2802

Swiss Benevolent Society Scholarship (See Chapter 12)

Chapter 47

Medical Awards and Scholarships in Florida

Medical students attending school in Florida are eligible for a number of scholarships, awards, and grants. We recommend starting with your Office of Financial Aid and your school's website. Donors have provided funds to each medical school, and you may be eligible for these school-specific internal awards and scholarships. Students may also benefit from reviewing scholarship and award opportunities posted on the websites of other Florida medical schools. Florida residents who are attending medical school in other states may also be eligible for scholarships posted on the financial aid websites of Florida medical schools. Below is a list of Florida medical schools along with their websites.

Financial Aid Websites of Florida Medical Schools	
Medical School	**Website**
Florida Atlantic University Charles E. Schmidt College of Medicine	http://med.fau.edu/students/financial_aid/
Florida International University Herbert Wertheim College of Medicine	http://medicine.fiu.edu/education/md/undergraduate-medical-education/office-of-student-affairs/fin-aid/index.html
Florida State University College of Medicine	http://med.fsu.edu/index.cfm?page=financialAid.home
Lake Erie College of Osteopathic Medicine	http://lecom.edu/financial-aid.php
Nova Southeastern University College of Osteopathic Medicine	http://www.nova.edu/financialaid/
University of Central Florida College of Medicine	http://med.ucf.edu/administrative-offices/student-affairs/financial-services/applying-for-aid/
University of Florida College of Medicine	http://finaid.med.ufl.edu/
University of Miami Leonard M. Miller School of Medicine	http://admissions.med.miami.edu/
University of South Florida College of Medicine	http://health.usf.edu/medicine/studentaffairs/financial_aid/md_students/application_process.htm

State medical associations often have information about scholarships and loans available for students from the state or attending school in the state:

Florida Medical Association
P.O. Box 10269
Tallahassee, FL 32302
(850) 224-6496
http://www.flmedical.org/Index.aspx

Inquiries with your county medical society or association are recommended as well. We also encourage you to check with community foundations in the area in which you live to see if you are eligible for scholarships. Community Foundations in the State of Florida are listed below.

Community Foundations in Florida

Bonita Springs
Community Foundation for Brevard
Community Foundation of Broward
Cape Coral Community Foundation
Central Florida Foundation
Charlotte Community Foundation
Community Foundation of Collier county
Community Foundation of East Central Florida
Community Foundation for Northeast Florida
Coral Gables Community Foundation
Community Foundation of Northwest Florida
Community Foundation of the Florida Keys
Community Foundation of North Central Florida
Gulf Coast Community Foundation
Indian River Community Foundation
Key Biscayne Community Foundation
Lake Community Foundation
Givewell Community Foundation
Mt. Dora Community Trust
Community Foundation of North Florida
Ocean Reef Community Foundation
Okaloosa Community Foundation
Community Foundation for Palm Beach & Martin Counties
Pinellas Community Foundation
Plantation Community Foundation
Community Foundation of Sarasota County
Community Foundation of South Lake County
Southwest Florida Community Foundation
South Shore Council Community Foundation
Community Foundation of Tampa Bay
Community Foundation of Ocala Marion County
Miami Foundation
Winter Park Community Foundation

Basil L. King Medical Scholarship

Description: The Basil L. King Scholarship Foundation administers this scholarship for medical students. Applicants must be St. Lucie County, Florida residents.
To Apply: Allopathic and osteopathic medical students are eligible to apply.
Deadline: The deadline is in May. For more information, visit:

http://www.blksf.org/

Brevard Heart Foundation, Inc. Scholarship

Description: Medical students who are residents of Brevard County or have graduated from high school while living in Brevard County may apply for this scholarship.
To Apply: The application includes transcripts, proof of residency, and three letters of reference. A letter stating who you are, your goals, and where you grew up in Brevard County is also required.
Deadline: The deadline is in June. For more information, visit:

http://brevardheartfoundation.org/docs/BHF_Scholarship-
Award_Application_2007.pdf

Dr. Robert C. Knapp Medical Student Award

Description: The Dr. Robert C. Knapp Medical Student Award allows medical students to shadow a gynecologic oncologist for a minimum of four weeks. At the end of the period, participants will submit a written description of the experience and preceptor. The award amount is $3,000.
To Apply: To be considered, you must be recommended by a medical school representative. Priority is given to Florida medical students.
Deadline: For more information, visit:

http://www.ovariancancerpbc.org/dr-robert-c-knapp-medical-student-award

Florida American Legion Medical School Scholarship

Description: Students entering their third year of medical school should consider applying for the Florida American Legion Medical School Scholarship. The award amount is $2,500. Two runners-up will each receive $1,500.
To Apply: To be considered, applicants must be entering their third year in one of Florida's allopathic medical schools. A nomination letter from the medical school dean or designate must be submitted. The letter should discuss the applicant's academic achievement, leadership ability in the first two years of medical school, awards and honors, research projects, and extracurricular activities.

Deadline: The application deadline is in April. For more information, visit:

http://www.floridalegion.org/Page%20Contents/Programs%20Content/Medical%20ScholarshipApp.pdf

Florida Medical Association Foundation Scholarship

Description: The Florida Medical Association Foundation offers the Foundation Scholarship. This is awarded to medical students who have shown commitment to organized medicine and public health initiatives. The award amount is $5,000.
To Apply: To be considered, applicants must attend one of Florida's six allopathic medical schools. One scholarship will be awarded for each school.
Deadline: For more information, visit:

http://www.flmedical.org/Medical_Students_-_Scholarships_and_Awards.aspx

Florida Medical Association Foundation Edward R. Annis, M.D. Scholarship

Description: The Florida Medical Association Foundation offers this award to medical students who have shown commitment to organized medicine and public health initiatives. The amount of the award is $1,000.
To Apply: To be considered, applicants must attend a U.S. allopathic medical school.
Deadline: For more information, visit:

http://www.flmedical.org/Medical_Students_-_Scholarships_and_Awards.aspx

Florida Medical Association Foundation Sanford A. Mullen, M.D. Award

Description: The Florida Medical Association Foundation offers this award to medical students who have demonstrated outstanding community service.
To Apply: To be considered, applicants must attend one of Florida's medical schools.
Deadline: For more information, visit:

http://www.flmedical.org/Medical_Students_-_Scholarships_and_Awards.aspx

Florida Osteopathic Medical Association Research Poster Competition

Description: The Florida Osteopathic Medical Association (FOMA) invites medical students, residents, and fellows to participate in the Research Poster Competition which takes place in conjunction with the Annual FOMA Convention in February. Applicants may enter in one of two categories – Experimental Research and Case Study. Three medical student winners are selected.
To Apply: For more information, visit the website below.
Deadline: For more information, visit:

http://www.foma.org/FOMA_PosterCompetition.htm

Hugh & Earle Fellows Memorial Loan Fund

Description: Medical students who are residents of Escambia, Santa Rosa, Okaloosa, and Walton County, Florida may apply for low-interest loans. Loans are interest free until four months of graduation.
To Apply: For more information, contact the organization below.
Deadline: For more information, contact:

Fellows Memorial Fund
c/o Ms. Virginia Santoni
Pensacola State College
1000 College Blvd.
Pensacola, FL 32504-8998
(850) 484-1682
Web: www.fellowsfund.org

Joanna F. Reed Memorial Scholarship (See Chapter 39)

Mary Jo and William Kirkley Scholarship

Description: Broward College graduates entering medical school may apply for the Mary Jo and William Kirkley Scholarship.
To Apply: To be considered, applicants must be a Broward College graduate who has been accepted into an accredited Florida medical school.
Deadline: For more information, visit:

http://www.broward.edu/sfs/

Pinellas Community Foundation Graham – Bowman Scholarship

Description: Graduates of Pinellas County high schools are eligible to apply for this scholarship.

To Apply: To be considered, medical school applicants must be graduates of Pinellas County high schools.
Deadline: For more information, visit:

http://www.pinellasccf.org/

Rotary Club of Miami: Thomas Brown McClelland Trust

Description: Through the Thomas Brown McClelland Trust, the Rotary Club of Miami provides scholarships to medical students who are permanent residents of Dade County, Florida.
To Apply: To be considered, applicants must be graduates of a Miami-Dade County High School and permanent residents of Dade County for at least the most recent five years. Criteria for selection include grades, positions held in extracurricular activities, and volunteer actions in the community.
Deadline: For more information, visit:

http://www.miamirotary.org

United Health Foundation/NMF Diverse Medical Scholars Program (See Chapter 13)

Chapter 48

Medical Awards and Scholarships in Georgia

Medical students attending school in Georgia are eligible for a number of scholarships, awards, and grants. We recommend starting with your Office of Financial Aid and your school's website. Donors have provided funds to each medical school, and you may be eligible for these school-specific internal awards and scholarships. Students may also benefit from reviewing scholarship and award opportunities posted on the websites of other Georgia medical schools. Georgia residents who are attending medical school in other states may also be eligible for scholarships posted on the financial aid websites of Georgia medical schools. Below is a list of Georgia medical schools along with their websites.

Financial Aid Websites of Georgia Medical Schools	
Medical School	**Website**
Emory University School of Medicine	https://www.med.emory.edu/education/financial/
Medical College of Georgia	http://www.gru.edu/finaid/
Mercer University School of Medicine	http://medicine.mercer.edu/student-services/financial-aid/
Morehouse School of Medicine	http://www.msm.edu/prospective_students/financial_aid.aspx
Philadelphia College of Osteopathic Medicine (Georgia Campus)	http://admissions.pcom.edu/costs-and-financial-aid/

State medical associations often have information about scholarships and loans available for students from the state or attending school in the state:

Medical Association of Georgia
1849 The Exchange, Ste. 200
Atlanta, GA 30339
(678) 303-9251
http://www.mag.org/

Inquiries with your county medical society or association are recommended as well. We also encourage you to check with community foundations in the area in which you live to see if you are eligible for scholarships. Community Foundations in the State of Georgia are listed below.

Community Foundations in Georgia

Greater Augusta Community Foundation
Community Foundation of Central Georgia
Community Foundation for the Central Savannah River Area
Community Foundation of the Chattahoochee Valley
Community Foundation for Greater Atlanta – Clayton Fund
Cobb Community Foundation
Community Foundation for Northeast Georgia
Coweta Community Foundation
Community Foundation for Greater Atlanta – Fayette Fund
Communities of Coastal Georgia Foundation
Community Foundation for Greater Atlanta – Morgan Fund
Community Foundation for Greater Atlanta – Newton Fund
Community Foundation for Greater Atlanta – NorthFulton Fund
North Georgia Community Foundation
Community Foundation of Northwest Georgia
Athens Area Community Foundation
Savannah Community Foundation
Community Foundation of Southwest Georgia
Community Foundation for Greater Atlanta
Community Foundation of West Georgia

G. Michael Shoffner, M.D. Scholarship

Description: Non-traditional medical students are eligible to apply for the G. Michael Shoffner, M.D. Scholarship. The award amount is $500 to $1,000. This is a renewable scholarship.

To Apply: To be considered, applicants must be at least 25 years of age, and enrolled in an accredited osteopathic or allopathic medical school in Georgia. Applicants must have lived and/or worked in Central Georgia for a minimum of 3 years prior to starting medical school. Counties in Central Georgia include Bibb, Baldwin, Butts, Coffee, Crawford, Houston, Jones, Lamar, Laurens, Monroe, Peach, Spalding, Taylor, Twiggs, Upson, and Wilkinson. The application includes resume and transcript.

Deadline: For more information, visit:

http://www.cfcga.org/page.aspx?pid=724

Georgia Chapter ACP Outstanding Medical Student in Volunteerism and Advocacy

Description: The Outstanding Medical Student in Volunteerism and Advocacy will be given to medical students in Georgia who have shown dedication to the service of others.
To Apply: Each medical school may nominate one outstanding medical student for this award. Preference is given to those with an interest in internal medicine.
Deadline: For more information, visit:

http://www.acponline.org/about_acp/chapters/ga/6-1-12.pdf

Georgia Osteopathic Medical Loan

Description: This student loan program is available to Georgia residents attending any accredited osteopathic institution in the U.S. This is a forgivable loan. Awardees must practice primary care medicine in underserved areas of Georgia following completion of training.
To Apply: For application information and instructions, visit the website below.
Deadline: For more information, visit:

http://www.gsfc.org

Samuel M. Goodrich M.D. Endowed Healthcare Scholarship

Description: Medical students are eligible to apply for the Samuel M. Goodrich M.D. Endowed Healthcare Scholarship. To be considered, the applicant must be a Georgia resident. Preference will be given to former and current residents of Baldwin, Georgia.
To Apply: The application includes an essay describing your vision for your career and how you will carry on the legacy of Dr. Samuel M. Goodrich. A CV and two letters of recommendation are also required.
Deadline: For more information, visit:

http://www.msm.edu/Libraries/Docs_Other/Samuel_M_Goodrich_Scholarhip_Application.sflb.ashx

Steve Dearduff Scholarship

Description: Medical students are eligible to apply for the Steve Dearduff Scholarship. The award amount is up to $2,500. Three scholarships are awarded annually.
To Apply: To be considered, applicants must be legal residents of Georgia. Criteria for judging include demonstrated history of commitment to community

service, potential for success in chosen field, minimum 2.0 GPA, and financial need.

Deadline: The application deadline is in March. For more information, visit:

http://www.cfgreateratlanta.org/grants-support/Scholarships/Steve-Dearduff-Scholarship-Fund-.aspx

Ty Cobb Scholarship Program

Description: This scholarship program was developed to support the education of Georgia residents, and medical students are eligible to apply. The award is renewable for one or more years, and can be used for education in any state.
To Apply: To be considered, applicants must be a Georgia resident. The application includes financial aid documents and letter of recommendation.
Deadline: For more information, visit:

http://www.msm.edu/Libraries/Docs_Other/Ty_Cobb_Educational_Foundation.sflb.ashx

United Health Foundation/NMF Diverse Medical Scholars Program (See Chapter 13)

Chapter 49

Medical Awards and Scholarships in Hawaii

Medical students attending school in Hawaii are eligible for a number of scholarships, awards, and grants. We recommend starting with your Office of Financial Aid and your school's website. Donors have provided funds to each medical school, and you may be eligible for these school-specific internal awards and scholarships. Hawaii residents who are attending medical school in other states may also be eligible for scholarships posted on the financial aid websites of Hawaii medical schools.

State medical associations often have information about scholarships and loans available for students from the state or attending school in the state:

Hawaii Medical Association
1360 Beretania St., 2nd Floor
Honolulu, HI 96814
(808) 536-7702
http://www.hmaonline.net/

Inquiries with your county medical society or association are recommended as well. We also encourage you to check with community foundations in the area in which you live to see if you are eligible for scholarships. Community Foundations in the State of Hawaii include the Hawai'i Community Foundation and Waipahu Community Foundation.

Cora Aguda Manayan Fund Scholarship

Description: This is a scholarship for medical students who are of Filipino ancestry. The program is administered by the Hawaii Community Foundation.
To Apply: The applicant must be a resident of the state of Hawaii. Preference is given to students studying in Hawaii. Criteria for selection include minimum GPA and demonstrated financial need.
Deadline: For more information, visit:

http://www.hawaiicommunityfoundation.org/search-scholarships

Dan & Pauline Lutkenhouse & Hawaii Tropical Botanical Garden Scholarship

Description: This is a scholarship available to residents of the Hilo Coast and the Hamakua Coast. To be eligible, the applicant must be a resident of the State of Hawaii. Undergraduate and graduate students, including medical students, may apply.
To Apply: Criteria for selection include minimum GPA and demonstrated financial need.
Deadline: For more information, visit:

http://www.hawaiicommunityfoundation.org

Dr. Hans and Clara Zimmerman Foundation Health Scholarship

Description: This is a scholarship available to residents of the State of Hawaii who are pursuing an education in a health field. Medical students are eligible to apply.
To Apply: Criteria for selection include minimum GPA and demonstrated financial need.
Deadline: For more information, visit:

http://www.hawaiicommunityfoundation.org

Edward J. and Norma Doty Scholarship Fund

Description: This is a scholarship available to residents of the State of Hawaii who are pursuing an education in medicine. Preference is given to students specializing in geriatric medicine or Alzheimer's disease.
To Apply: Criteria for selection include minimum GPA and demonstrated financial need.
Deadline: For more information, visit:

http://www.hawaiicommunityfoundation.org

George & Lucille Cushnie Scholarship

Description: This is a scholarship available to residents of the State of Hawaii who are pursuing an education in a medical-related field. Preference is given to students from the Island of Hawaii.
To Apply: Criteria for selection include minimum GPA, personal statement, and demonstrated financial need. The personal statement should describe the applicant's community service and how a future career may benefit the lives of Hawaii residents and/or advance Native Hawaiian culture.
Deadline: For more information, visit:

http://www.hawaiicommunityfoundation.org

Hokuli'a Foundation Scholarship

Description: This is a scholarship available to residents of the State of Hawaii who are pursuing an education in healthcare, education, or social work. The applicant must be a resident of North or South Kona. Preference is given to students who demonstrate an emphasis in advancing Native Hawaiian culture.
To Apply: Criteria for selection include minimum GPA and demonstrated financial need.
Deadline: For more information, visit:

http://www.hawaiicommunityfoundation.org

Robanna Fund Scholarship

Description: This is a scholarship available to residents of the State of Hawaii who are pursuing an education in medicine.
To Apply: Criteria for selection include minimum GPA and demonstrated financial need.
Deadline: For more information, visit:

http://www.hawaiicommunityfoundation.org

Chapter 50

Medical Awards and Scholarships in Idaho

State medical associations often have information about scholarships and loans available for students from the state:

Idaho Medical Association
305 W. Jefferson
Boise, ID 83702
(208) 344-7888
http://www.idmed.org/idaho/

Inquiries with your county medical society or association are recommended as well. We also encourage you to check with community foundations in the area in which you live to see if you are eligible for scholarships. Community Foundations in the State of Idaho include the Community Foundation of Teton Valley and Idaho Community Foundation.

Northwest Osteopathic Medical Association Scholarships

Description: The Northwest Osteopathic Medical Association Scholarships are awarded to medical students from Alaska, Idaho, Montana, Oregon, and Washington.
To Apply: Osteopathic medical students from Alaska, Idaho, Montana, Oregon, and Washington are eligible to apply. Applicants must be in their second, third, or fourth year of medical school. Priority is given to applicants who are committed to practicing primary care medicine in the Northwest.
Deadline: The application deadline is in May. Please see the following link for further information:

http://www.nwosteo.org/scholarship/

Osteopathic Foundation of Central Washington Scholarship (See Chapter 17)

Osteopathic Foundation of Yakima Scholarship (See Chapter 17)

Chapter 51

Medical Awards and Scholarships in Illinois

Medical students attending school in Illinois are eligible for a number of scholarships, awards, and grants. We recommend starting with your Office of Financial Aid and your school's website. Donors have provided funds to each medical school, and you may be eligible for these school-specific internal awards and scholarships. Students may also benefit from reviewing scholarship and award opportunities posted on the websites of other Illinois medical schools. Illinois residents who are attending medical school in other states may also be eligible for scholarships posted on the financial aid websites of Illinois medical schools. Below is a list of Illinois medical schools along with their websites.

Financial Aid Websites of Illinois Medical Schools	
Medical School	**Website**
Loyola University Chicago Stritch School of Medicine	http://www.stritch.luc.edu/admission/tuition-and-financial-aid
Midwestern University Chicago College of Osteopathic Medicine	http://www.midwestern.edu/programs-and-admission/student-financial-services.html
Northwestern University Feinberg School of Medicine	http://www.feinberg.northwestern.edu/admissions/tuition/
Rosalind Franklin University - Chicago Medical School	http://www.rosalindfranklin.edu/prospectivestudents/Student FinancialServices/financialaid.aspx
Rush Medical College	http://www.rushu.rush.edu/servlet/Satellite?c=RushUnivLev el1Page&cid=1206970210739&pagename=StudentServices %2FRushUnivLevel1Page%2FLevel_1_Student_Services_ Area_Home_Page
Southern Illinois University School of Medicine	http://www.siumed.edu/studentaffairs/financialaid.html
University of Chicago Pritzker School of Medicine	http://pritzker.uchicago.edu/admissions/financialaid/
University of Illinois School of Medicine	http://www.medicine.uic.edu/finaid

State medical associations often have information about scholarships and loans available for students from the state or attending school in the state:

Illinois State Medical Society
20 N. Michigan Ave., Suite 700
Chicago, IL 60602
(312) 782-1654
https://www.isms.org/home/

Inquiries with your county medical society or association are recommended as well. We also encourage you to check with community foundations in the area in which you live to see if you are eligible for scholarships. Community Foundations in the State of Illinois are listed below.

Community Foundations in Illinois	
Barrington Area Community Foundation	Highland Park Community Foundation
Boone County Community Foundation	Illinois Prairie Community Foundation
Community Foundation of Central Illinois	Community Foundation of Kankakee River Valley
Chicago Community Trust	
Community Foundation for the Land of Lincoln	Lake County Community Foundation
Community Foundation of Decatur/Macon County	McHenry County Community Foundation
	Metamora Community Foundation
DeKalb County Community Foundation	Moline Community Foundation
DuPage Community Foundation	Community Foundation of Grundy County
Community Foundation of East Central Illinois	Morton Community Foundation
Edgar County Community Foundation	Community Foundation of Northern Illinois
Greater Edwardsville Area Community Foundation	Oak Park – River Forest Community Foundation
	Community Foundation Serving W. Central Illinois & NE Missouri
Evanston Community Foundation	
Community Foundation of the Fox River Valley	Rochelle Area Community Foundation
Freeport Community Foundation	Southeastern Illinois Community Foundation
Galesburg Community Foundation	Southern Illinois Community Foundation
Geneseo is For Tomorrow (GIFT) Foundation	Will County Community Foundation

Advocate Good Shepherd Hospital Scholarship

Description: This is a scholarship for medical students who live in the hospital service area and will be attending school in Illinois.

To Apply: The applicant must reside in the hospital service area of Advocate Good Shepherd Hospital and attend school in Illinois. Criteria for selection include leadership, attitude, education, citizenship, personality, and financial need.

Deadline: The deadline is in April. For more information, visit:

www.advocatehealth.com/gshp/scholarships

Aetna Foundation/NMF Healthcare Leadership Program (See Chapter 13)

Central DuPage Auxiliary Scholarship

Description: This is a scholarship for medical students who reside in the Central DuPage Hospital core service area (Bartlett, Batavia, Bloomingdale, Carol Stream, Geneva, Glen Ellyn, Glendale Heights, Hanover Park, Lisle, Lombard, Naperville, North Aurora, Roselle, St. Charles, Villa Park, Warrenville, Wayne, West Chicago, Wheaton, and Winfield). Criteria for selection include minimum GPA, academic record, and strong interest in pursuing a healthcare career.
To Apply: For application information, visit the website below.
Deadline: The deadline is in March. For more information, visit:

http://www.cdh.org/About-Us/Auxiliary/Scholarship.aspx

Dr. David Monash/John Caldwell Scott Medical Student Scholarship (See Chapter 13)

DuPage Medical Society Foundation Scholarship

Description: Medical students who are residents of DuPage County in Illinois may apply for the DuPage Medical Society Foundation Scholarship.
To Apply: To be eligible, the applicant must be a resident of DuPage County.
Deadline: For more information, contact:

DuPage Medical Society Foundation
800 Roosevelt Road
Building B, Suite 300
Glen Ellyn, Illinois 60137
(708) 858 - 9603

Edward Arthur Mellinger Educational Foundation Graduate Loan

Description: This scholarship program is offered to graduate school applicants who are residents of Fulton, Henderson, Knox, McDonough, Mercer or Warrant County in Illinois. The award amount is up to $2,500.
To Apply: For application information, contact the organization below.
Deadline: The deadline is in May. For more information, contact Edward Arthur Mellinger Educational Foundation, Inc., 1025 East Broadway, Monmouth, Il 61462 or call (309) 734-2419.

Hugo Avalos Endowed Scholarship

Description: This is a scholarship for medical students who live in the hospital service area of Morris Hospital. The award amount is $5,000.
To Apply: The applicant must reside in the hospital service area of Morris Hospital, and live in Illinois. Criteria for selection include academic

performance, individual character, and overall merit. Preference may be given to students with military or Peace Corps background.
Deadline: The deadline is in April. For more information, visit:

http://www.morrishospital.org/foundation/scholarships/

Illinois Hospital Association Scholarship

Description: Medical students who are residents of Illinois may apply for the Illinois Hospital Association Scholarship. The award amount is $500.
To Apply: To be eligible, the applicant must be a resident of Illinois.
Deadline: For more information, contact:

Illinois Hospital Association & Health Systems Association
1151 East Warrenville Road
PO Box 3015
Naperville, IL 60566
(630) 505 - 7777

Iroquois County Scholarship

Description: Medical students who are residents of Iroquois County may apply for this scholarship. The award amount is $250 to $500.
To Apply: To be eligible, the applicant must be a resident of Iroquois County in Illinois.
Deadline: For more information, contact:

Iroquois County Medical Society
Director of Volunteer Services
Iroquois Memorial Hospital
Watseka, IL 60970
Phone: 815-432-7712

Jewish Federation of Metropolitan Chicago Academic Scholarship

Description: Scholarships are available for Jewish college and graduate students. Each year, $500,000 is made available to support full-time students.
To Apply: Applicants must be Jewish. To be eligible, applicants must have been born or raised in Cook County, Chicago metropolitan area, or Northwest Indiana. Exceptions to this rule will be made for applicants who have worked full-time in these areas for a period of one year prior to beginning professional education. Applicants must demonstrate desire to stay in the area after completing school. Criteria for judging include career promise and financial need.
Deadline: The application deadline is in February. For more information, visit:

http://jvschicago.org/scholarship/

Knights of Dabrowski Crusade for Education (See Chapter 12)

LaSalle County Medical Society Special Education Fund

Description: Medical students who are residents of LaSalle County in Illinois may apply for this award.
To Apply: To be eligible, the applicant must be a junior medical student. The applicant must be or have been a resident of LaSalle County at the time of admission.
Deadline: The application deadline is in April. For more information, contact:

Janet Beck Jakupcak, M.D., ABFP
151 Washington St.
Marseilles, IL 61341
Phone: 815-795-2171
Email: docbeck151@hotmail.com

McFarland Medical Education Foundation Scholarship

Description: Medical students who are from the Havana, Illinois area may apply for this scholarship.
To Apply: To be eligible, the applicant must agree to return to the Havana area and practice two years for each year of funding.
Deadline: For more information, contact:

McFarland Medical Education Foundation
The Havana National Bank
Trustee – Linda M. Butler
112 South Orange St.
P.O. Box 200
Havana, IL 62644
(309) 543 – 3361

Memorial Hospital Medical Student Grant Program

Description: Grant funds are available to allopathic and osteopathic students pursuing one of the following specialties: primary care, orthopaedic surgery, or cardiology. In return, recipients agree to practice medicine in the Belleville, Illinois area or a mutually agreed upon within Memorial Hospital's extended area. The grant amount is $12,000.
To Apply: For application information and instructions, contact the organization below.
Deadline: The deadline is in November. For more information, contact Stephanie Walter, Medical Student Grant Program, Memorial Hospital, Medical Directors Office, 4500 Memorial Drive, Belleville, IL 62226 or call (618) 257-5644 Ext. 6154.

Memorial Hospital of Carbondale Auxiliary Scholarship

Description: Medical students who are permanent residents of southern Illinois may apply for this scholarship.
To Apply: The application includes two letters of recommendation, transcripts, and one page essay describing the reasons for choosing your career and why you believe you should receive this scholarship.
Deadline: The application deadline is in May. For more information, contact Peggy Henson, Volunteer Services/Auxiliary Scholarship Program, Memorial Hospital of Carbondale, 405 West Jackson Street, Carbondale, IL 62901 or call (618) 549-0721.

Nesbitt Medical Student Foundation Scholarship

Description: Medical students who are residents of Illinois may apply for the Nesbitt Medical Student Foundation Scholarship.
To Apply: To be eligible, the applicant must be a resident of Illinois. Preference is given to women and former or current residents of DeKalb County who intend to practice family medicine in either DeKalb County or another county in Illinois with a population less than 50,000.
Deadline: The application deadline is in April. For more information, contact:

Nesbit Medical Student Foundation
c/o Trust Department
National Bank and Trust Co. of Sycamore
230 West State Street
Sycamore, IL 60178

Skelton Scholarship

Description: Medical students who are high school graduates and residents of Sangamon County in Illinois may apply for this scholarship.
To Apply: For application information and instructions, contact the organization below.
Deadline: The application deadline is in March. For more information, contact Mary Beth Anderson or Heather A. Smith at JPMorgan – IL2-8283, 1 East Old State Capital Plaza, Floor 3, Springfield, IL 62701-1320 or call (217) 525-9737.

Springfield Noon Lions Club Scholarship

Description: Healthcare students who are residents of Sangamon County in Illinois may apply for this scholarship. Medical students are eligible but preference will be given to sight and hearing oriented program students. The award amount is $1,000.
To Apply: For application information and instructions, contact the organization below.
Deadline: The application deadline is in April. For more information, contact John Albers, 532 Linden Lane, Williamsville, IL 62693.

St. Elizabeth Health Foundation Scholarship

Description: Medical students who are residents of Madison County or St. Clair County, Illinois are eligible to apply for this scholarship. The award amount is up to $15,000.
To Apply: For application information and instructions, contact the organization below.
Deadline: The application deadline is in May. For more information, contact Carmel Hobbs, Program Manager for the St. Elizabeth Health Foundation Scholarship Program at (507) 931-1682 or visit:

http://sms.scholarshipamerica.org/saintelizabeth/index.html

William E. McElroy Charitable Trust Scholarship

Description: Medical students who are male graduates of an accredited or private high school in Sangamon County, Illinois may apply for this scholarship. Preference is given to pre-medical, medical, and science students. Criteria for selection include high aptitude and interest in careers relating to heart disease and cancer.
To Apply: For application information and instructions, contact the organization below.
Deadline: The application deadline is in April. For more information, contact William E. McElroy Charitable Foundation College Education Grant/Loan US Bank, NA-Trust Department, P.O. Box 19264, Springfield, IL 62794-9264 or call (217) 753-7362.

William H. Walton, MD Student Scholarship

Description: This scholarship program is sponsored by the Southern Illinois Medical Association, and is offered to medical students from Southern Illinois. The award amount is $2,000. Three awards will be granted per year.
To Apply: For application information and instructions, contact the organization below.
Deadline: For more information, contact SIMA, Kathy Swafford, MD, 115 N. Main St., Anna, IL 62906 or call (618) 833-9355.

Chapter 52

Medical Awards and Scholarships in Indiana

Medical students attending school in Indiana are eligible for a number of scholarships, awards, and grants. We recommend starting with your Office of Financial Aid and your school's website. Donors have provided funds, and you may be eligible for these school-specific internal awards and scholarships.

State medical associations often have information about scholarships and loans available for students from the state or attending school in the state:

Indiana State Medical Assn.
322 Canal Walk, Canal Level
Indianapolis, IN 46202-3268
(317) 261-2060
http://www.ismanet.org/

Inquiries with your county medical society or association are recommended as well. We also encourage you to check with community foundations in the area in which you live to see if you are eligible for scholarships. Community Foundations in the State of Indiana are listed on the following page.

Dr. Ferrell W. Dunn Memorial Scholarship

Description: This is a scholarship for medical students who are graduates of high schools in Delaware County, Indiana.
To Apply: Criteria for selection include aptitude and desire to study and practice medicine, scholastic achievement, and financial need. One letter of recommendation is required. For application information and instructions, contact the organization below.
Deadline: The deadline is in April. For more information, visit:

http://cms.bsu.edu/-
/media/WWW/DepartmentalContent/Financial%20Aid/PDFs/DunnScholarship
.pdf

Community Foundations in Indiana	
Adams County Community Foundation	Legacy Fund Community Foundation
Benton Community Foundation	Community Foundation of Madison and
Blackford County Community Foundation	Jefferson County
Community Foundation of Bloomington and	Madison County Community Foundation
Monroe County	Marshall County Community Foundation
Blue River Community Foundation	Miami County Community Foundation
Community Foundation of Boone county	Montgomery County Community Foundation
Brown County Community Foundation	Community Foundation of Morgan County
Cass County Community Foundation	Community Foundation of Muncie & Delaware
Community Foundation Alliance	County
Community Foundation of Greater Fort Wayne	Newton County Community Foundation
Community Foundation of Switzerland County	Noble County Community Foundation
Community Foundation Partnership	Northern Indiana Community Foundation
Community Foundation of Crawford County	Ohio County Community Foundation
Crown Point Community Foundation	Orange County Community Foundation
Daviess County Community Foundation	Owen County Community Foundation
Dearborn Community Foundation	Parke County Community Foundation
Decatur County Community Foundation	Perry County Community Foundation
DeKalb County Community Foundation	Pike County Community Foundation
Dubois County Community Foundation	Porter County Community Foundation
Elkhart County Community Foundation	Portland Foundation
Fayette County Community Foundation	Posey County Community Foundation
Franklin County Community Foundation	Pulaski County Community Foundation
Gibson County Community Foundation	Putnam County Community Foundation
Community Foundation of Grant County	Community Foundation of Randolph County
Greene County Foundation	Ripley County Community Foundation
Hancock County Community Foundation	Rush County Community Foundation
Harrison County Community Foundation	Scott County Community Foundation
Hendricks County Community Foundation	South Madison Community Foundation
Henry County Community Foundation	Community Foundation of Southern Indiana
Heritage Fund – the Community Foundation of	Spencer County Community Foundation
Bartholomew County	Community Foundation of St. Joseph County
Huntington County Community Foundation	Steuben County Community Foundation
Community Foundation of Howard County	Tipton County Foundation
Huntingburg Foundation	Union County Foundation
Central Indiana Community Foundation	Unity Foundation of La Porte county
Western Indiana Community Foundation	Vanderburgh Community Foundation
Indianapolis Foundation	Vermillion County Community Foundation
Community Foundation of Jackson County	Community Foundation of Wabash County
Jasper Foundation Community Foundation	Wabash Valley Community Foundation
Jennings County Community Foundation	Warrick County Community Foundation
Johnson County Community Foundation	Washington County Community Foundation
Knox County Community Foundation	Wayne County, Indiana Foundation
Kosciusko County Community Foundation	Wells County Foundation
Community Foundation of Greater Lafayette	White County Community Foundation
LaGrange County Community Foundation	Whitley County Community Foundation

Dr. Higgins Scholarship

Description: This scholarship is available to students pursuing a medical degree. The amount of the scholarship is $10,000. It is awarded by the Community Foundation of Boone County, and may be used at any medical school in the U.S. To be eligible, the applicant must be a Boone or Tippecanoe County resident.

To Apply: For application information and instructions, visit the website below.

Deadline: The deadline is in May. For more information, visit:

http://www.communityfoundationbc.org/dr-higgins-scholarship-available-for-medical-students/

Dr. Leslie M. Baker Memorial Scholarship

Description: This scholarship is available to students pursuing a medical degree. It is awarded by the Dearborn Community Foundation. To be eligible, the applicant must be a resident of Dearborn, Ohio or Switzerland counties. Preference is given to students at the Indiana University School of Medicine.
To Apply: For application information and instructions, visit the website below.
Deadline: The deadline is in July. For more information, visit:

http://www.dearborncf.org

Indiana Association of Osteopathic Physicians and Surgeons Scholarship

Description: This scholarship is open to Indiana medical students who are in their first or second year at any osteopathic medical school.
To Apply: For application information and instructions, contact the organization below.
Deadline: For more information, contact the organization at (800) 942 – 0501.

Jewish Federation of Metropolitan Chicago Academic Scholarship (See Chapter 51)

Kelly-Prentiss Scholarship

Description: This scholarship is open to medical students who are residents of La Porte County.
To Apply: Criteria for selection include residency in La Porte County. To be eligible, applicants must have completed 3 years of education in an accredited medical institution.
Deadline: The deadline is in April. For more information, visit:

http://www.laportecountylife.com/community/serving/28293-unity-foundation-community-scholarship-applications-available-now

Michiana Osteopathic Medical Foundation Loan

Description: The Michiana Osteopathic Medical Foundation offers forgivable loans to medical students from Michigan or Indiana who are interested in practicing in the Michiana Indiana area.
To Apply: For application information, visit the website below.
Deadline: The application deadline is in May. For more information, visit:

http://www.omfmichiana.org

Motyka Dannin Osteopathic Educational Foundation Loan

Description: This is a forgivable loan available to students from Indiana. Applicants must be current first- or second-year osteopathic medical students interested in returning to Indiana to practice.
To Apply: Criteria for selection include good moral character and financial need. For application information, contact the organization below.
Deadline: The deadline is in December. For more information, contact dcoyle@inosteo.org or call (800) 942-0501

Peter V. Westhaysen Medical Education Trust Scholarship

Description: This scholarship is open to medical students who are residents of Lake County, Indiana.
To Apply: Criteria for selection include residency in Lake County, outstanding scholastic ability, and financial need.
Deadline: The deadline is in June. For more information, visit:

http://uflc.net/funds/contribute-online/kelly-prentiss-scholarship-fund/

Ronald D. Roberts Memorial Medical Scholarship

Description: This scholarship is available to medical students residing in southern Indiana. Preference is given to residents of Bartholomew, Monroe, and contiguous counties. The award amount is $4,000.
To Apply: The applicant must be currently enrolled in medical school and demonstrate financial need.
Deadline: For more information, visit:

http://www.crh.org/community-involvement/scholarships-and-loans.aspx

Westview Hospital Foundation, Inc. Forgivable Loan Program

Description: This loan program is available to third- or fourth-year osteopathic students who plan to return to Westview Hospital to practice osteopathic medicine. Students at any accredited osteopathic school may apply.
To Apply: For application information and instructions, contact the organization below.
Deadline: For more information, call (317) 923-0942 or contact Westview Hosptial Foudnation, Inc., Ruth Nisenshal, Executive Director, 3630 Guion Road, Indianapolis, IN 26222.

Chapter 53

Medical Awards and Scholarships in Iowa

Medical students attending school in Iowa are eligible for a number of scholarships, awards, and grants. We recommend starting with your Office of Financial Aid and your school's website. Donors have provided funds to each medical school, and you may be eligible for these school-specific internal awards and scholarships. Students may also benefit from reviewing scholarship and award opportunities posted on the websites of other Iowa medical schools. Iowa residents who are attending medical school in other states may also be eligible for scholarships posted on the financial aid websites of Iowa medical schools. Below is a list of Iowa medical schools along with their websites.

Financial Aid Websites of Iowa Medical Schools	
Medical School	Website
University of Iowa Carver College of Medicine	http://www.medicine.uiowa.edu/md/financial/
Des Moines College of Osteopathic Medicine	http://www.dmu.edu/financial-aid/tuition-and-budget-information/doctor-of-osteopathic-medicine/

State medical associations often have information about scholarships and loans available for students from the state or attending school in the state:

Iowa Medical Society
1001 Grand Ave.
West Des Moines, IA 50265
(515) 223-1401
http://www.iowamedical.org/

Inquiries with your county medical society or association are recommended as well. We also encourage you to check with community foundations in the area in which you live to see if you are eligible for scholarships. Community Foundations in the State of Iowa are listed on the next page.

Community Foundations in Iowa	
Akron Community Foundation	Greater Greenfield Community Foundation
Allamakee County Community Foundation	Hardin County Community Endowment
Buchanan Community Foundation	Foundation
Community Foundation of Carroll County	Ida County Community Betterment Foundation
Community Foundation of Cedar County	Greater Jefferson County Foundation
Greater Cedar Rapids Community Foundation	Community Foundation of Johnson County
Clarinda Foundation	Louisa County Community Foundation
Clay County Community Foundation	Community Foundation of Lyon County
Clayton County Community Foundation	Community Foundation of Greater Muscatine
Community Foundation of Greater Story County	Community Foundation of North Lee County
Greater Delaware County Community	Okoboji Foundation
Foundation	Pella Community Foundation
Foundation for the Future of Delaware County	Community Foundation of Greater Plymouth
Community Foundation of Greater Des Moines	County
DeWitt Area Community Foundation	Pottawattamie County Community Foundation
Community Foundation of Greater Dubuque	River Bluff Community Foundation
Dyersville Area Foundation for the Future	Siouxland Community Foundation
Empowering Adair County Foundation	South Central Iowa Community Foundation
Fort Dodge Community Foundation	Traer Community Foundation
Foundation for the Enhancement of Mitchell	Community Foundation of Van Buren County
County	Wakefield Community Foundation
Community Foundation of the Great River Bend	Community Foundation of Washington County
Greater Poweshiek Community Foundation	Community Foundation of Northeast Iowa
Greene County Community Foundation	

Des Moines Women's Club Liselotte Gurau Memorial Scholarship

Description: This scholarship is awarded to a female student pursuing a degree in healthcare. To be eligible, the applicant must be a legal resident of Polk, Boone, Dallas, Jasper, Madison, Marion, Story, or Warren counties in Iowa.
To Apply: Criteria for selection include essay and three letters of recommendation.
Deadline: The deadline is in January. For more information, visit:

http://www.desmoineswomensclub.org

Des Moines Women's Club Lois Dell Memorial Scholarship

Description: This scholarship is awarded to a female student pursuing a degree in an academic field. To be eligible, the applicant must be a legal resident of Polk, Boone, Dallas, Jasper, Madison, Marion, Story, or Warren counties in Iowa.
To Apply: Criteria for selection include essay and three letters of recommendation.
Deadline: The deadline is in January. For more information, visit:

http://www.desmoineswomensclub.org

Dr. George and Eunice Tice Scholarship

Description: This scholarship is awarded to medical students who are from the eight counties surrounding Mason City in Iowa. The award amount is $3,000.
To Apply: For application information, visit the website below.
Deadline: The deadline is in January. For more information, visit:

http://www.mercynorthiowa.com/workfiles/Tice_application14.pdf

Dr. William Walker Memorial Scholarship

Description: The Community Foundation of the Ozarks presents the Dr. William Walker Memorial Scholarship to students entering their final year of medical school in Iowa or Missouri. The award amount is $5,000.
To Apply: Criteria for selection include academic achievement (top 15% of class), superior clinical skills, and ability to communicate with patients effectively with empathy. The application includes two letters of recommendation.
Deadline: The deadline is in June. For more information, visit:

http://www.cfozarks.org/scholarship-tool.php

Kathie J. Lyman Scholarship

Description: The Polk County Medical Society Board administers the Kathie J. Lyman Scholarship. To be eligible, the applicant must be a legal resident of Iowa at the time of medical school application and attending an accredited medical or osteopathic school in Iowa. Two scholarships of $1,000 will be awarded.
To Apply: Criteria for selection include academic achievement (top 15% of class), superior clinical skills, and ability to communicate with patients effectively with empathy. The application includes two letters of recommendation, transcript, and essay indicating the reasons for selecting a career in medicine.
Deadline: The deadline is in November. For more information, contact the organization at (512) 288 – 0172 or visit:

http://pcms.org/KJlyman_Scholarship.html

Kathleen Fields Scholarship and Loan

Description: The Greene County Medical Center awards this scholarship/loan. Recipients will receive up to $5,000. Half of the amount will be a scholarship. The other half will be a loan. To be eligible, the applicant must be from Greene, Carroll, Calhoun, Webster, Boone, Dallas, or Guthrie counties in Iowa. Preference may be given to medical students at Creighton University and the Carver College of Medicine.

To Apply: Criteria for selection include good academic standing and financial need.
Deadline: The deadline is in July. For more information, contact:

Kathleen Fields Medical Scholarship Fund
c/o Greene County Medical Center
1000 West Lincolnway
Jefferson, IA 50129

United Health Foundation/NMF Diverse Medical Scholars Program (See Chapter 13)

Chapter 54

Medical Awards and Scholarships in Kansas

Medical students attending school in Kansas are eligible for a number of scholarships, awards, and grants. We recommend starting with your Office of Financial Aid and your school's website. Donors have provided funds to each medical school, and you may be eligible for these school-specific internal awards and scholarships. Kansas residents who are attending medical school in other states may also be eligible for scholarships posted on the financial aid websites of Kansas medical schools.

State medical associations often have information about scholarships and loans available for students from the state or attending school in the state:

Kansas Medical Society
623 SW 10th Ave.
Topeka, KS 66612
(785) 235-2383
http://www.kmsonline.org/

Inquiries with your county medical society or association are recommended as well. We also encourage you to check with community foundations in the area in which you live to see if you are eligible for scholarships. Community Foundations in the State of Kansas are listed below.

Community Foundations in Kansas	
Atchison Community Foundation	Kansas Rural Community Foundation
Central Kansas Community Foundation	Community Foundation of Southeast Kansas
Coffeyville Area Community Foundation	Legacy, A Regional Community Foundation
Columbus Community Foundation	McPherson County Community Foundation
Central Kansas Community Foundation – Butler County	Parsons Area Community Foundation
Council Grove Area Foundation	Rice County Community Foundation
Derby Community Foundation	Rossville Community Foundation
Community Foundation of Dickinson County	Greater Salina Community Foundation
Douglas County Community Foundation	Scott Community Foundation
Emporia Community Foundation	South Central Community Foundation
Golden Belt Community Foundation	Community Foundation of Southwest Kansas
Greater Manhattan Community Foundation	Thomas County Community Foundation
Hutchinson Community Foundation	Topeka Community Foundation
Jackson County Community Foundation	Western Kansas Community Foundation
Kansas Association of Community Foundations	Wichita Community Foundation

Kansas Osteopathic Medical Service Scholarship

Description: This scholarship program was developed to encourage primary care physicians to practice in rural parts of Kansas. Osteopathic students attending any accredited school are eligible to receive $15,000 per year. Preference is given to first-year students. In return, recipients agree to practice one year for each year of assistance provided.
To Apply: For application information and instructions, contact the organization below.
Deadline: For more information, contact Kansas Board of Regents, 1000 SW Jackson St, Suite 520, Topeka, KS 66612-1368 or call (785) 296-3518.

Mingenback Family Scholarship

Description: The Mingenback Family Scholarship is open to medical students from Barton County in Kansas. Preference is given to students attending school in Kansas.
To Apply: For application information and instructions, visit the website below.
Deadline: The application deadline is in March. For more information, contact:

http://www.goldenbeltcf.org/scholarships.php

United Health Foundation/NMF Diverse Medical Scholars Program (See Chapter 13)

Zola N. and Lawrence R. Nell Educational Trust Scholarship Program

Description: Medical or dental students who are graduates of high schools in Sedgwick County in Kansas may apply. To be eligible, applicants must agree to practice in Sedgwick County or the State of Kansas for a specified period of time.
To Apply: For application information and instructions, contact the organization below.
Deadline: The application deadline is in April. For more information, contact The Commerce Trust Company, Attn: Brian Adams, CTFA, Assistant Vice President, P.O. Box 637, Wichita, KS 67201-0637 or call (800) 627-6808 Ext. 3682.

Chapter 55

Medical Awards and Scholarships in Kentucky

Medical students attending school in Kentucky are eligible for a number of scholarships, awards, and grants. We recommend starting with your Office of Financial Aid and your school's website. Donors have provided funds to each medical school, and you may be eligible for these school-specific internal awards and scholarships. Students may also benefit from reviewing scholarship and award opportunities posted on the websites of other Kentucky medical schools. Kentucky residents who are attending medical school in other states may also be eligible for scholarships posted on the financial aid websites of Kentucky medical schools. Below is a list of Kentucky medical schools along with their websites.

Financial Aid Websites of Kentucky Medical Schools	
Medical School	**Website**
University of Kentucky College of Medicine	https://meded.med.uky.edu/financial-aid
University of Louisville School of Medicine	http://louisville.edu/medicine/financialaid
Pikeville Kentucky College of Osteopathic Medicine	http://www.upike.edu/College-of-Osteopathic-Medicine/financial_aid

State medical associations often have information about scholarships and loans available for students from the state or attending school in the state:

Kentucky Medical Association
4965 U.S. Hwy 42, Ste. 2000
Louisville, KY 40222-6301
(502) 426-6200
https://www.kyma.org/content.asp

Inquiries with your county medical society or association are recommended as well. We also encourage you to check with community foundations in the area in which you live to see if you are eligible for scholarships. Community Foundations in the State of Kentucky are listed on the next page.

Community Foundations in Kentucky	
Blue Grass Community Foundation	Community Foundation of Owensboro-Daviess
Central Kentucky Community Foundation	County
Foundation for Appalachian Kentucky	Shelby County Community Foundation
Community Foundation of Northern Kentucky	Community Foundation of South Central
Green River Area Community Foundation	Kentucky
Hardin County Community Foundation	Foundation for the Tri-State Community
Lake Area Community Foundation	Community Foundation of West Kentucky
Community Foundation of Louisville	Wilderness Trace Community Foundation
Community Foundation of Nelson County	

Baptist Regional Medical Center Medical Staff Academic Scholarship

Description: This scholarship program is open to students accepted or currently enrolled in an accredited health care program. To be eligible, the applicant must be a resident of Laurel, Whitley, or Knox County in Kentucky. The award amount is $1,500.
To Apply: For application information, visit the website below.
Deadline: The application deadline is in June. For more information, visit:

http://www.baptistregional.com/Left+Navigation/Community/Scholarships

Ephraim McDowell Health Scholarship

Description: Ephraim McDowell Health awards scholarships to students pursuing careers in health care. To be eligible, the applicant must be from Boyle and surrounding counties.
To Apply: For application information, contact the organization below.
Deadline: For more information, contact Stephen C. Kincer, Mountain Comprehensive Health Corporation, 226 Medical Plaza Lane, Whitesburg, KY 41858, phone 606.633.4823, email at skincer@ mtncomp.org.

Mountain Comprehensive Health Corporation Medical Resident Scholarship

Description: This scholarship program is open to fourth-year medical students and residents. The award amount is $20,000.
To Apply: For application information and instructions, contact the organization below.
Deadline: For more information, visit:

http://www.emhealth.org/index.php/aboutus/emh-news/816-ephraim-mcdowell-health-offers-health-care-scholarship

United Health Foundation/NMF Diverse Medical Scholars Program (See Chapter 13)

Chapter 56

Medical Awards and Scholarships in Louisiana

Medical students attending school in Louisiana are eligible for a number of scholarships, awards, and grants. We recommend starting with your Office of Financial Aid and your school's website. Donors have provided funds to each medical school, and you may be eligible for these school-specific internal awards and scholarships. Students may also benefit from reviewing scholarship and award opportunities posted on the websites of other Louisiana medical schools. Louisiana residents who are attending medical school in other states may also be eligible for scholarships posted on the financial aid websites of Louisiana medical schools. Below is a list of Louisiana medical schools along with their websites.

Financial Aid Websites of Louisiana Medical Schools	
Medical School	**Website**
Tulane University School of Medicine	http://tulane.edu/financialaid/hsc/
LSU School of Medicine (New Orleans)	http://www.lsuhsc.edu/financialaid/
LSU School of Medicine (Shreveport)	http://www.lsuhscshreveport.edu/FinancialAid/StudentFinancialAidCostofAttendance.aspx

State medical associations often have information about scholarships and loans available for students from the state or attending school in the state:

Louisiana State Medical Society
6767 Perkins Rd.
Baton Rouge, LA 70808
(225) 763-8500
http://www.lsms.org/site/

Inquiries with your county medical society or association are recommended as well. We also encourage you to check with community foundations in the area in which you live to see if you are eligible for scholarships. Community Foundations in the State of Louisiana are listed on the next page.

Community Foundations in Louisiana	
Community Foundation of Acadiana	Northshore Community Foundation
Baton Rouge Area Foundation	Community Foundation of Southwest Louisiana
Central Louisiana Community Foundation	Community Foundation of North Louisiana
Greater New Orleans Foundation	

United Health Foundation/NMF Diverse Medical Scholars Program (See Chapter 13)

Chapter 57

Medical Awards and Scholarships in Maine

State medical associations often have information about scholarships and loans available for students from the state:

Maine Medical Association
P.O. Box 190
Manchester, ME 04351
(207) 622-3374
http://www.mainemed.com/

Inquiries with your county medical society or association are recommended as well. We also encourage you to check with community foundations in the area in which you live to see if you are eligible for scholarships. Community Foundations in the State of Maine include the Maine Community Foundation and North Haven Foundation.

Beale Family Memorial Scholarship

Description: This scholarship is administered by the Maine Osteopathic Association. To be eligible, the applicant must be an osteopathic medical student who has been a resident of the State of Main for at least three years. Preference is given to applicants from Bangor, Maine. Students in their second, third, or fourth year of osteopathic education at any school in the U.S who have an interest in returning to Maine to practice may apply.
To Apply: For application information and instructions, contact the organization below.
Deadline: For more information, visit:

http://www.mainedo.org

Ryu Family Foundation Scholarship (See Chapter 12)

United Health Foundation/NMF Diverse Medical Scholars Program (See Chapter 13)

Chapter 58

Medical Awards and Scholarships in Maryland

Medical students attending school in Maryland are eligible for a number of scholarships, awards, and grants. We recommend starting with your Office of Financial Aid and your school's website. Donors have provided funds to each medical school, and you may be eligible for these school-specific internal awards and scholarships. Students may also benefit from reviewing scholarship and award opportunities posted on the websites of other Maryland medical schools. Maryland residents who are attending medical school in other states may also be eligible for scholarships posted on the financial aid websites of Maryland medical schools. Below is a list of Maryland medical schools along with their websites.

Financial Aid Websites of Maryland Medical Schools	
Medical School	**Website**
University of Maryland School of Medicine	http://www.umaryland.edu/fin/index.html
Johns Hopkins University School of Medicine	http://www.hopkinsmedicine.org/financialaid

State medical associations often have information about scholarships and loans available for students from the state or attending school in the state:

MedChi,
The Maryland State Medical Society
1211 Cathedral St
Baltimore, MD 21201
(410) 539-0872
http://www.medchi.org/

Inquiries with your county medical society or association are recommended as well. We also encourage you to check with community foundations in the area in which you live to see if you are eligible for scholarships. Community Foundations in the State of Maryland are listed on the next page.

Community Foundations in Maryland	

Baltimore Community Foundation
Community Foundation of Carroll County
Community Foundation of Southern Maryland
Community Foundation of Anne Arundel
  County
Community Foundation of Howard County
Community Foundation of Harford County
Community Foundation of the Eastern Shore
Foundation for Community Partnerships
	Community Foundation of Frederick County,
	  MD
	Mid-Shore Community Foundation
	Community Foundation for Montgomery
	  County
	Community Foundation for Prince George's
	  County
	Community Trust Foundation
	Community Foundation of Washington County
	  Maryland

ACAP – MAC Julian Cheng Hu Scholarship

Description: This scholarship is offered to Chinese American medical students whose primary residence is in Maryland, Virginia, or District of Columbia.
To Apply: Medical students at all levels can apply for the loan. Criteria for judging include academic achievement, community service involvement, and financial need.
Deadline: The application deadline is in December. For more information, contact:

Mark Li, M.D.
1721 University Blvd
Silver Spring, MD 20902

Baltimore City Medical Society Foundation Scholarship

Description: The Baltimore City Medical Society offers this award to medical students whose permanent residence is Baltimore city.
To Apply: To be eligible, applicants must have completed at least one year of medical school at any accredited allopathic or osteopathic institution. Applicants must have lived in Baltimore City for at least three years while attending high school. Criteria for judging include academic achievement, personal qualities, and financial need
Deadline: The application deadline is in June. For more information, visit:

Lisa B. Williams, Executive Director
Tel: 410- 625-0022
Email: info@bcmsdocs.org

Daniel R. Miller Trust Fund for Education (See Chapter 76)

Edith SeVille Coale Scholarship

Description: The Zonta Club of Washington, D.C. administers this scholarship program. The award amount is $5,000 to $8,000.

To Apply: To be eligible, applicants must be attending Georgetown University, George Washington University, Johns Hopkins University, or Howard University. Only female medical students who are entering their second or third year may apply. Criteria for judging include academic performance and financial need. Applicants must submit their application through their school's Financial Aid Office.

Deadline: The application deadline is in March. For more information, visit:

http://www.zontawashingtondc.org/scholarship-edith-seville-coale-medical.html

North Charles/Wyman Park Medical Staff Scholarship

Description: The Baltimore City Medical Society offers this award to medical students whose permanent residence is in Maryland.

To Apply: To be eligible, applicants must have completed at least one year of medical school either at Johns Hopkins University or University of Maryland. Applicants must have lived in the state for at least three years while attending high school.

Deadline: The application deadline is in June. For more information, contact:

Lisa B. Williams, Executive Director
Tel: 410- 625-0022
Email: info@bcmsdocs.org

Chapter 59

Medical Awards and Scholarships in Massachusetts

Medical students attending school in Massachusetts are eligible for a number of scholarships, awards, and grants. We recommend starting with your Office of Financial Aid and your school's website. Donors have provided funds to each medical school, and you may be eligible for these school-specific internal awards and scholarships. Students may also benefit from reviewing scholarship and award opportunities posted on the websites of other Massachusetts medical schools. Massachusetts residents who are attending medical school in other states may also be eligible for scholarships posted on the financial aid websites of Massachusetts medical schools. Below is a list of Massachusetts medical schools along with their websites.

Financial Aid Websites of Massachusetts Medical Schools	
Medical School	**Website**
Harvard Medical School	http://hms.harvard.edu/departments/financial-aid-harvard-medical-school
Tufts University School of Medicine	http://medicine.tufts.edu/Who-We-Are/Administrative-Offices/Office-of-Financial-Aid
Boston University School of Medicine	http://www.bumc.bu.edu/osfs/med/
University of Massachusetts Medical School	http://www.umassmed.edu/financialaid/

State medical associations often have information about scholarships and loans available for students from the state or attending school in the state:

Massachusetts Medical Society
860 Winter St.
Waltham, MA 02451-1411
(781) 893-4610
http://www.massmed.org/

Inquiries with your county medical society or association are recommended as well. We also encourage you to check with community foundations in the area in which you live to see if you are eligible for scholarships. Community Foundations in the State of Massachusetts are listed on the next page.

Community Foundations in Massachusetts	
Berkshire Taconic Community Foundation	Permanent Endowment Fund for Martha's
Boston Foundation	Vineyard Philanthropic Initiative
Brookline Community Foundation	Skillworks: Partners for a Productive Workforce
Cambridge Community Foundation	South Shore & Neponset Valley Community
Cape Cod Foundation	Foundation
Essex County Community Foundation	Community Foundation of Southeastern
Foundation for MetroWest	Massachusetts
Greater Lowell Community Foundation	Watertown Community Foundation
Community Foundation for Nantucket	Community Foundation of Western
Community Foundation of North Central	Massachusetts
Massachusetts	Woods Hole Community Foundation
	Greater Worcester Community Foundation

Berkshire District Medical Society Revolving Scholarship Loan

Description: The Berkshire District Medical Society offers this medical scholarship loan to students who are residents of Berkshire County in Massachusetts. The award amount is up to $5,000 per year, and is renewable. This is a loan at zero percent interest, and payment of the loan is not required until graduation. After graduation, repayment is required at a minimum of $100 per month.

To Apply: Allopathic and osteopathic medical students in the U.S. and Canada may apply. The application includes four letters of reference and transcript. Financial need is a consideration. A personal statement describing your concept of medicine and motivation to attend medical school and enter the medical profession is required.

Deadline: The deadline for the application is in April. For more information, visit:

http://www.massmed.org/Governance-and-Leadership/Districts-and-Regions/Berkshire-District-Medical-Society/#.U46rOHxOVtQ

Charles River District Medical Society Dr. George G. Katsas Scholarship Fund

Description: The Charles River District Medical Society Program offers this scholarship to a medical student who is a legal resident of one of five towns in the district (see below).

To Apply: Applicants must be a legal resident of one of five towns: Needham, Newton, Waltham, Wellesley, or Weston. To be considered, applicants must submit a CV, statement of personal goals, financial aid form, letter from medical school financial aid officer, statement of academic standing, and letter of recommendation from a district society member or faculty member. Students in their sophomore or junior years may apply. Sophomore scholarship award winners may be able to renew their scholarship for their junior year. Applicants are eligible if they attend any U.S. medical school.

Deadline: The application deadline is in December. For more information, visit:

http://www.massmed.org/Medical-Students/Scholarships-and-Financial-Resources/Massachusetts-Medical-Society-Scholarships-and-Grants/

Community Foundation of Western Massachusetts Scholarship

Description: The Community Foundation of Western Massachusetts offers numerous scholarships primarily to residents of Western Massachusetts. Some of these scholarships are for medical students.
To Apply: For more information, visit the organization below.
Deadline: For more information, visit:

http://www.communityfoundation.org

Dr. Marie E. Zakrewski Medical Scholarship (See Chapter 11)

Dr. Thomas P. and Edwina H. Devlin Medical Scholarship

Description: Medical students who have established residency in Melrose, North Reading, Reading, Stoneham, Wakefield, Wilmington, Winchester, or Woburn are eligible to apply. The award amount ranges from $500 to $4,000.
To Apply: To be eligible, applicants must be residents of one of the areas indicated above. Criteria for judging include scholastic standing, character, and financial need.
Deadline: The application deadline is in June. For more information, visit:

http://devlinmedicalscholarship.org/history.html

Edward Banks Kelley and Elza Kelley Foundation Scholarship

Description: Medical students who are residents of Barnstable County in Massachusetts are eligible to apply for this scholarship. Students who are not residents but have significant ties to the county will also be considered. The award amount ranges from $500 to $2,000. Preference is given to applicants who plan to return to the area and contribute to the health of county residents.
To Apply: Criteria for selection include merit and need.
Deadline: The application deadline is in April. For more information, visit http://kelleyfoundation.org/funding.html or contact:

Henry L. Murphy, Jr.
20 North Main Street
South Yarmouth, MA 02664
(508)775-3117

Edwards Scholarship

Description: This scholarship is only open to Boston residents who are attending medical school and under the age of 25. The award amount ranges from $250 to $5,000.
To Apply: Criteria for selection include scholastic ability, good character, and financial need.
Deadline: The application deadline is in March. For more information, contact the organization at (617) 426 – 4434 or:

Edwards Scholarship Fund
Ten Post Office Square, South
12th floor
Boston, MA 02109

Essex South District Medical Society Medical Student Scholarship Program

Description: Medical students who have established residency in an Essex South community may be considered for this award. These communities include Beverly, Danvers, Essex, Gloucester, Hamilton, Ipswich, Lynn, Lynnfield, Manchester, Marblehead, Middleton, Nahant, Peabody, Rockport, Salem, Saugus, Swampscott, Topsfield, and Wenham.
To Apply: Applicants must be Massachusetts Medical Society members who have established residency in an Essex South Community. The application includes CV, statement of academic standing from medical school, letter of recommendation from a district society member, and statement of personal goals. Preference is given to applicants with a desire to practice in the area.
Deadline: The application deadline is in January. For more information, visit:

http://www.massmed.org/Medical-Students/Scholarships-and-Financial-Resources/Massachusetts-Medical-Society-Scholarships-and-Grants/

Franklin District Medical Society Percy W. Wadman, M.D. Scholarship

Description: The Franklin District Medical Society offers this scholarship to medical student residents of Franklin County. The usual amount of this award is $1,000 to 1,500.
To Apply: Applicants must be Massachusetts Medical Society members who have established residency in Franklin County. Applicants whose family resides in the county are also eligible. The application includes letter of matriculation from medical school, copy of federal tax return, letter of recommendation submitted to medical school from undergraduate school. Criteria for judging include merit and financial need.
Deadline: The application deadline is in April. For more information, visit:

http://www.massmed.org/Medical-Students/Scholarships-and-Financial-Resources/Massachusetts-Medical-Society-Scholarships-and-Grants/

Hampshire District Medical Society and the Rollin M. Johnson, M.D. Student Grants Program

Description: Medical students residing in Western Massachusetts may be considered for this $2,000 award.

To Apply: Applicants must be full-time medical students who live or have lived in Western Massachusetts for at least five consecutive years. A completed application includes letter of matriculation from the medical school, and a copy of the letter of recommendation submitted to the medical school from the undergraduate school.

Deadline: The application deadline is in April. For more information, visit:

http://www.massmed.org/Medical-Students/Scholarships-and-Financial-Resources/Massachusetts-Medical-Society-Scholarships-and-Grants/

Massachusetts Medical Society Scholars Award Program

Description: The Massachusetts Medical Society offers the Scholars Award Program to medical students at Boston University, Harvard Medical School, Tufts University, and University of Massachusetts. Four fourth-year medical students from these schools will each receive $10,000.

To Apply: Applicants must be members of the Massachusetts Medical Society. Applications are available at each school's Office of Student Affairs.

Deadline: For more information, visit:

http://www.massmed.org/Medical-Students/Scholarships-and-Financial-Resources/Massachusetts-Medical-Society-Scholarships-and-Grants/

Massachusetts Medical Society Medical Information Technology Awards

Description: The Massachusetts Medical Society (MMS) annually offers the Medical Information Technology Award to one medical student and one resident/fellow physician for the creation of information technology solutions for medicine. Award recipients will receive $3,000.

To Apply: To be eligible, applicants must be MMS members enrolled in medical school or residency program at Harvard University, Tufts University, Boston University, or University of Massachusetts. Semi-finalists will be invited to present their projects to the Committee on Information Technology.

Deadline: The deadline is in November. For more information, visit:

http://www.massmed.org/Medical-Students/Scholarships-and-Financial-Resources/Massachusetts-Medical-Society-Scholarships-and-Grants/

Massachusetts Medical Society International Health Studies Grant Program

Description: The Massachusetts Medical Society (MMS) offers grants to defray the costs associated with study abroad. Four grants of $2,000 are available.
To Apply: To be eligible, applicants must be MMS members. Candidates who plan to serve underprivileged populations in the future are given preference.
Deadline: The application deadline is in September. For more information, visit:

http://www.massmed.org/Medical-Students/Scholarships-and-Financial-Resources/Massachusetts-Medical-Society-Scholarships-and-Grants/

Middlesex Central District Medical Society Scholarships

Description: Medical students living in certain towns in Massachusetts (see below) may apply for this scholarship. The award amount is $2,000 annually, and is given to one student from each of the four Massachusetts medical schools.
To Apply: To be eligible, applicants must be members of the Massachusetts Medical Society (MMS), and attend Boston University, Tufts University, Harvard University, or University of Massachusetts. Applicants must be legal residents of Acton, S. Acton, W. Acton, Bedford, Boxboro, Carlisle, Concord, W. Concord, Lincoln, S. Lincoln, Littleton, Maynard, or Stow.
Deadline: The application deadline is in December. For more information, visit:

http://www.massmed.org/Medical-Students/Scholarships-and-Financial-Resources/Massachusetts-Medical-Society-Scholarships-and-Grants/

Middlesex North District Medical Society Dr. Hugh Mahoney Scholarship Fund

Description: Medical students living in certain towns in Massachusetts (see below) may apply for this scholarship. The award amount is $1,000 to $1,250 annually.
To Apply: To be eligible, applicants must be members of the Massachusetts Medical Society (MMS). Only applicants who have completed one year of medical school in U.S. or Canada may apply. Applicants must be legal residents of Billerica, Chelmsford, Dracut, Dunstable, Groton, Lowell, Pepperell, Tewksbury, Tyngsboro, or Westford.
Deadline: The application deadline is in April. For more information, visit:

http://www.massmed.org/Medical-Students/Scholarships-and-Financial-Resources/Massachusetts-Medical-Society-Scholarships-and-Grants/

Norfolk District Medical Society Medical Student Scholarship Grant

Description: Medical students who are residents of the state of Massachusetts may apply for this scholarship.
To Apply: To be eligible, applicants must be members of the Massachusetts Medical Society (MMS) and the Norfolk District. Only applicants who have completed two years of medical school at one of the four Massachusetts medical schools may apply. Applicants must have been a legal resident of Massachusetts for five years.
Deadline: The application deadline is in March. For more information, visit:

http://www.massmed.org/Medical-Students/Scholarships-and-Financial-Resources/Massachusetts-Medical-Society-Scholarships-and-Grants/

Norfolk South District Medical Society Scholarship Program

Description: Medical students who are legal residents of any towns in this Massachusetts district (see below) may apply for this scholarship. The award amount is $500 to $1,000 annually.
To Apply: Only applicants who are enrolled in medical school in the U.S. may apply. Applicants must be legal residents of one of the towns in the district.
Deadline: The application deadline is in April. For more information, visit:

http://www.massmed.org/Medical-Students/Scholarships-and-Financial-Resources/Massachusetts-Medical-Society-Scholarships-and-Grants/

Profile of a Winner

James Besante, a second-year student at the University of New Mexico School of Medicine, was a recent recipient of the Nicholas Skala Student Activist Award. For several years, he has been advocating for a state constitutional amendment that would recognize health care as a fundamental right. He has attended hearings at the State Capitol where he served as an expert witness, and worked tirelessly to advance the bill through legislative committees.

His advocacy efforts have led to endorsements by numerous organizations, including the New Mexico Public Health Association, Network of Health Professionals for a National Health Program, and the New Mexico Health Equity Working Group.

He received his award at the PNHP Annual Meeting.[1]

Plymouth District Medical Society Scholarship

Description: Medical students who are legal residents of any towns in this Massachusetts district (see below) may apply for this scholarship. The award amount is $500 to $1,000 annually.
To Apply: Applicants must be legal residents of one of the towns in the district.
Deadline: The application deadline is in December. For more information, visit:

http://www.massmed.org/Medical-Students/Scholarships-and-Financial-Resources/Massachusetts-Medical-Society-Scholarships-and-Grants/

Rocco D. LaPenta Scholarship (See Chapter 45)

Roland Jackson Medical Scholarship

Description: Medical students who are graduates of either Swampscott or Marblehead High School in Massachusetts are eligible to apply for this scholarship. Residents of Swampscott and Marblehead who attended other schools will also be considered.
To Apply: Financial need is a consideration.
Deadline: The application deadline is in June. For more information, contact:

The Reverend Dean Pedersen
Jackson Medical Scholarship Committee
40 Monument Ave.
Swampscott, MA 01907
(781) 592-6081

Ryu Family Foundation Scholarship (See Chapter 12)

Suffolk District Medical Society Scholarship

Description: Medical student members of Massachusetts Medical Society and Suffolk District Medical Society may apply for this award. The award amount is $2,000, and three awards are available each year.
To Apply: Applicants must be members of the Massachusetts Medical Society (MMS) and Suffolk District Medical Society. The completed application includes cover letter with statement of personal goals, CV, statement of academic standing from medical school, and letter of recommendation from a MMS member. Selection criteria are quality of personal statement, academic and literary achievements, and interest in community service or advocacy.
Deadline: The application deadline is in December. For more information, visit:

http://www.massmed.org/Medical-Students/Scholarships-and-Financial-Resources/Massachusetts-Medical-Society-Scholarships-and-Grants/

Worcester District Medical Society Scholarship Fund

Description: Medical students who are legal residents of Central Massachusetts may apply for this scholarship.

To Apply: Applicants must be members of the Massachusetts Medical Society (MMS) and legal residents of Central Massachusetts. Only second, third, or fourth-year medical students enrolled in allopathic or osteopathic schools may apply.

Deadline: The application deadline is in December. For more information, visit:

http://www.massmed.org/Medical-Students/Scholarships-and-Financial-Resources/Massachusetts-Medical-Society-Scholarships-and-Grants/

Chapter 60

Medical Awards and Scholarships in Michigan

Medical students attending school in Michigan are eligible for a number of scholarships, awards, and grants. We recommend starting with your Office of Financial Aid and your school's website. Donors have provided funds to each medical school, and you may be eligible for these school-specific internal awards and scholarships. Students may also benefit from reviewing scholarship and award opportunities posted on the websites of other Michigan medical schools. Michigan residents who are attending medical school in other states may also be eligible for scholarships posted on the financial aid websites of Michigan medical schools. Below is a list of Michigan medical schools along with their websites.

Financial Aid Websites of Michigan Medical Schools	
Medical School	Website
University of Michigan Medical School	http://medicine.umich.edu/medschool/education/md-program/financial-aid
Michigan State University College of Human Medicine	http://mdadmissions.msu.edu/faq/pages/financialAid_faq.php
Michigan State University College of Osteopathic Medicine	http://www.com.msu.edu/Students/Financial_Aid/Financial_Aid.htm
Wayne State University School of Medicine	http://financialaid.med.wayne.edu/
Oakland University William Beaumont School of Medicine	https://www.oakland.edu/?id=29735&sid=340
Central Michigan University College of Medicine	https://www.cmich.edu/colleges/cmed/students/Pages/Financial%20Aid.aspx
Western University Homer Stryker MD School of Medicine	http://med.wmich.edu/education/students/future-students/your-finances-and-financial-aid

State medical associations often have information about scholarships and loans available for students from the state or attending school in the state:

Michigan State Medical Society
120 W. Saginaw St.
East Lansing, MI 48823
(517) 336-5768
http://www.msms.org/

Inquiries with your county medical society or association are recommended as well. We also encourage you to check with community foundations in the area in which you live to see if you are eligible for scholarships. Community Foundations in the State of Michigan are listed below.

Community Foundations in Michigan

Albion Community Foundation
Alger Regional Community Foundation
Allegan County Community Foundation
Ann Arbor Area Community Foundation
Athens Area Community Foundation
Baraga County Community Foundation
Barry Community Foundation
Battle Creek Community Foundation
Bay Area Community Foundation
Bedford Community Foundation
Berrien Community Foundation
Branch County Community Foundation
Cadillac Area Community Foundation
Canton Community Foundation
Capital Region Community Foundation
Cascade Community Foundation
Charlevoix County Community Foundation
Chippewa County Community Foundation
Community Foundation for Delta County
Dickinson Area Community Foundation
East Grand Rapids Community Foundation Trust
Community Foundation of Greater Flint
Four County Community Foundation
Greater Frankenmuth Area Community Foundation
Fremont Area Community Foundation
Grand Haven Area Community Foundation
Grand Rapids Community Foundation
Grand Traverse Regional Community Foundation
Gratiot County Community Foundation
Hillsdale County Community Foundation
Community Foundation of the Holland/Zeeland Area
Homer Area Community Foundation
Huron County Community Foundation
Jackson Community Foundation
Kalamazoo Community Foundation
Keweenaw Community Foundation
Lake County Community Foundation
Lapeer County Community Foundation

Leelanau Township Community Foundation
Lenawee Community Foundation
Les Cheneaux Community Foundation
Lowell Area Community Fund
M & M Community Foundation
Mackinac Island Community Foundation
Manistee County Community Foundation
Marquette County Community Foundation
Marshall Community Foundation
Mecosta County Community Foundation
Michigan Gateway Community Foundation
Midland Area Community Foundation
Community Foundation of Monroe County
Mt. Pleasant Area Community Foundation
Community Foundation for Muskegon County
Community Foundation for Northeast Michigan
Oakland County Community Trust
Community Foundation for Oceana County
Ontonagon County Community Foundation
Osceola County Community Foundation
Otsego County Community Foundation
Petoskey-Harbor Springs Area Community Foundation
Community Foundation of Greater Rochester
Roscommon County Community Foundation
Saginaw Community Foundation
Sanilac County Community Foundation
Shelby Community Foundation
Shiawassee Community Foundation
South Haven Community Foundation
Community Foundation for Southeast Michigan
Southeast Ottawa Community Foundation
Southfield Community Foundation
Sparta Community Foundation
Community Foundation of St. Clair County
Sturgis Area Community Foundation
Three Rivers Area Foundation
North Woodward Community Foundation
Tuscola County Community Foundation
Community Foundation of the Upper Peninsula
Wyoming Community Foundation Fund

Bernard F. and Melissa Anne Bailey Family Fund Healthcare Scholarship

Description: The Bernard F. and Melissa Anne Bailey Family Fund Healthcare Scholarship is administered by MidMichigan Health. Applicants must be residents or have immediate family living in one of the following mid-Michigan counties: Bay, Clare, Gladwin, Gratiot, Isabella, Midland, Montcalm, Ogemaw, Roscommon, and Saginaw.
To Apply: For application information, visit the website below.
Deadline: The application deadline is in March. For more information, visit:

https://www.midmichigan.org/careers/EducationOpportunities/ScholarshipsFinancialAid/bailey-scholarships/

Blue Cross Blue Shield of Michigan Foundation Excellence in Research Award for Students

Description: Medical students who publish research papers that contribute to health policy or clinical care are eligible for this award. The award amount is $1,000 for first place, $750 for second place, and $500 for third place.
To Apply: Applicants must be attending medical school in Michigan. To be eligible, the applicant must be nominated by a faculty member at the student's institution. A copy of the research article must be submitted with the application.
Deadline: The application deadline is in January. For more information, visit:

https://www.bcbsm.com/content/microsites/foundation/en/grants.html

Blue Cross Blue Shield of Michigan Foundation Student Award Program

Description: Medical students who research health care topics are encouraged to apply for this award. The award amount is $3,000.
To Apply: Applicants must be attending medical school in Michigan. The completed application includes research proposal, letter of endorsement from faculty member, transcript, resume, and biographical sketch.
Deadline: The application deadline is in April. For more information, visit:

https://www.bcbsm.com/content/microsites/foundation/en/grants.html

Michiana Osteopathic Medical Foundation Loan (See Chapter 52)

Muskegon County Medical Society Scholarship

Description: This scholarship is open to residents of one of the 12 local constituent school districts of the Muskegon Area Intermediate School District and graduates of a Muskegon County public or private school.

To Apply: Applicants must be attending medical school in Michigan. The completed application includes research proposal, letter of endorsement from faculty member, transcript, resume, and biographical sketch.

Deadline: The application deadline is in March. For more information, contact Marcy Joy, Program Officer, Scholarships, 425 W. Western Ave., Suite 200, Muskegon, MI 49440 or call (231) 332-4538.

Muskegon General Osteopathic Foundation Loan

Description: Through this forgivable loan program, medical students who live in the geographical area of the Western Michigan Osteopathic Association may receive $10,000 per year. Applicants attending any accredited osteopathic institution may apply.

To Apply: For application information and instructions, contact the organization below.

Deadline: For more information, contact Muskegon General Osteopathic Foundation, 110 W. Colby St., Whitehall, MI 49461-2004 or call (231) 894-5211.

S. Rudolph Light Medical Education Scholarship

Description: The S. Rudolph Light Medical Education Scholarship provides financial assistance to medical, dental, and nursing students. The award amount is up to $2,500. To be eligible, the applicant must have been a resident of Kalamazoo County while attending high school or a graduate of a Kalamazoo County high school applying to or admitted to a health professions school.

To Apply: The application includes an essay addressing why you merit consideration for this scholarship. Other components of the application include two letters of recommendation, transcript, and proof of admission if you are an accepted student. Financial need is a consideration.

Deadline: The application deadline is in March. For application information and instructions, visit:

http://www.kalfound.org/Scholarships/ScholarshipSearch/tabid/230/s/1328/Default.aspx

Saginaw County Medical Society Loans

Description: Low interest loans are provided to medical students by the Saginaw County Medical Society (SCMS). Loan amounts vary from $1,000 to $10,000. The interest is forgiven if the recipient establishes practice in Saginaw County following completion of residency.

To Apply: To be eligible, medical students must have ties to the Saginaw area. Preference is given to students who are past their first year of medical school.

Deadline: The application deadline is in March. For more information, contact SCMS at (989) 790 – 3590 or email Jamie Chamberlin at jdchamberlin@sbcglobal.net.

Chapter 61

Medical Awards and Scholarships in Minnesota

Medical students attending school in Minnesota are eligible for a number of scholarships, awards, and grants. We recommend starting with your Office of Financial Aid and your school's website. Donors have provided funds to each medical school, and you may be eligible for these school-specific internal awards and scholarships. Students may also benefit from reviewing scholarship and award opportunities posted on the websites of other Minnesota medical schools. Minnesota residents who are attending medical school in other states may also be eligible for scholarships posted on the financial aid websites of Minnesota medical schools. Below is a list of Minnesota medical schools along with their websites.

Financial Aid Websites of Minnesota Medical Schools	
Medical School	**Website**
Mayo Medical School	http://www.mayo.edu/mms/programs/md/tuition-and-financial-aid
University of Minnesota Medical School	http://www.meded.umn.edu/financial/

State medical associations often have information about scholarships and loans available for students from the state or attending school in the state:

Minnesota Medical Association
Chief Executive Officer
1300 Godward St. NE, Ste. 2500
Minneapolis, MN 55413
(612) 378-1875
http://www.mnmed.org/

Inquiries with your county medical society or association are recommended as well. We also encourage you to check with community foundations in the area in which you live to see if you are eligible for scholarships. Community Foundations in the State of Minnesota are listed on the following page.

Community Foundations in Minnesota	
Bloomington Community Foundation	Northfield Area Foundation
Central Minnesota Community Foundation	Northwest Minnesota Foundation
	Rochester Area Foundation
Duluth Superior Area Community Foundation	Saint Paul Foundation
	Southwest Initiative Foundation
Eden Prairie Community Foundation	St. Anthony Park Community Foundation
Grand Rapids Area Community Foundation	Stillwater Area Foundation
	Community Foundation for Carver County
Initiative Foundation	
Luverne Area Community Foundation	Virginia Community Foundation
Minneapolis Foundation	Walker Area Foundation
Minnesota Community Foundation	Wayzata Community Foundation
North Suburban Community Foundation	Winona Community Foundation

Affiliated Community Health Foundation (ACHF) Medical Student Scholarship

Description: This scholarship program was established to encourage medical students to practice in rural Minnesota communities. The award amount is $1,000. Allopathic and osteopathic students may apply. To be eligible, the applicant must demonstrate permanent residency within the service area of an ACMC affiliate clinic. This includes Benson, Granite Falls, Hancock, Litchfield, New London/Spicer, Marshall, Redwood Falls, and Willmar.
To Apply: The application includes two letters of reference. For application information and instructions, visit the website below.
Deadline: The application deadline is in June. For more information, visit:

http://www.acmc.com/scholarships/

Hugh J. Anderson Memorial Scholarship (See Chapter 13)

Minnesota Heart Research Scholarships

Description: This scholarship program offers three medical student awards to support heart research. The scholars are selected by the American Heart Association Midwest Affiliate Committee. Only medical students in Minnesota are eligible.
To Apply: For application information and instructions, visit the website below.
Deadline: The application deadline is in May. For more information, visit:

http://www.heart.org/HEARTORG/General/Minnesota-Heart-Research-Scholarships_UCM_316166_Article.jsp

Chapter 62

Medical Awards and Scholarships in Mississippi

Medical students attending school in Mississippi are eligible for a number of scholarships, awards, and grants. We recommend starting with your Office of Financial Aid and your school's website. Donors have provided funds to each medical school, and you may be eligible for these school-specific internal awards and scholarships. Students may also benefit from reviewing scholarship and award opportunities posted on the websites of other Mississippi medical schools. Mississippi residents who are attending medical school in other states may also be eligible for scholarships posted on the financial aid websites of Mississippi medical schools. Below is a list of Mississippi medical schools along with their websites.

Financial Aid Websites of Mississippi Medical Schools	
Medical School	**Website**
University of Mississippi School of Medicine	http://www.umc.edu/financialaid/
William Carey University College of Osteopathic Medicine	http://www.wmcarey.edu/financial-aid-wcucom

State medical associations often have information about scholarships and loans available for students from the state or attending school in the state:

Mississippi State Medical Association
P.O. Box 2548
Ridgeland, MS 39158-2548
601.853.6733
http://www.msmaonline.com/

Inquiries with your county medical society or association are recommended as well. We also encourage you to check with community foundations in the area in which you live to see if you are eligible for scholarships. Community Foundations in the State of Mississippi are listed on the following page.

Community Foundations in Mississippi

CREATE Foundation, Inc.
Community Foundation of East Mississippi
Greater PineBelt Community Foundation
Gulf Coast Community Foundation
Greater PineBelt Community Foundation
Community Foundation of Greater Jackson
Lowndes Community Foundation
Foundation for the Mid South, Inc.
Community Foundation of Northwest Mississippi
West Point Community Foundation

SREB Osteopathy Loan/Scholarship

Description: This scholarship program is open to osteopathic medical students enrolled in out-of-state schools. In return, recipients agree to practice osteopathic medicine the State of Mississippi. To be eligible, the applicant must be a current legal resident of Mississippi.

To Apply: For application information and instructions, visit the website below.

Deadline: For more information, visit:

http://riseupms.com/state-aid/sreb-osteopathy/

Chapter 63

Medical Awards and Scholarships in Missouri

Medical students attending school in Missouri are eligible for a number of scholarships, awards, and grants. We recommend starting with your Office of Financial Aid and your school's website. Donors have provided funds to each medical school, and you may be eligible for these school-specific internal awards and scholarships. Students may also benefit from reviewing scholarship and award opportunities posted on the websites of other Missouri medical schools. Missouri residents who are attending medical school in other states may also be eligible for scholarships posted on the financial aid websites of Missouri medical schools. Below is a list of Missouri medical schools along with their websites.

Financial Aid Websites of Missouri Medical Schools	
Medical School	**Website**
Washington University School of Medicine	http://wumsfinaid.wustl.edu/
Saint Louis University School of Medicine	http://www.slu.edu/student-financial-services-x48030
University of Missouri – Columbia School of Medicine	http://medicine.missouri.edu/financial/
University of Missouri – Kansas City School of Medicine	http://www.sfa.umkc.edu/site2/health_profess ionals.cfm?info_pane=3
A.T. Still University Kirksville College of Osteopathic Medicine	http://www.atsu.edu/kcom/programs/osteopat hic_medicine/financial_aid.htm
Kansas City University of Medicine and Biosciences College of Osteopathic Medicine	http://www.kcumb.edu/admissions/financial-aid/tuition-fees/

State medical associations often have information about scholarships and loans available for students from the state or attending school in the state:

Missouri State Medical Association
113 Madison Street
P.O. Box 1028
Jefferson City, Missouri 65102
800-869-6762
http://www.msma.org/mx/hm.asp?id=home#.VC2q6Hx0xtQ

Inquiries with your county medical society or association are recommended as well. We also encourage you to check with community foundations in the area in which you live to see if you are eligible for scholarships. Community Foundations in the State of Missouri are listed below.

Community Foundations in Missouri

Community Capital Fund
Community Foundation of Central Missouri
Community Foundation of Northwest Missouri, Inc.
Greater Kansas City Community Foundation
Northeast Missouri Community Foundation
Community Foundation of the Ozarks
Greater Saint Louis Community Foundation
Community Foundation of Steelville, MO
Truman Heartland Community Foundation
Willow Springs Community Foundation

Boone County Medical Society Scholarship

Description: The Boone County Medical Society awards this scholarship to medical students who have completed the first semester of their third year of medical school. The award amount is $2,000. To be eligible, the applicant must have graduated from high school in Boone, Cooper, or Howard County in Missouri.

To Apply: The application includes letter of support from Dean of Students and two letters of reference. Financial need is not a consideration.

Deadline: The application deadline is in January. For more information, contact Beverly Wilcox at (573) 814-1894 or write to: Beverly Wilcox, Executive Director, Boone County Medical Society, PO Box 196, Columbia, MO 65205.

Cole County Medical Society Scholarship

Description: The Cole County Medical Society awards this scholarship to medical students who have completed the first semester of their third year of medical school. The award amount is $3,000. To be eligible, the applicant must have graduated from high school in Cole, Moniteau, or Osage County in Missouri. Only applicants attending medical school in Missouri will be considered. Criteria for selection include scholastic achievement, community involvement, and financial need.

To Apply: For application information and instructions, contact the organization below.

Deadline: The application deadline is in January. For more information, contact Jackie Trippensee at (573) 636-4759 or write to: Jackie Trippensee, Cole County Medical Society, 1020 Satinwood Ct., Jefferson City, MO 65102.

Doctor William Jones McElhiney M.D. Scholarship

Description: This scholarship program is sponsored by the St. Charles-Lincoln County Medical Society, and is offered to medical students that graduated from high school in Saint Charles or Lincoln County, Missouri. The applicant must be attending medical school in Missouri. Criteria for selection include academic achievement, volunteerism, and financial need. The award amount is $5,000.
To Apply: For application information and instructions, contact the organization below.
Deadline: The deadline is in February. For more information, contact Martin L. Wilman, M.D., President, 4790 Executive Center Parkway, St. Peters, MO 63376 or call (636) 441-3100.

Dr. William Walker Memorial Scholarship (See Chapter 53)

Fannie Johnson Pitman Memorial Fund

Description: Medical students from the Springfield or Buffalo, Missouri area are eligible to apply. The award amount is 3,000 to $10,400.
To Apply: For application information and instructions, contact the organization below.
Deadline: The application deadline is in November. For more information, contact Maria Botelho, AVP, Philanthropic Service Officer, M.S. RI1-102-M1-02, 111 Westminster St., Providence, RI 02903 or call (866) 461-7287.

Glenn Medical Scholarship

Description: Medical students who reside in the State of Missouri within 100 mile radius of the City of Springfield, Missouri are eligible to apply. Financial need is a consideration. The award amount is $3,650 to $6,000.
To Apply: The application includes an essay describing the student's career and educational goals.
Deadline: The deadline is in September. For more information, contact Maria Botelho, AVP, Philanthropic Service Officer, M.S. RI1-102-M1-02, 111 Westminster St., Providence, RI 02903 or call (866) 461-7287.

Greater Lee's Summit Healthcare Foundation Scholarship

Description: This scholarship program is offered to applicants who have lived in Lee's Summit for a period of at least five years, or have graduated from an area high school. The award amount is $5,000.

To Apply: For application information and instructions, contact the organization below.

Deadline: The deadline is in March. For more information, contact The Greater Lee's Summit Healthcare Foundation, P.O. Box 571, Lee's Summitt, MO 64063.

Jayne M. Perkins Memorial Scholarship (See Chapter 18)

Missouri State Medical Association Scholarship

Description: With the support of the Missouri State Medical Foundation, scholarships in the amount of $2,500 are given to five students in each of the medical schools in Missouri.

To Apply: To be considered, applicants must be first- or second-year medical students attending school in Missouri. Applicants must have attended high school in Missouri. Financial need is also a consideration. There is no application form for this scholarship.

Deadline: For more information, visit:

http://www.msma.org/mx/hm.asp?id=MSMFoundation

Northeast Missouri County Medical Society Scholarship

Description: Medical students who have graduated from high school in Northeast Missouri are eligible to apply for this scholarship. Criteria for selection include interest in rural medicine, scholastic achievement, community involvement, and financial need. The award amount is $1,000.

To Apply: For application information and instructions, contact the organization below.

Deadline: The deadline is in March. For more information, contact Dr. Bryson McHardy, 100 Medical Drive, P.O. Box 311, Hannibal, MO 63401 or call (573) 221-5250.

Smith-Glynn-Callaway Med School Scholarship

Description: This scholarship program is sponsored by the Community Foundation of the Ozarks, and is offered to medical students accepted in a Missouri medical school. Preference is given to applicants who completed undergraduate education in a Missouri institution. Applicants from Southwest Missouri are preferred. Financial need is a consideration. The award amount is $5,000.

To Apply: For application information and instructions, contact the organization below.

Deadline: The deadline is in June. For more information, contact Judith Billins, Grants & Scholarships Coordinator, P.O. Box 8960, Springfield, MO 65801 or call (417) 864-6199.

Texas County Memorial Hospital Healthcare Foundation Scholarship

Description: The Texas County Memorial Hospital Healthcare Foundation in Missouri offers scholarships to medical students. To be eligible, medical students must be accepted to or currently enrolled in an accredited medical school. Only residents of Texas County and Mountain Grove who have graduated from area high schools may apply.

To Apply: The application includes an essay describing the student's career and educational goals.

Deadline: The deadline is in July. For more information, visit:

www.tcmhfoundation.org.

Chapter 64

Medical Awards and Scholarships in Montana

State medical associations often have information about scholarships and loans available for students from the state:

Montana Medical Association
2021 Eleventh Avenue, Suite 1
Helena, MT 59601
Phone: 406-443-4000
http://www.mmaoffice.org/

Inquiries with your county medical society or association are recommended as well. We also encourage you to check with community foundations in the area in which you live to see if you are eligible for scholarships. Community Foundations in the State of Montana are listed below.

Community Foundations in Montana	
Absarokee Community Foundation	Central Montana Foundation
Billings Community Foundation	Montana Community Foundation
Blackfeet Community Endowment Fund	Park County Community Foundation
Blaine County Community Foundation	Phillips County Community Foundation
Bozeman Area Community Foundation	Powder River Community Endowment
Broadwater Community Foundation	Fund
Butte-Silver Bow Community Foundation	Powell County Foundation
Carter County Community Foundation	Prairie Benefits
Columbus Community Foundation	Redwater Community Foundation
Community Foundation for a Better	Richland County Community Foundation
Bigfork	Roosevelt County Community Foundation
Culbertson Area Community Foundation	FAIR Community Foundation of Northern
Darby Town Endowment Fund	Rosebud County
Flathead Community Foundation	Ruby Valley Foundation
Greater Glendive Community Foundation	Sheridan County Community Foundation
Grass Range Community Foundation	Stevensville Community Foundation
Great Falls Area Community Foundatoin	Sunburst Community Foundation
Greater Polson Community Foundation	Sweet Grass Health and Wellness
Hill County Community Endowment	Foundation
Jefferson Valley Community Foundation	Three Mile Lone Rock Community
Joliet Area Community Foundation	Foundation
Helena Area Community Foundation	Tobacco Valley Community Foundation
Lincoln County Community Foundation	Valley County Community Foundation
Lincoln Valley Community Foundation	West Yellowstone Foundation
Lower Flathead Valley Community Foundation	Whitefish Community Foundation
Mineral County Community Foundation	Wibaux Endowment Foundation

Northwest Osteopathic Medical Association Scholarships (See Chapter 17)

Osteopathic Foundation of Central Washington Scholarship (See Chapter 17)

Thomas R. Johnson, M.D. Medical Scholarship

Description: The Thomas R. Johnson, M.D. Medical Scholarship is awarded to a medical student who has graduated from a Montana high school. Medical students in their second (second semester), third, and fourth years will be considered.

To Apply: The application includes a letter of intent with the answers to five questions and a faculty letter of reference.

Deadline: The application deadline is in April. Please see the following link for further information:

http://www.svfoundation.org/sections/scholarship/johnson_scholarship_2008.pdf

Chapter 65

Medical Awards and Scholarships in Nebraska

Medical students from Nebraska and/or attending school in Nebraska are eligible for a number of scholarships, awards, and grants. We recommend starting with your Office of Financial Aid and your school's website. Donors have provided funds to each medical school, and you may be eligible for these school-specific internal awards and scholarships. Students may also benefit from reviewing scholarship and award opportunities posted on the websites of other Nebraska medical schools. Nebraska residents who are attending medical school in other states may also be eligible for scholarships posted on the financial aid websites of Nebraska medical schools. Below is a list of Nebraska medical schools along with their websites.

Financial Aid Websites of Nebraska Medical Schools	
Medical School	**Website**
University of Nebraska Medical Center	http://www.unmc.edu/financialaid/
Creighton University School of Medicine	http://medschool.creighton.edu/medicine/admin/staffairs/financial/

State medical associations often have information about scholarships and loans available for students from the state or attending school in the state:

Nebraska Medical Association
233 South 13th Street
Suite 1200
Lincoln, Nebraska 68508-2091
(402) 474 – 4472
http://www.nebmed.org/Default.aspx

Inquiries with your county medical society or association are recommended as well. We also encourage you to check with community foundations in the area in which you live to see if you are eligible for scholarships. Community Foundations in the State of Nebraska are listed on the following page.

Community Foundations in Nebraska	
Bennington Community Foundation	Merrick Foundation, Inc.
Blair Area Community Foundation	Mid-Nebraska Community Foundation
Custer County Foundation	Nebraska Community Foundation
Fremont Area Community Foundation	Omaha Community Foundation
Grand Island Community Foundation, Inc.	Oregon Trail Community Foundation
Hamilton Community Foundation (NE)	Phelps County Community Foundation
Hastings Community Foundation, Inc.	Waverly Community Foundation
Kearney Area Community Foundation	West Point Community Foundation
La Vista Community Foundation	Western Nebraska Community
Lexington Community Foundation	Foundation
Lincoln Community Foundation, Inc.	York Community Foundation

Community Hospital Health Career Scholarship

Description: The Community Hospital in McCook, Nebraska offers scholarships to students pursuing a career in a health related field. Two programs are available. The General Assistance Program is a forgivable loan that requires applicants to work at Community Hospital following training. The Scholarship Assistance Program does not require repayment or forgiveness.
To Apply: For application information, visit the website below.
Deadline: The deadlines are in March and September. Please see the following link for further information:

http://chmccook.org/assets/files/Educational%20Loan%20Program%208x11.pdf

DeRoin Scholarship

Description: The Nebraska Academy of Family Physicians presents this award annually to a student attending either Creighton University or the University of Nebraska. A strong interest in family medicine and financial need are major considerations. The award amount is $1,000.
To Apply: For application information, visit the website below.
Deadline: Please see the following link for further information:

http://www.nebrafp.org/foundation/foundation_programs/foundation_scholarships.html

Fay Smith Scholarship

Description: The Nebraska Academy of Family Physicians presents this award annually to a fourth-year student attending the University of Nebraska who has chosen to pursue a career in family medicine. The award amount is $500.
To Apply: Students apply for this scholarship through the University of Nebraska Medical Center.
Deadline: Please see the following link for further information:

http://www.nebrafp.org/foundation/foundation_programs/foundation_scholarships.html

Haiti Mission Trip Scholarship

Description: The Nebraska Academy of Family Physicians presents this award to students or residents with a strong interest in family medicine who wish to participate in a medical mission trip to Haiti. The award amount is $1,000.
To Apply: For application information and instructions, visit the website below.
Deadline: Please see the following link for further information:

http://www.nebrafp.org/foundation/foundation_programs/foundation_scholarships.html

Kathleen Fields Scholarship and Loan (See Chapter 53)

Medical Mission Trip Educational Grant

Description: The Nebraska Academy of Family Physicians presents this award to students interested in family medicine who are participating in medical mission trips. The award amount is $500.
To Apply: For application information and instructions, visit the website below.
Deadline: Please see the following link for further information:

http://www.nebrafp.org/foundation/foundation_programs/foundation_scholarships.html

Michael Haller Scholarship

Description: The Nebraska Academy of Family Physicians presents this award annually to a fourth-year student attending Creighton University who has chosen to pursue a career in family medicine. The award amount is $500.
To Apply: Students apply for this scholarship through the Creighton University Department of Family Medicine.
Deadline: Please see the following link for further information:

http://www.nebrafp.org/foundation/foundation_programs/foundation_scholarships.html

Chapter 66

Medical Awards and Scholarships in Nevada

Medical students from Nevada and/or attending school in Nevada are eligible for a number of scholarships, awards, and grants. We recommend starting with your Office of Financial Aid and your school's website. Donors have provided funds to each medical school, and you may be eligible for these school-specific internal awards and scholarships. Students may also benefit from reviewing scholarship and award opportunities posted on the websites of other Nevada medical schools. Nevada residents who are attending medical school in other states may also be eligible for scholarships posted on the financial aid websites of Nevada medical schools. Below is a list of Nevada medical schools along with their websites.

Financial Aid Websites of Nevada Medical Schools	
Medical School	Website
University of Nevada Reno School of Medicine	http://www.unr.edu/financial-aid/medical-students
Touro University College of Osteopathic Medicine	http://tun.touro.edu/current-students/student-services/financial-aid/

State medical associations often have information about scholarships and loans available for students from the state or attending school in the state:

Nevada State Medical Association - Reno
3660 Baker Lane #101
Reno, NV 89509
Phone: 775-825-6788
http://www.nsmadocs.org/

Nevada State Medical Association – Las Vegas
2590 Russell Road
Las Vegas, Nevada 89120

Inquiries with your county medical society or association are recommended as well. We also encourage you to check with community foundations in the area in which you live to see if you are eligible for scholarships. Community Foundations in the State of Nevada are listed on the following page.

Community Foundations in Nevada

Henderson Community Foundation
Lake Tahoe Community Trust
Nevada Community Foundation
Parasol Tahoe Community Foundation
Community Foundation of Western Nevada

Nevada State Medical Association Scholarship

Description: The Nevada State Medical Association offers grants to medical students who are legal Nevada residents attending accredited U.S. medical schools.
To Apply: For application information and instructions, contact the organization below.
Deadline: The deadline is in July. For more information, visit:

Cynthia Rambo
Nevada State Medical Association
3660 Baker Lane #101
Reno, NV 89509
(702) 825-6788

Northwest Osteopathic Medical Association Scholarships (See Chapter 17)

Sierra Nevada Region Fellowships for Graduate Women in Doctoral Programs

Description: The Sierra Nevada Region of Soroptimist International offers this fellowship for women who are enrolled in a doctoral graduate school program.
To Apply: To be eligible, female applicants must be attending school in the Sierra Nevada Region (University of California Davis or University of Nevada at Reno). The application includes brief autobiographical sketch, statement of financial need, and two letters of reference.
Deadline: The deadline is in March. For more information, visit:

http://soroptimistsnr.org/pages/projects/scholarships.html

Chapter 67

Medical Awards and Scholarships in New Hampshire

Medical students from New Hampshire and/or attending school in New Hampshire are eligible for a number of scholarships, awards, and grants. We recommend starting with your Office of Financial Aid and your school's website. Donors have provided funds, and you may be eligible for these school-specific internal awards and scholarships.

State medical associations often have information about scholarships and loans available for students from the state or attending school in the state:

New Hampshire Medical Society
7 North State Street, Concord, NH 03301-4018
(603) 224-1909
http://www.nhms.org/

Inquiries with your county medical society or association are recommended as well. We also encourage you to check with community foundations in the area in which you live to see if you are eligible for scholarships. Community Foundations in the State of New Hampshire include the New Hampshire Charitable Foundation.

Alice M. Yarnold and Samuel Yarnold Scholarhsip

Description: Medical students who are New Hampshire residents may apply for this scholarship.
To Apply: To be eligible, applicants must be residents of New Hampshire. The application includes transcript, two letters of recommendation, and FAFSA.
Deadline: The deadline is in May. For more information, visit:

http://financialaid.unh.edu/forms/Yarnold%20Schol.PDF

Rocco D. LaPenta Scholarship (See Chapter 45)

Ryu Family Foundation Scholarship (See Chapter 12)

Seacoast Health Foundation Scholarship

Description: The Seacoast Health Foundation offers this scholarship to students pursuing an undergraduate or graduate degree in a health-related field of study. To be eligible, applicants must have a primary residence in Portsmouth, Rye, Newcastle, Greenland, Newington, and North Hampton in New Hampshire or Kittery, Elliott, and York in Maine.

To Apply: Criteria for selection includes scholastic aptitude and performance, personal achievements, leadership, and community involvement.

Deadline: The application deadline is in March. For more information, visit:

http://www.ffsh.org/sites/default/files/PDFs/ScholApp-generic_0.pdf

Chapter 68

Medical Awards and Scholarships in New Jersey

Medical students from New Jersey and/or attending school in New Jersey are eligible for a number of scholarships, awards, and grants. We recommend starting with your Office of Financial Aid and your school's website. Donors have provided funds to each medical school, and you may be eligible for these school-specific internal awards and scholarships. Students may also benefit from reviewing scholarship and award opportunities posted on the websites of other New Jersey medical schools. New Jersey residents who are attending medical school in other states may also be eligible for scholarships posted on the financial aid websites of New Jersey medical schools. Below is a list of New Jersey medical schools along with their websites.

Financial Aid Websites of New Jersey Medical Schools	
Medical School	**Website**
Cooper Medical School of Rowan University	http://www.rowan.edu/coopermed/students/financial_aid/
Rowan University School of Osteopathic Medicine	http://www.rowan.edu/som/financialaid/
Rutgers New Jersey Medical School	http://njms.rutgers.edu/education/student_affairs/student_life/financial_aid.cfm
Rutgers Robert Wood Johnson Medical School	http://rwjms.rutgers.edu/education/current_students/student_life/financial_aid.html

State medical associations often have information about scholarships and loans available for students from the state or attending school in the state:

New Jersey Medical Society
2 Princess Road
Lawrenceville, NJ 08646
info@msnj.org
(609) 896-1766
http://www.msnj.org/

Inquiries with your county medical society or association are recommended as well. We also encourage you to check with community foundations in the area in which you live to see if you are eligible for scholarships. Community Foundations in the State of New Jersey are listed on the following page.

Community Foundations in New Jersey

Community Foundation of South Jersey
Englewood Area Community Foundation
Jewish Community Foundation
Community Foundation of New Jersey
Northern New Jersey Community Foundation
Princeton Area Community Foundation
The Westfield Foundation

Aetna Foundation/NMF Healthcare Leadership Program (See Chapter 13)

Camden County AAUW Scholarship

Description: This scholarship is open to female medical students who are residents of Camden or Burlington County in New Jersey.
To Apply: For application information and instructions, visit the website below.
Deadline: The deadline is in May. For more information, visit:

http://www.ccaauw.org/

Ferdinand C. Valentine Medical Student Research Grant in Urology (See Chapter 38)

Frank & Louise Groff Foundation Medical Scholarship

Description: The Frank and Louise Groff Foundation offers this award to medical students who have graduated from a public high school within Monmouth County in New Jersey. Scholarships may be renewed for four years.
To Apply: To be eligible, applicants must have attended public high school in Monmouth County. Criteria for selection include financial need, transcripts, and test scores.
Deadline: The deadline is in March. For more information, visit:

http://groff-foundation.org/medical.aspx

Hellenic Medical Society of New York Scholarship (See Chapter 12)

Hellenic University Club of Philadelphia Scholarship (See Chapter 12)

Henry I. Russek Travel Awards for FITs and Medical Students (See Chapter 70)

Howard G. Lapsley Memorial Scholarship

Description: The goal of this scholarship is to provide financial support to recipients for the study of medicine, osteopathy, or dentistry. The award is open to students who were raised in certain counties (see below).

To Apply: To be considered, applicants must have attended elementary or secondary school in Union County, Somerset County, or Middlesex County. Allopathic and osteopathic medical students in the first through fourth years of medical school can apply. Financial need is a consideration. A personal interview may be required.

Deadline: The application deadline is in May. For more information, visit:

http://jfkmc.org/pdf/LapsleyScholarship_Brochure.pdf

Ida Foreman Fleisher Fund (See Chapter 12)

Margaret Yardley Fellowship

Description: The New Jersey State Federation of Women's Clubs administers the Margaret Yardley Fellowship. This scholarship is open to female medical students who are residents of New Jersey. The award amount is $1,000.

To Apply: Female medical students who are residents of New Jersey are eligible to apply. Criteria for judging include scholastic achievement, career service potential, and charitable endeavors.

Deadline: The deadline is in March. For more information, visit:

www.njsfwc.org

Middlesex County Medical Society Foundation Scholarhsip

Description: The Middlesex County Medical Society Foundation offers scholarships to medical students who are residents of Middlesex County in New Jersey. Applicants must have been residents of the county for at least five years.

To Apply: Allopathic and osteopathic medical students are eligible to apply. Criteria for selection include academic achievement and financial need.

Deadline: For more information, visit:

www.msnj.org/

New Jersey Osteopathic Education Scholarship (See Chapter 17)

NJCFSA Medical Student Scholarship

Description: The New Jersey Chronic Fatigue Syndrome Association (NJCFSA) offers the Chronic Fatigue Syndrome Medical Student Scholarship to a second-year medical student in the State of New Jersey. The award amount is $3,000.
To Apply: Applicants must submit an essay on a chronic fatigue syndrome related subject. Only second-year medical students will be considered.
Deadline: For more information, visit:

http://njcfsa.org/medschol.html

Polish University Club of New Jersey Scholarship (See Chapter 12)

Ryu Family Foundation Scholarship (See Chapter 12)

Swiss Benevolent Society Scholarship (See Chapter 12)

William F. Grupe Foundation Scholarship

Description: The William F. Grupe Foundation provides scholarships to medical students who are residents of certain counties in New Jersey.
To Apply: Allopathic and osteopathic medical students who are permanent residents of Hudson, Bergen, or Essex counties are eligible to apply.
Deadline: For more information, contact:

William F. Grupe Foundation, Inc.
Attn: President
PO Box 775
Livingston, NJ 07039
(973) 428 - 1190

Chapter 69

Medical Awards and Scholarships in New Mexico

Medical students from New Mexico and/or attending school in New Mexico are eligible for a number of scholarships, awards, and grants. We recommend starting with your Office of Financial Aid and your school's website. Donors have provided funds, and you may be eligible for these school-specific internal awards and scholarships.

State medical associations often have information about scholarships and loans available for students from the state or attending school in the state:

New Mexico Medical Society
316 Osuna Road, NE Suite 501
Albuquerque, NM 87107
505.828.0237
http://www.nmms.org/

Inquiries with your county medical society or association are recommended as well. We also encourage you to check with community foundations in the area in which you live to see if you are eligible for scholarships. Community Foundations in the State of New Mexico are listed below.

Community Foundations in New Mexico

Albuquerque Community Foundation
Carlsbad Foundation
Community Foundation of Chaves County
New Mexico Community Foundation
Santa Fe Community Foundation
Community Foundation of Southern New Mexico
Taos Community Foundation, Inc.

Osteopathic Medical Student Loan for Service Program

Description: The New Mexico Commission on Higher Education established this program to increase the number of osteopathic physicians in underserved parts of the state. As a condition of the loan, the recipient promises to practice as an osteopathic physician in a designated area. The award amount is $12,000. To be eligible, the applicant must be a New Mexico resident attending an accredited osteopathic institution in the U.S.

To Apply: For application information and instructions, visit the website below.

Deadline: For more information, visit:

http://www.hed.state.nm.us

Chapter 70

Medical Awards and Scholarships in New York

Medical students from New York and/or attending school in New York are eligible for a number of scholarships, awards, and grants. We recommend starting with your Office of Financial Aid and your school's website. Donors have provided funds to each medical school, and you may be eligible for these school-specific internal awards and scholarships. Students may also benefit from reviewing scholarship and award opportunities posted on the websites of other New York medical schools. On the following page is a list of New York medical schools along with their websites. State medical associations often have information about scholarships and loans available for students from the state or attending school in the state:

Medical Society of the State of New York
865 Merrick Avenue
Westbury, NY 11590
(516) 488-6100
http://www.mssny.org/

Inquiries with your county medical society or association are recommended as well. We also encourage you to check with community foundations in the area in which you live to see if you are eligible for scholarships. Community Foundations in the State of New York are listed below.

Community Foundations in New York	
Adirondack Foundation	The Glens Falls Foundation
Allegany County Area Foundation	The Community Foundation of Herkimer & Oneida Counties
Attica Area Community Foundation	
Brooklyn Community Foundation	Long Island Community Foundation
Community Foundation for Greater Buffalo	New York Community Trust
Community Foundation for the Greater Capital Region	Northern New York Community Foundation
	Greater Olean Community Foundation
Cattaraugus Region Community Foundation	Community Foundation of Orange County, Inc.
Central New York Community Foundation, Inc.	Rochester Area Community Foundation
Northern Chautauqua Community Foundation	Rockland Community Foundation
Chautauqua Region Community Foundation	The Community Foundation for South Central New York, Inc.
Community Foundations of the Hudson Valley	
Community Foundation of Dutchess County	Community Foundation of Tompkins County
Community Foundation of Putnam County	Community Foundation of Ulster County
Cortland Community Foundation	Community Foundation of Unadilla
Community Foundation of the Elmira-Corning and the Finger Lakes	Westchester Community Foundation

Financial Aid Websites of New York Medical Schools	
Medical School	**Website**
Albany Medical College	http://www.amc.edu/Academic/Undergraduate/Financial Aid.cfm
Albert Einstein College of Medicine at Yeshiva University	http://www.einstein.yu.edu/education/md-program/financial-aid/
Columbia University College of Physicians & Surgeons	http://cumc.columbia.edu/student/finaid/
Hofstra University – North Shore LIJ School of Medicine	http://medicine.hofstra.edu/financialaid/financialaid_faq.html
Icahn School of Medicine at Mt. Sinai	http://icahn.mssm.edu/education/student-resources/financial-aid
New York Institute of Technology College of Osteopathic Medicine	http://www.nyit.edu/medicine/financialaid/financial_aid_home/
New York Medical College	https://www.nymc.edu/AdmissionsAndFinancialAid/
New York University School of Medicine	http://school.med.nyu.edu/admissions/fees-and-financial-aid
Stony Brook University School of Medicine	http://medicine.stonybrookmedicine.edu/som/financialaid
State University of New York Upstate University	http://www.upstate.edu/currentstudents/financial_resources/finaid/
State University of New York Downstate Medical Center College of Medicine	http://sls.downstate.edu/financial_aid/
Touro College of Osteopathic Medicine	http://legacy.touro.edu/med/financial.html
University of Buffalo School of Medicine	http://financialaid.buffalo.edu/graduate/medschool.php
University of Rochester School of Medicine	http://www.urmc.rochester.edu/education/financial-aid/
Weill Cornell Medical College	http://weill.cornell.edu/education/admissions/app_fin_aid.html

Aetna Foundation/NMF Healthcare Leadership Program (See Chapter 13)

Community Foundation for Greater Buffalo Scholarship

Description: The Community Foundation for Greater Buffalo has a limited number of scholarships for medical students.
To Apply: To be eligible, the applicant must be a current resident of one of the eight counties of western New York. For application information and instructions, visit the website below.
Deadline: For more information, visit:

http://www.cfgb.org/for-scholarships/

Dr. Abraham R. Bullis Medical Scholarship

Description: This scholarship is open to medical students who are graduates of Palmyra-Macedon Central School. The award amount is at least $2,000.
To Apply: For application information and instructions, visit the website below.
Deadline: For more information, contact:

http://www.racf.org/Scholarships/CollegeScholarshipSearch/tabid/282/Default.aspx

Dr. John A. Burn Scholarship

Description: This scholarship is awarded by the Wilson Central School District for a male graduate.
To Apply: Criteria for selection includes aptitude for successful graduate work, character, and financial need. For application information and instructions, contact the organization below.
Deadline: The application deadline is in March. For more information, contact:

Daniel O'Connor
Superintendent of Schools
Wilson Central School District
412 Lake Street
PO Box 648
Wilson NY 14172

Dr. Matthew Krupp Memorial Medical Scholarship

Description: This scholarship is awarded by the Central New York Community Foundation for medical students who have demonstrated both academic achievement and the ability to overcome adversity.
To Apply: For application information and instructions, visit the website below.
Deadline: For more information, visit:

https://www.cnycf.org/sslpage.aspx?pid=793

Dr. U.R. Plante Medical Scholarship

Description: This scholarship is awarded annually to a medical student who is a resident (or has lived there for at least two years) of one of the following New York counties: Adirondack Park, St. Lawrence, Franklin, Clinton, Essex, or Hamilton County. The award amount is $10,000.

To Apply: The applicant must be willing to return to the area or another underserved area to practice. For application information and instructions, visit the website below. Only allopathic medical students are eligible to apply.
Deadline: For more information, visit:

https://www.generousact.org/granting/apply-scholarship/scholarship-applications/dr-ur-plante-medical-scholarship-fund

Empire State Medical Association Student Research Poster Competition

Description: The Empire State Medical Association sponsors a student poster research competition for undergraduate and medical students of African descent. Monetary prizes are given.
To Apply: Posters are judged on the basis of quality, significance to the field, thoroughness, and clarity of presentation.
Deadline: For more information, visit:

http://www.nyesma.org/student-research-poster-competition/

Ferdinand C. Valentine Medical Student Research Grant in Urology (See Chapter 38)

Hellenic Medical Society of New York Scholarship (See Chapter 12)

Henry I. Russek Travel Awards for FITs and Medical Students

Description: This scholarship provides funding for five medical students with interest in cardiovascular medicine to attend the New York Cardiovascular Symposium. Recipients will be given $800 to cover the cost of travel and registration.
To Apply: To be eligible, applicants must be attending medical schools in New York, New Jersey, or Connecticut. For more information, visit the website below.
Deadline: For more information, visit:

http://www.cardiosource.org/en/ACC/About-ACC/Awards-Program/Travel-Awards.aspx

Medical Societies of the Counties of Chenango and Osnego, NY Scholarship Loan

Description: The Medical Societies of the Counties of Chenango and Osnego, New York offer the Lee C. Van Wagner Scholarship Loan to medical students who are legal residents of these counties. Recipients agree to practice medicine in one of these counties for one year.

To Apply: For more information, contact the organization below.
Deadline: For more information, visit:

Kathleen E. Dyman, Executive Vice President
Medical Society of the County of Chenango
4311 Middle Settlement Road, New Hartford, NY 13413-5317
kdyman@medsocieties.com
315-735-2204

Glorney-Raisbeck Student Fellowship in Cardiovascular Research (See Chapter 24)

New York City Health Department HRTP (See Chapter 10)

New York State Osteopathic Medical Society Poster Competition

Description: The New York State Osteopathic Medical Society has a poster competition open to medical students.
To Apply: For poster submission information, visit the website below.
Deadline: For more information, visit:

http://www.nysoms.org/news/viewarticle.asp?a=2293

NYS Regents Health Care Opportunity Scholarship

Description: This scholarship is awarded annually to medical students who are attending school in New York. The award amount is $10,000 a year for up to 4 years. Following completion of training, students must work 1 year for each annual payment received in an underserved area of New York. Note that the minimum service requirement is 2 years.
To Apply: To be eligible, the applicant must be a resident of the state of New York. Criteria for selection include the following:

- Those who are economically disadvantaged
- Those who are members of a minority group historically underrepresented in the chosen profession.
- Those who are enrolled in or graduates of the following opportunity programs: SEEK, College Discovery, EOP, or HEOP

For application information and instructions, contact the organization below.
Deadline: For more information, contact:

NYS Education Department
Office of K-16 Initiatives and Access Programs
Scholarships and Grants Administration Unit
Room 1078 Education Building Addition
Albany, NY 12234
Phone: (518) 486-1319

Ryu Family Foundation Scholarship (See Chapter 12)

Swiss Benevolent Society Scholarship (See Chapter 12)

United Health Foundation/NMF Diverse Medical Scholars Program (See Chapter 13)

Wayne Anthony Butts Scholarship (See Chapter 13)

Western New York Osteopathic Medical Society Scholarship

Description: This scholarship is open to fourth-year osteopathic medical students who have either lived in Western New York for at least 4 years or who have done clinical rotations in the area. Counties in Western New York include Erie, Niagara, Genesee, Orleans, Wyoming, Allegheny, Chautauqua, and Cattaraugus. The award amount is $500.

To Apply: For application information and instructions, visit the website below.

Deadline: The deadline for the application is in July. For more information, contact:

Dr. Michael Pusatier
295 Essjay Rd.
Williamsville, NY 14221
(716) 877 - 3007

Chapter 71

Medical Awards and Scholarships in North Carolina

Medical students from North Carolina and/or attending school in North Carolina are eligible for a number of scholarships, awards, and grants. We recommend starting with your Office of Financial Aid and your school's website. Donors have provided funds to each medical school, and you may be eligible for these school-specific internal awards and scholarships. Students may also benefit from reviewing scholarship and award opportunities posted on the websites of other North Carolina medical schools. North Carolina residents who are attending medical school in other states may also be eligible for scholarships posted on the financial aid websites of North Carolina medical schools. Below is a list of North Carolina medical schools along with their websites.

Financial Aid Websites of North Carolina Medical Schools	
Medical School	**Website**
University of North Carolina School of Medicine	http://www.med.unc.edu/ome/finaid
Wake Forest University School of Medicine	http://www.wakehealth.edu/financialaid/
Brody School of Medicine at East Carolina University	http://www.ecu.edu/cs-dhs/bsomstudentaffairs/Brody-School-of-Medicine-Financial-Aid.cfm
Duke University School of Medicine	http://medschool.duke.edu/education/financial-aid-office

State medical associations often have information about scholarships and loans available for students from the state or attending school in the state:

North Carolina Medical Society
PO Box 27167
Raleigh, NC 27611
(919) 833-3836
http://www.ncmedsoc.org/

Inquiries with your county medical society or association are recommended as well. We also encourage you to check with community foundations in the area in which you live to see if you are eligible for scholarships. Community Foundations in the State of North Carolina are listed on the following page.

Community Foundations in North Carolina	
Northern Albemarle Community Foundation	Johnston County Community Foundation
Alleghany County Community Foundation	Jones County Community Foundation
Anson County Community Foundation	Lee County Community Foundation
Ashe County Community Foundation	Lenoir County Community Foundation
Avery County Community Foundation	Lexington Area Community Foundation
Beaufort County Community Foundation	Macon County Community Foundation
Bertie-Hertford Community Foundation	Madison County Community Foundation
Black Mountain - Swannanoa Valley Foundation	Martin County Community Foundation
	The McDowell Foundation
Brunswick County Community Foundation	Montgomery County Fund
Community Foundation of Burke County	Moore County Community Foundation
Cabarrus County Community Foundation	Mount Airy Community Foundation
Capital Community Foundation, Inc.	North Carolina Community Foundation
Foundation For The Carolinas	Northampton County Community Foundation
Carteret Community Foundation	Northern Albemarle Community Foundation
Cary Community Foundation	Onslow County Community Foundation
Catawba Valley Community Foundation	Outer Banks Community Foundation
Cherokee County Community Foundation	Pamlico County Community Foundation
Chowan County Community	Pender County Community Foundation
Clay County Community Foundation	Person County Community Foundation
Cleveland County Community Foundation	Pitt County Community Foundation
Columbus County Community Foundation	The Polk County Community Foundation, Inc.
Craven County Community Foundation	Randolph County Community Foundation
Cumberland Community Foundation, Inc.	Robeson County Community Foundation
Currituck-Dare Community Foundation	Rockingham County Community Foundation
Davie Community Foundation, Inc.	Salisbury Community Foundation
Duplin County Community Foundation	Sampson County Community Foundation
Edenton-Chowan Community Foundation	Swain County Community Foundation
Edgecombe County Community Foundation	The Greater Greenville Community Foundation
Foundation For Richmond County	The High Point Community Health Fund
Franklin County Community Foundation	Thomasville Community Foundation, Inc.
Community Foundation of Gaston County, Inc.	Transylvania Endowment
Graham County Community Foundation	Triangle Community Foundation
Granville County Community Foundation	Vance County Community Foundation
Greater Rocky Mount Community Foundation	Wake County Community Foundation
Community Foundation of Greater Greensboro	Watauga County Community Foundation
Halifax County Community Foundation	Wayne Community Foundation
Harnett County Community Foundation	Wayne County Community Foundation
Haywood County Community Foundation	The Community Foundation of Western North Carolina
The Fund for Haywood County	
Community Foundation of Henderson County	Wilkes County Community Foundation
High Point Community Foundation	Wilson County Community Foundation
Highlands Community Foundation	The Winston-Salem Foundation
Hoke County Community Foundation	Yadkin County Community Foundation
Iredell County Community Foundation	Yancey Foundation
Jackson County Community Foundation	

Albermale Hospital Volunteer Scholarship

Description: This scholarship is available for medical students residing in one of the following counties: Camden, Chowan, Currituck, Dare, Gates, Pasquotank, and Perquimans. The award amount is $5,000.
To Apply: For application information and instructions, contact the organization below.
Deadline: For more information, contact (252) 384 – 4676.

Dr. Grover White Scholarship

Description: The Community Foundation of Gaston County administers the Dr. Grover White Scholarship. Medical students who are residents of Gaston, Cleveland, or Lincoln County in North Carolina or York County in South Carolina are eligible to apply. The award amount is up to $1,500.
To Apply: Applicants must attend medical school in North or South Carolina. For application information and instructions, contact the organization below.
Deadline: The deadline for the application is in March. For more information, visit:

http://www.cfgastron.org

Dr. Henderson D. Mabe, Jr. Scholarship

Description: This scholarship is available for medical students who graduated from a public high school in Harnett County in North Carolina. Preference is given to those from Erwin area.
To Apply: For application information and instructions, contact the organization below.
Deadline: For more information, visit:

http://nccommunityfoundation.org/Scholarship?county=32

Gertrude B. Elion Mentored Medical Student Research Award

Description: The Triangle Community Foundation administers this award to support one female medical student in the amount of $10,000. The award is for health-related research.
To Apply: To be eligible, female applicants must be nominated by either Duke University Medical Center or University of North Carolina at Chapel Hill School of Medicine.
Deadline: The deadline for the application is in March. For more information, visit:

http://www.trianglecf.org/grants_support/view_scholarships/gertrude_b._elion_mentored_medical_student_research_award/

NCAFP Foundation Loan/Scholarship Program

Description: The North Carolina Academy of Family Physicians Foundation offers scholarships to medical students based in North Carolina. The award amount is up to $2,000.
To Apply: To be eligible, applicants must be seeking a career as a family physician. Financial need is also a consideration. For application information and instructions, visit the website below.

Deadline: The deadline for the application is in May. For more information, visit:

http://www.ncafp.com/residents_and_newfps/scholarships

NCAFP Research Poster Presentation

Description: The North Carolina Academy of Family Physicians Foundation invites medical students to submit original research not yet published or presented elsewhere. Exceptions are made for work presented at medical schools or student "Research Days."

To Apply: Research presentations may address any topic relevant to Family Medicine. For application information and instructions, visit the website below.

Deadline: For more information, visit:

http://www.ncafp.com/residents_and_newfps/scholarships

Robert A. Team Scholarship

Description: This scholarship is available to medical students with an interest in delivering primary health care of a direct and personal nature. Preference is given to residents of Lexington/Davidson County area in North Carolina.

To Apply: For application information and instructions, contact the organization below.

Deadline: For more information, visit:

https://www.davidsonccc.edu/sites/default/files/downloads/pdfs/TEAM%20app
lication%202013-14%20(2).pdf

Chapter 72

Medical Awards and Scholarships in North Dakota

Medical students from North Dakota and/or attending school in North Dakota are eligible for a number of scholarships, awards, and grants. We recommend starting with your Office of Financial Aid and your school's website. Donors have provided funds, and you may be eligible for these school-specific internal awards and scholarships.

State medical associations often have information about scholarships and loans available for students from the state or attending school in the state:

North Dakota Medical Assn
P.O. Box 1198
Bismarck, ND 58502-1198
(701) 223-9475
http://ndmed.org/

Inquiries with your county medical society or association are recommended as well. We also encourage you to check with community foundations in the area in which you live to see if you are eligible for scholarships. Community Foundations in the State of North Dakota are listed below

---

Community Foundations in North Dakota

Devils Lake Area Foundation
Fargo-Moorhead Area Foundation
Grand Forks Community Foundation/Bremer
Community Foundation of Grand Forks, East Grand Forks, & Region
Minot Area Community Foundation
North Dakota Community Foundation
Saint Joseph's Community Health Foundation

RuralMed

Description: This scholarship program is sponsored by the state of North Dakota, and was developed to increase providers practicing in rural parts of the state. Students will have their tuition paid through this program. In return, students agree to practice in rural areas. Students must be enrolled at the University of North Dakota, and enter a family medicine residency following medical school. Within six months of completing residency, scholarship recipients must establish a full-time medical practice, and practice for at least five years.

To Apply: For application information and instructions, visit the website below.

Deadline: For more information, visit:

http://www.med.und.edu/student-affairs-admissions/financial-
aid/ruralmed2013.pdf

Chapter 73

Medical Awards and Scholarships in Ohio

Medical students from Ohio and/or attending school in Ohio are eligible for a number of scholarships, awards, and grants. We recommend starting with your Office of Financial Aid and your school's website. Donors have provided funds to each medical school, and you may be eligible for these school-specific internal awards and scholarships. Students may also benefit from reviewing scholarship and award opportunities posted on the websites of other Ohio medical schools. Ohio residents who are attending medical school in other states may also be eligible for scholarships posted on the financial aid websites of Ohio medical schools. Below is a list of Ohio medical schools along with their websites.

Financial Aid Websites of Ohio Medical Schools	
Medical School	**Website**
Boonshoft School of Medicine at Wright State University	http://www.med.wright.edu/admiss/financialaid
Case Western Reserve University School of Medicine	http://casemed.case.edu/financial_aid/
Cleveland Clinic Lerner College of Medicine	http://portals.clevelandclinic.org/cclcm/TuitionFinancial Aid/tabid/7336/Default.aspx
Northeast Ohio Medical University	http://www.neomed.edu/students/es/finaid/financial-aid
Ohio State University College of Medicine	http://medicine.osu.edu/students/financial_services/pages/ index.aspx
Ohio University Heritage College of Osteopathic Medicine	http://www.oucom.ohiou.edu/Aid/
University of Cincinnati College of Medicine	http://med2.uc.edu/studentservices/FinancialServices.aspx
University of Toledo College of Medicine	http://www.utoledo.edu/financialaid/hsc/sfamed.html

State medical associations often have information about scholarships and loans available for students from the state or attending school in the state:

Ohio State Medical Association
3401 Mill Run Dr.
Hilliard, OH 43026
(614) 527-6762
https://www.osma.org/

Inquiries with your county medical society or association are recommended as well. We also encourage you to check with community foundations in the area in which you live to see if you are eligible for scholarships. Community Foundations in the State of Ohio are listed below

Community Foundations in Ohio

Akron Community Foundation
Alliance Community Foundation
Foundation for Appalachian Ohio
Archbold Area Foundation
Ashland County Community Foundation
Athens Foundation
Barberton Community Foundation
Belpre Area Community Development Foundation
Bowling Green Community Foundation
Bratenahl Community Foundation
Brown County Foundation
Bryan Area Foundation
Community Foundation for Crawford County
Chillicothe-Ross Community Foundation
Greater Cincinnati Foundation
Cleveland Foundation
Clinton County Foundation
Columbiana Community Foundation
Columbus Foundation
Coshocton Foundation
Dayton Foundation
Defiance Area Foundation
Community Foundation of Delaware County
Dublin Foundation
East Liverpool Fawcett Community Foundation
Edgerton Area Foundation
Fairfield Community Foundation
Fairfield County Foundation
Fayette County Charitable Foundation
Findlay-Hancock County Community Foundation
Granville Foundation
Greater Alliance Community Foundation
Greene County Community Foundation
Hamilton Community Foundation
Hardin County Community Foundation
Henry County Community Foundation
Hudson Community Foundation
Fund for Huron County Community Foundation
Northern Kentucky Fund
Lake County Foundation
Licking County Foundation

Lisbon Community Foundation
London Community Foundation
Community Foundation of Lorain County
Community Foundation of the Mahoning Valley
Marietta Community Foundation
Marion Community Foundation
Medina County Women's Endowment Fund
Mercer County Civic Foundation
Middletown Community Foundation
Monroe Area Community Foundation
Montpelier Area Foundation
Morrow County Foundation
Community Foundation of Mount Vernon & Knox County
Muskingum County Community Foundation
New Bremen Foundation
Oxford Community Foundation
Paulding County Area Foundation
Pickaway County Community Foundation
Piqua Community Foundation
Portage Foundation
Richland County Foundation
Salem Community Foundation
Erie County Community Foundation
Scioto County Area Foundation
Sebring West Branch Area Community Foundation
Sharon Community Trusts
Community Foundation of Shelby County
Springfield Foundation
St. Clair Foundation
Stark Community Foundation
Tiffin Charitable Foundation
Toledo Community Foundation
Troy Foundation
Union County Foundation
Urbana Foundation
Wapakoneta Area Community Foundation
Warren County Foundation
Wayne County Foundation
Community Foundation of West Chester/Liberty
Yellow Springs Community Foundation
Youngstown Foundation

Academy of Medicine Education Foundation Scholarship

Description: The Academy of Medicine Education Foundation awards scholarships to third- and fourth-year medical students who are, or were, residents of Cuyahoga, Ashtabula, Geauga, Lake, Lorain, Portage, or Summit County.

To Apply: The applicant must be attending one of the following schools: Case Western Reserve University, Cleveland Clinic, Northeast Ohio Medical University, or Ohio University College of Medicine. Criteria for judging include involvement in organized medicine, community activities, leadership, and academic achievement.

Deadline: The deadline for the application is in January. For more information, visit:

http://www.amcno.org/index.php?id=70

Charles Fox Medical Scholarship

Description: This scholarship is open to medical students who are graduates of Salem High School.

To Apply: To be eligible, applicants must have completed one year in medical school. Criteria for judging include minimum GPA.

Deadline: The deadline for the application is in April. For more information, visit:

http://www.salemohioalumni.org/scholarships/postsecondary-alumni-scholarships.html

Columbus Medical Association Alliance Scholarship

Description: This scholarship is open to fourth-year medical students at the Ohio State University College of Medicine.

To Apply: Criteria for judging include academic achievement (top ten percent of the class), leadership, and community service.

Deadline: For more information, visit:

http://columbusmedicalassociationalliance.weebly.com/uploads/2/5/5/9/2559600/m4_applicationform2014.pdf

Choose Ohio First Scholarship

Description: This scholarship program was developed to increase the number of primary care practitioners in underserved areas of Ohio. Medical students may receive $30,000 per year if they meet the following requirements:

- Commitment to community service before and during medical school

- Intent to complete residency in family medicine, internal medicine, pediatrics or med-peds in Ohio
- Commitment to practice in Ohio for no less than three years
- Willingness to accept Medicaid patients while in practice

To Apply: The applicant must be a student at one of the following schools: Wright State University, University of Toledo, Northeast Ohio Medical University, Case Western Reserve University, Ohio State University, University of Cincinnati, and Ohio University. Preference will be given to first-generation, low-income or disadvantaged students.
Deadline: For more information, visit:

https://www.chooseohiofirst.org/press/new-choose-ohio-first-scholarships-target-primary-care-physicians

College Club West Scholarships

Description: This scholarship provides funding to support the education of women over the age of 25 who live in the Cleveland, Ohio region.
To Apply: The applicant must be at least 25 years of age, and reside in the Cleveland, Ohio West Shore area of Avon, Avon Lake, Bay Village, Berea, Brookpark, Columbia Station, Fairview Park, Lakewood, Middleburg Heights, North Olmstead, No. Ridgeville, No. Royalton, Olmstead, Parma, Parma Heights, Rocky River, Strongsville, Westlake, or the west side of Cleveland (west of W. 25th Street).
Deadline: For more information, contact:

College Club West Scholarships
c/o Mrs. Virginia Kazimer
14 Nantucket Row
Rocky River, Ohio 44116

Dr. A. L. Berman and Family Medical Scholarship

Description: This scholarship is sponsored by the Community Foundation of Greater Lorain County, and is offered to persons residing or employed in Lorain County. Medical students are eligible to apply.
To Apply: For application information and instructions, contact the organization below.
Deadline: The deadline is in March. For more information, contact Community Foundation of Greater Lorain County, Ramona Grigsby, Special Projects Coordinator, 9080 Leavitt Rd., Elyria, OH 44035 or call (440) 984-7390.

Dr. Frederick A. Prescott Medical Scholarship (See Chapter 76)

Gabriel A. Sabga M.D. Memorial Scholarship

Description: This scholarship is sponsored by the Community Foundation of Greater Lorain County, and is offered to college students residing in Lorain County who are attending medical school.
To Apply: For application information, contact the organization below.
Deadline: The deadline is in March. For more information, contact Community Foundation of Greater Lorain County, Ramona Grigsby, Special Projects Coordinator, 9080 Leavitt Rd., Elyria, OH 44035 or call (440) 984-7390.

Dr. Leslie M. Baker Memorial Scholarship (See Chapter 52)

Harry T. and Dorothy Zahars Memorial Scholarship

Description: This scholarship is sponsored by the Community Foundation of Greater Lorain County, and is offered to past male graduates of high schools in Elyria, Ohio pursuing education in engineering, medicine, or in the sciences.
To Apply: For application information and instructions, contact the organization below.
Deadline: The deadline is in March. For more information, contact Community Foundation of Greater Lorain County, Ramona Grigsby, Special Projects Coordinator, 9080 Leavitt Rd., Elyria, OH 44035 or call (440) 984-7390.

Jerome Kowal Award

Description: The Ohio Geriatrics Society offers the Jerome Kowal Award for up to 3 students to attend the American Geriatrics Society Conference. The award amount is up to $750.
To Apply: For application information and instructions, contact the organization.
Deadline: For more information, contact Dr. Donald Mack at donald.mack@osumc.edu.

John L. Flaherty Trust

Description: The John L. Flaherty Trust offers loans to residents of Cuyahoga County and surrounding areas. Repayment of the loan begins one year after graduation in the amount of $100 per month.
To Apply: For application information and instructions, contact the organization.
Deadline: For more information, contact:

Senior Trust Officer
Ameritrust Co.
PO Box 5937
Cleveland, OH 44101
(216) 737 - 5244

Licking County Foundation Medical Scholarship

Description: The Licking County Foundation offers several medical scholarships to students who are from Licking County.
To Apply: For application information and instructions, contact the organization.
Deadline: For more information, visit:

http://www.thelcfoundation.org/scholarships/availablescholarships/

Lorain County Medical Society Scholarship

Description: The Lorain County Medical Society offers scholarships to medical students who are residents of Lorain County.
To Apply: To be eligible, the applicant must be enrolled in or formally admitted to an accredited medical school. Criteria for judging include academic competence and financial need. For application information and instructions, contact the organization.
Deadline: For more information, visit:

http://www.lcmedicalsociety.com/pages/guidelines.html

Marion Community Foundation Scholarship

Description: The Marion Community Foundation offers several scholarships to students pursuing careers in medicine.
To Apply: For application information and instructions, visit the website below.
Deadline: For more information, visit:

https://www.marioncommunityfoundation.org/mcf/tabId/394/itemId/154/Scholarship-Funds.aspxZelma Gray Scholarship

Mary J. and Paul J. Kopsch Memorial Scholarship

Description: This scholarship is sponsored by the Community Foundation of Greater Lorain County, and is offered to students who have been accepted into osteopathic or allopathic medical school.
To Apply: For application information and instructions, contact the organization below.
Deadline: The deadline is in March. For more information, contact Community Foundation of Greater Lorain County, Ramona Grigsby, Special Projects Coordinator, 9080 Leavitt Rd., Elyria, OH 44035 or call (440) 984-7390.

Miami Community Foundation Scholarship

Description: The Miami Community Foundation offers several scholarships to students pursuing careers in medicine.
To Apply: To be eligible, the applicant must be a resident of Miami or Darke County. For application information and instructions, visit the website below.
Deadline: For more information, visit:

http://www.miamicountyfoundation.org/scholarships

Miami County Medical Society Scholarship

Description: The Troy Community Foundation offers the Miami County Medical Society Scholarship.
To Apply: To be eligible, the applicant must be a resident of Miami County. For application information and instructions, visit the website below.
Deadline: For more information, visit:

https://thetroyfoundation.academicworks.com/opportunities/56

Ohio Osteopathic Poster Contest

Description: The Ohio Osteopathic Symposium provides an opportunity for osteopathic medical students, interns, and residents to present their work. In 2013, the symposium featured entries from five states, including Ohio, Illinois, Pennsylvania, Washington, and West Virginia. Over 90 abstracts were submitted. Posters were judged in two categories – case reports and biomedical/clinical. First and second place winners in each category received $1,000 and $500, respectively.
To Apply: For more information, visit the website below.
Deadline: For more information, visit:

http://www.ooanet.org/aws/OOSA/pt/sp/research_poster

Physician Memorial Scholarship

Description: This scholarship is available to an incoming or current student at an accredited allopathic or osteopathic medical school. To be eligible, the applicant must be a Shelby County high school graduate. The award amount is $2,000.
To Apply: For application information and instructions, visit the Wilson Memorial Hospital website below.
Deadline: For more information, visit:

http://www.wilsonhospital.com/

Roy E. Hayes, M.D. Memorial Scholarship

Description: This scholarship is sponsored by the Community Foundation of Greater Lorain County, and is offered to college students residing in Lorain County who are attending medical school.
To Apply: For application information and instructions, contact the organization below.
Deadline: The deadline is in March. For more information, contact Community Foundation of Greater Lorain County, Ramona Grigsby, Special Projects Coordinator, 9080 Leavitt Rd., Elyria, OH 44035 or call (440) 984-7390.

Stark County Medical Society Scholarship

Description: The Stark County Medical Society offers scholarships to health care students who are residents of Stark County.
To Apply: To be eligible, the applicant must be a resident of Stark County and enrolled in an accredited health care program in Ohio. Preference is given to students who are within one to two years of completing their education. For application information and instructions, visit the website below.
Deadline: The deadline is in May. For more information, visit:

http://www.scms-a.org/pdfs/scmsa_scholarship_application.pdf

Zelma Gray Scholarship

Description: This scholarship provides funding to cover tuition and others costs for medical students who are permanent or current residents of Guernsey County.
To Apply: The applicant must be current or permanent resident of Guernsey County, Ohio, have graduated from high school in the county, and have a parent residing in the county. The application includes college transcript, MCAT scores, and financial aid form.
Deadline: The deadline is in March. For more information, visit:

http://www.appalachianohio.org/upload_files/files/Zelma%20Gray%20Medical
%20School%20Scholarship%20Application.pdf

Chapter 74

Medical Awards and Scholarships in Oklahoma

Medical students from Oklahoma and/or attending school in Oklahoma are eligible for a number of scholarships, awards, and grants. We recommend starting with your Office of Financial Aid and your school's website. Donors have provided funds to each medical school, and you may be eligible for these school-specific internal awards and scholarships. Students may also benefit from reviewing scholarship and award opportunities posted on the websites of other Oklahoma medical schools. Oklahoma residents who are attending medical school in other states may also be eligible for scholarships posted on the financial aid websites of Oklahoma medical schools. Below is a list of Oklahoma medical schools along with their websites.

Financial Aid Websites of Oklahoma Medical Schools	
Medical School	**Website**
University of Oklahoma College of Medicine	http://www.ouhsc.edu/financialservices/SFA/
Oklahoma State University College of Osteopathic Medicine	http://www.healthsciences.okstate.edu/com/financialaid/

State medical associations often have information about scholarships and loans available for students from the state or attending school in the state:

Oklahoma State Medical Assn
601 NW Grand Blvd.
Oklahoma City, OK 73118
(405) 843-9571
http://www.o-c-m-s.org/

Inquiries with your county medical society or association are recommended as well. We also encourage you to check with community foundations in the area in which you live to see if you are eligible for scholarships. Community Foundations in the State of Oklahoma are listed on the next page.

Community Foundations in Oklahoma

Bartlesville Community Foundation
Blackwell Community Foundation
Broken Arrow Community Foundation
Cherokee Strip Community Foundation
Kirkpatrick Family Fund
Oklahoma City Community Foundation
Communities Foundation of Oklahoma
Tulsa Community Foundation
Woodward Community Foundation

Catholic Foundation of Oklahoma Medical Scholarship

Description: The Catholic Foundation of Oklahoma awards scholarships to undergraduate and graduate students who are Catholics in the Archdiocese of Oklahoma City. Two scholarships in the amount of $1,000 are given annually.
To Apply: To be eligible, applicants must be attending medical school at the University of Oklahoma. Criteria for judging include merit, need, and church affiliation.
Deadline: The application deadline is in March. For more information, visit:

Oklahoma Educational Foundation for Osteopathic Medicine Scholarship

Description: The Oklahoma Educational Foundation for Osteopathic Medicine offers scholarships to medical students who are residents of Oklahoma.
To Apply: To be eligible, applicants must be residents of Oklahoma currently enrolled in an osteopathic medical school. Criteria for judging include class standing and cumulative GPA. Preference will be given to applicants who have completed their first two years of medical school and express an interest to practice in the state.
Deadline: The application deadline is in February. For more information, visit:

http://www.okosteo.org/displaycommon.cfm?an=1&subarticlenbr=33

Rural Medical Education Scholarship Loan Program

Description: The State of Oklahoma administers this scholarship program. Financial assistance is given to state residents currently enrolled in medical school who desire to practice primary care medicine in rural Oklahoma. Recipients must agree to devote one year of practice in a rural community for each year of scholarship support. A minimum of two years of practice is required.

To Apply: To be eligible, applicants must be accepted into or currently enrolled in medical school. Only state residents who intend to complete a residency in a primary care specialty will be considered.

Deadline: For more information, visit:

http://www.pmtc.ok.gov/ruraspecs.htm

Tulsa County Medical Society Education Assistance Award

Description: The Tulsa County Medical Society offers the Educational Assistance Award to medical students who are residents of the Tulsa Metropolitan area.

To Apply: The applicant must be a legal resident of the Tulsa Metropolitan area for at least the past five years. Students must be enrolled in the University of Oklahoma College of Medicine or the Oklahoma State University College of Osteopathic Medicine. Only second-, third-, and fourth-year medical students may apply.

Deadline: For more information, visit:

http://tcmsok.org/

Chapter 75

Medical Awards and Scholarships in Oregon

Medical students from Oregon and/or attending school in Oregon are eligible for a number of scholarships, awards, and grants. We recommend starting with your Office of Financial Aid and your school's website. Donors have provided funds to each medical school, and you may be eligible for these school-specific internal awards and scholarships. We also recommend that you visit the Oregon Student Access Commission which administers a number of scholarships for a variety of organizations:

http://www.getcollegefunds.org/scholarships.aspx

Students may also benefit from reviewing scholarship and award opportunities posted on the websites of other Oregon medical schools. Below is a list of Oregon medical schools along with their websites.

Financial Aid Websites of Oregon Medical Schools	
Medical School	Website
Oregon Health Sciences University	http://www.ohsu.edu/xd/education/student-services/financial-aid/
COMP - Northwest	http://www.westernu.edu/northwest/northwest-about/

State medical associations often have information about scholarships and loans available for students from the state or attending school in the state:

Oregon Medical Association
11740 SW 68th Pkwy, Ste. 100
Portland, OR 97223-9038
(503) 619-8000
http://www.theoma.org/

Inquiries with your county medical society or association are recommended as well. We also encourage you to check with community foundations in the area in which you live to see if you are eligible for scholarships. Community Foundations in the State of Oregon are listed on the next page.

Community Foundations in Oregon

Benton County Foundation
Cottage Grove Community Foundation
Four Way Community Foundation
Gorge Community Foundation
Mt. Angel Community Foundation
Newberg Community Foundation
Oregon Community Foundation
Salem Foundation
Western Lane Community Foundation

Franz Stenzel M.D. and Kathryn Stenzel Scholarship

Description: This scholarship is sponsored by the Oregon Student Access Commission, and is offered to graduates of Oregon high schools pursuing a medical degree. Applicants may attend any institution in the U.S. Financial need is a consideration.
To Apply: For application information and instructions, contact the organization below.
Deadline: The deadline is in February. For more information, contact Oregon Student Access Commission, Scholarships, Grants and Access Programs, 500 Valley River Dr., Suite 100, Eugene, OR 97401 or call (541) 687-7395.

Gayle and Harvey Rubin Scholarship

Description: This scholarship is sponsored by the Oregon Student Access Commission, and is offered to Oregon residents pursuing a MD, JD, or DDM degree. Applicants may attend any institution in the U.S. Financial need is a consideration.
To Apply: For application information and instructions, contact the organization below.
Deadline: The deadline is in February. For more information, contact Oregon Student Access Commission, Scholarships, Grants and Access Programs, 500 Valley River Dr., Suite 100, Eugene, OR 97401 or call (541) 687-7395.

James R. Naibert, M.D., Scholarship

Description: The James R. Naibert, M.D., Scholarship is offered by The Corvallis Clinic.
To Apply: To be eligible, the applicant must be a college sophomore or above who is studying in a health-related profession. Medical student applicants will only be considered if they are graduates of a high school in Linn or Benton County. Applicants must also have lived in the mid-valley for at least three years while working in a healthcare field with direct patient care.

Deadline: The deadline is in June. For more information, visit:

http://archive.constantcontact.com/fs172/1101832407064/archive/1113488922393.html

John Shonerd, DO Osteopathic Student Leadership Award

Description: The John Shonerd, DO Osteopathic Student Leadership Award is offered by the Oregon Osteopathic Foundation. The scholarship recognizes outstanding osteopathic medical student leaders.
To Apply: To be eligible, the applicant must be in good standing at an accredited osteopathic medical school in the U.S. The applicant must be entering his third or fourth year of medical school, and have the intent to practice in Oregon. The applicant must be a resident of Oregon or have lived in the state for a minimum of two years.
Deadline: For more information, visit:

http://www.opso.org/?page=Medical_Students

Myra E. Otterdale Memorial Scholarship

Description: The Myra E. Otterdale Memorial Scholarship is open to medical students who are or were residents of Oregon. The award amount ranges from $5,000 to $9,000.
To Apply: To be eligible, the applicant must have successfully completed the first year of medical school. Preference is given to applicants who lived in Jackson County (Oregon) prior to medical school matriculation. Criteria for selection include financial need, motivation, and commitment to medicine.
Deadline: The deadline is in May. For more information, visit:

http://www.faqs.org/tax-exempt/OR/Myrta-E-Otterdale-Memorial-Scholarship-Fund-2458100.html

Northwest Osteopathic Medical Association Scholarships

Description: The Northwest Osteopathic Medical Association Scholarships are awarded to medical students from Alaska, Idaho, Montana, Oregon, and Washington.
To Apply: Osteopathic medical students from Alaska, Idaho, Montana, Oregon, and Washington are eligible to apply. Applicants must be in their second, third, or fourth year of medical school. Priority is given to applicants who are committed to practicing primary care medicine in the Northwest.
Deadline: The application deadline is in May. Please see the following link for further information:

http://www.nwosteo.org/scholarship/

Osteopathic Foundation of Central Washington Scholarship (See Chapter 17)

Osteopathic Foundation of Yakima Scholarship (See Chapter 17)

Salem Hospital Foundation Scholarship

Description: The Salem Hospital Foundation offers numerous scholarships to students pursuing careers in medicine.
To Apply: To be eligible, the applicant must be a resident of Marion or Polk County.
Deadline: The deadline is in May. For more information, contact Greta Mauze at (503) 561 – 5576 or greta.mauze@salemhealth.org.

Chapter 76

Medical Awards and Scholarships in Pennsylvania

Medical students from Pennsylvania and/or attending school in Pennsylvania are eligible for a number of scholarships, awards, and grants. We recommend starting with your Office of Financial Aid and your school's website. Donors have provided funds to each medical school, and you may be eligible for these school-specific internal awards and scholarships. Students may also benefit from reviewing scholarship and award opportunities posted on the websites of other Pennsylvania medical schools. Pennsylvania residents who are attending medical school in other states may also be eligible for scholarships posted on the financial aid websites of Pennsylvania medical schools. Below is a list of Pennsylvania medical schools along with their websites.

Financial Aid Websites of Pennsylvania Medical Schools	
Medical School	**Website**
The Commonwealth Medical College	http://www.thecommonwealthmedical.com/financialaid
Drexel University College of Medicine	http://www.drexelmed.edu/Home/Admissions/MDProgram/FinancialPlanningServices.aspx
Jefferson Medical College at Thomas Jefferson University	http://www.jefferson.edu/university/academic-affairs/tju/academic-services/financial_aid/process/apply_jmc.html
Penn State University College of Medicine	http://www.pennstatehershey.org/web/md/financialaid
Lake Erie College of Osteopathic Medicine	http://lecom.edu/financial-aid.php
Perelman School of Medicine at University of Pennsylvania	http://www.med.upenn.edu/financialaid/
Philadelphia College of Osteopathic Medicine	http://www.pcom.edu/Financial_Aid/financial_aid.html
Temple University School of Medicine	http://www.temple.edu/medicine/education/student_affairs.htm
University of Pittsburgh School of Medicine	http://www.medadmissions.pitt.edu/

State medical associations often have information about scholarships and loans available for students from the state or attending school in the state:

Pennsylvania Medical Society
777 E. Park Drive
Harrisburg, PA 17111-2753
(717) 558-7750
http://pennsylvaniamedicalsociety.net/

Inquiries with your county medical society or association are recommended as well. We also encourage you to check with community foundations in the area in which you live to see if you are eligible for scholarships. Community Foundations in the State of Pennsylvania are listed below.

Community Foundations in Pennsylvania	

Adams County Community Foundation
Community Foundation for the
  Alleghenies
Armstrong County Community
  Foundation
Beaver County Foundation
Berks County Community Foundation
Bridge Builders Community Foundation
Bucks County Foundation
Central Susquehanna Community
  Foundation
Centre Foundation
Chester County Community Foundation
Clinton County Community Foundation
Crawford Heritage Community
  Foundation
Danville Area Community Foundation
Delaware County Community Foundation
Elk County Community Foundation
Erie Community Foundation
Community Foundation of Fayette County
First Community Foundation Partnership
  of Pennsylvania
Foundation for Enhancing Communities
Community Foundation of Greene County
Lancaster County Community Foundation
Lehigh Valley Community Foundation
	Luzerne Foundation
	Montgomery County Foundation
	Mt. Lebanon Community Endowment
	North East Community Foundation
	Central Pennsylvania Community
	  Foundation
	Philadelphia Foundation
	Pittsburgh Foundation
	Schuylkill Area Community Foundation
	Scranton Area Foundation
	Community Foundation of Western
	  Pennsylvania & Eastern O
	Community Foundation of the Endless
	  Mountains
	Triskeles Foundation
	Community Foundation for the Twin
	  Tiers
	Union County Foundation
	Venango Area Community Foundation
	Community Foundation of Warren County
	Washington County Community
	  Foundation
	Community Foundation of Westmoreland
	  County
	Williamsport-Lycoming Community
	  Foundation
	York County Community Foundation

A Archie Feinstein Scholarship

Description: This scholarship is available to Pennsylvania residents who will be starting their third or fourth year of osteopathic medical school. The applicant may be attending any college of osteopathic medicine in the U.S.

To Apply: For application information and instructions, contact the organization.
Deadline: For more information, contact the Pennsylvania Osteopathic Medical Association (POMA) Foundation.

Addison H. Gibson Foundation Loan

Description: The Addison H. Gibson Foundation offers low interest loans to medical students whose family home is located in western Pennsylvania.
To Apply: For application information and instructions, contact the organization.
Deadline: For more information, contact the organization at (412) 261 – 1611 or ldunbar@gibson-fnd.org.

Aetna Foundation/NMF Healthcare Leadership Program (See Chapter 13)

Alfred A. Grilli Scholarship

Description: This scholarship is available to Western Pennsylvania residents who will be starting their fourth year of osteopathic medical school. The applicant may be attending any college of osteopathic medicine in the U.S.
To Apply: For application information and instructions, contact the organization.
Deadline: For more information, contact the Pennsylvania Osteopathic Medical Association (POMA) Foundation.

Allegheny County Medical Society Medical Student Scholarship

Description: The Foundation of the Pennsylvania Medical Society administers this award. Residents of certain counties are eligible. Two medical students will each receive $2,000.
To Apply: Medical students who are residents of one of the following counties may apply: Allegheny, Armstrong, Beaver, Butler, Washington, and Westmoreland. Applicants must be in or entering their third or fourth year of medical school. The application includes two reference letters (one must be from a medical school professor or physician) and an essay. Questions that should be addressed in the essay include:

- How do you hope to be involved in your community beyond clinical care of patients?
- In what ways would you hope to demonstrate leadership as a physician in your community?

Deadline: The application deadline is in September. For more information, visit:

http://www.foundationpamedsoc.org/SFS/Scholarships/Allegheny.aspx

Alliance Medical Education Scholarship Fund

Description: The Foundation of the Pennsylvania Medical Society administers this award. Residents of Pennsylvania attending medical school in the state are eligible. The award amount is $2,000.
To Apply: Medical students who are in their second or third years of medical school may apply. Applicants must be Pennsylvania residents and U.S. citizens. At the time of application, the applicants must be second- or third-year medical students. The application includes two reference letters and an essay describing the applicant's vision for the future of Pennsylvania medicine. An interview may be required.
Deadline: The application deadline is in February. For more information, visit:

http://www.foundationpamedsoc.org/SFS/Scholarships/Allegheny.aspx

Apollo Scholarship

Description: The Cambria County Medical Society awards the Apollo Scholarship to medical students who agree to practice in the Cambria-Somerset region.
To Apply: For application information and instructions, visit the website below.
Deadline: For more information, visit:

http://www.ccmsociety.org/organizational-structure-of-the-ccms

Blair County Medical Society Scholarship

Description: The Foundation of the Pennsylvania Medical Society administers this award. Residents of Blair County are eligible. Two medical students will each receive $2,000.
To Apply: Medical students who are residents of Blair County may apply. Applicants must be enrolled in a Pennsylvania medical school as a second-, third-, or fourth-year medical student. Previous award winners are not eligible.
Deadline: For more information, visit:

http://www.foundationpamedsoc.org/SFS/Scholarships/Allegheny.aspx

Chester County Medical Society Horace P. Darlington Award

Description: The Chester County Medical Society encourages medical students who are residents of Chester County to apply for this award. The award amount is $1,000.
To Apply: For application information and instructions, contact the organization.
Deadline: The application deadline is in April. For more information, contact:

Chester County Medical Society
Carol Dot
P.O. Box 859
Kimberton, PA 19422
(610) 827 – 1543
Email: caroldot@erols.com

Chester County Medical Society Scholarship

Description: The Chester County Medical Society encourages medical students who are residents of Chester County to apply for this award. The award amount is $500. The scholarship is renewable for up to four years.
To Apply: For application information and instructions, contact the organization.
Deadline: The application deadline is in April. For more information, contact:

Chester County Medical Society
Carol Dot
P.O. Box 859
Kimberton, PA 19422
(610) 827 – 1543
Email: caroldot@erols.com

Daniel R. Miller Trust Fund for Education

Description: This scholarship is open to medical students who are residents of Pine Grove Borough and Pine Grove Township in Pennsylvania and Clear Spring in Maryland.
To Apply: For application information and instructions, contact the organization below.
Deadline: The application deadline is in April. For more information, contact:

Wachovia Bank
Daniel R. Miller Trust Fund for Education
Attn: Sally King
100 North Main Street
Winston – Salem, NC 27150
(864) 268 – 3363
http://www.wachoviascholars.com

DCMS Presidential Scholarship

Description: The Foundation of the Pennsylvania Medical Society administers this award. The award amount is $1,500. Medical students who have been residents of Pennsylvania for at least 12 months before beginning medical school may apply.

To Apply: Applicants must be in their second year of medical school at Penn State College of Medicine. The application includes two reference letters and an essay describing the person or event that most influenced the decision to become a physician. The essay should also include a description of how the applicant sees himself leading others into medicine.

Deadline: The application deadline is in April. For more information, visit:

http://www.foundationpamedsoc.org/SFS/Scholarships/Allegheny.aspx

District VIII Scholarship

Description: This scholarship is available to medical students who are Pennsylvania residents of District VIII of the Pennsylvania Osteopathic Medical Association. These include the following counties: Allegheny, Armstrong, Beaver, Bedford, Blair, Cambria, Fayette, Greene, Indiana, Somerset, Washington, and Westmoreland. Only osteopathic medical students entering their third or fourth year of medical school are eligible.

To Apply: For application information and instructions, visit the website below.

Deadline: For more information, visit:

http://studentservices.tu.edu/_resources/docs/financialaid/POMA_District_VIII _Scholarship_Application.pdf

Dr. Arthus J. and Helen M. Horvart Foundation Scholarship

Description: This is a scholarship administered by the Center for Scholarship Administration. Medical school applicants must have resided in Duryea or surrounding areas for at least one year before high school graduation.

To Apply: For application information and instructions, visit the website below.

Deadline: The deadline is in April. For more information, visit:

https://www.csascholars.org/horvat/

Dr. Frederick A. Prescott Medical Scholarship

Description: This is a scholarship given to medical students who have completed one year of medical school. Only applicants who are graduates of Elizabeth Forward High School in Allegheny County or Ohio Northern University are eligible.

To Apply: For application information and instructions, contact the organization below.

Deadline: For more information, contact:

Mrs. Joan R. Macdonald, Administrator
Medical Scholarship Fund

17 Koch Drive, McKeesport, PA 15135
412-751-5477

Dr. H. William Knab Medical Scholarship

Description: This is a scholarship for third- and fourth-year medical students who are residents of Allegheny, Armstrong, Butler, or Westmoreland County in Pennsylvania.
To Apply: The application must include a letter explaining why the applicant should be awarded the grant. For application information and instructions, contact the organization.
Deadline: For more information, contact:

Knab Medical Scholarship Grant Colonial Clinic, P.C.
P.O. Box 256
706 Ekastown Road
Sarver, PA 16055

Dr. John Garrott Memorial Scholarship

Description: This is a scholarship for medical students who are residents of Armstrong County or students who have graduated from Karns City High School. The scholarship is administered by the Cowansville Area Health Center Board of Directors. The award amount is $2,500.
To Apply: A personal essay is required. For application information and instructions, contact the organization.
Deadline: For more information, visit:

http://www.accfound.org/grants-scholarships/scholarships/scholarship-funds/dr-john-garrott-memorial-scholarship-fund/

Dr. W. R. Walter Trust Scholarship

Description: This is a scholarship offered to medical students who graduated from a public high school in Dauphin or Cumberland County, Pennsylvania.
To Apply: For application information and instructions, visit the website below.
Deadline: For more information, visit:

https://www.csascholars.org/walt/index.php

Endowment for South Asian Students of Indian Descent Scholarship

Description: The Foundation of the Pennsylvania Medical Society administers this award. The amount of the award is $2,000. Medical students who are of South Asian Indian descent may apply. Applicants must be Pennsylvania residents and enrolled full-time as a second-, third-, or fourth-year medical student in the state of Pennsylvania.

To Apply: The application includes two reference letters and an essay indicating the reasons that led the applicant to pursue a medical career and the contributions he/she expects to make in the field.

Deadline: The application deadline is in September. For more information, visit:

http://www.foundationpamedsoc.org/SFS/Scholarships/Allegheny.aspx

Hellenic Medical Society of New York Scholarship (See Chapter 12)

Hellenic University Club of Philadelphia Scholarship (See Chapter 12)

Ida Foreman Fleisher Fund (See Chapter 12)

Joseph A. Williams Medical Scholarship

Description: This scholarship is offered by the Elk County Community Foundation. Medical students who are graduates of any St. Marys PA high school may apply.

To Apply: Students accepted by or currently attending an accredited medical institution are eligible to apply. For application information and instructions, contact the organization.

Deadline: The application deadline is in April. For more information, visit:

http://www.elkcountyfoundation.com

J.B. Lowman Scholarship

Description: This scholarship is offered by the Cambria County Medical Society. Medical students who are residents of Cambria County may apply.

To Apply: Students must be accepted into an accredited medical school. For application information and instructions, contact the organization.

Deadline: The application deadline is in April. For more information, visit:

http://www.ccmsociety.org/Lowman

Lancaster Medical Society Scholarship

Description: The Lancaster Medical Society Scholarship Foundation provides financial assistance to Lancaster County residents attending medical school.

To Apply: Allopathic and osteopathic medical students are eligible to apply. Criteria for selection include academic excellence, good character, motivation, and financial need. The application includes cover letter explaining why the applicant has chosen medicine as a career, copy of income tax form (individual or parents), and transcript.

Deadline: The deadline is in July. For more information, visit:nor

http://lancastermedicalsociety.com/Content/lancastermedicalsocietyfoundation. asp

Lehigh County Medical Auxiliary's Scholarship and Education Fund Scholarship

Description: The Foundation of the Pennsylvania Medical Society administers this award. The award amount is $2,500. Medical students who are residents of Lehigh County are eligible. Applicants must be U.S. citizens and enrolled full time in an accredited U.S. medical school.

To Apply: The completed application must include two reference letters (one from a medical school professor or physician) and an essay addressing goals and expectations in medicine.

Deadline: The application deadline is in September. For more information, visit:

http://www.foundationpamedsoc.org/SFS/Scholarships/Allegheny.aspx

Lycoming County Medical Society Scholarship

Description: The Foundation of the Pennsylvania Medical Society administers this award. The award amount is $2,500. Medical students who are residents of Lycoming County are eligible. The applicant must be a resident of the county at least 12 months prior to beginning medical school.

To Apply: Full-time allopathic and osteopathic students will be considered for the award. The application includes two reference letters and an essay indicating the reasons for becoming a physician and contributions the applicant would like to make in the future.

Deadline: The application deadline is in September. For more information, visit:

http://www.foundationpamedsoc.org/SFS/Scholarships/Allegheny.aspx

Marian J. Wettrick Charitable Foundation Scholarship

Description: The Marian J. Wettrick Charitable Foundation offers scholarships to female medical students who have graduated from college in Pennsylvania. The award amount ranges from $5,000 to $35,000.

To Apply: Female medical students who have graduated from college in Pennsylvania and have continued their education in a Pennsylvania medical school are eligible to apply. This scholarship program is open to allopathic and osteopathic students.

Deadline: The deadline is in March. For more information, contact eileenb@cnbankpa.com.

Montgomery County Medical Society Scholarship

Description: The Foundation of the Pennsylvania Medical Society administers this award. The award amount is $1,000. Medical students who are residents of Montgomery County are eligible. The applicant must be a resident of the county for at least 4 years prior to beginning medical school. Exceptions to this rule are nonresident applicants who graduated from high school in the county.
To Apply: Applicants must be in or entering their first year of medical school. The application includes two reference letters and an essay indicating the reasons for becoming a physician, personal goals, and future plans.
Deadline: The application deadline is in September. For more information, visit:

http://www.foundationpamedsoc.org/SFS/Scholarships/Allegheny.aspx

Meadville Medical Center Medical Staff Memorial Scholarship

Description: The Crawford Heritage Foundation administers this scholarship. To be eligible, the applicant must have been a resident of the central or western section of Crawford County in Pennsylvania for at least one year. Allopathic and osteopathic medical students may apply.
To Apply: For application information and instructions, contact the organization below.
Deadline: For more information, visit:

http://www.crawfordheritage.org/scholarshipapply.html

Myrtle Siegfried, MD, and Michael Vigilante, MD, Scholarship

Description: The Foundation of the Pennsylvania Medical Society administers this award. The award amount is $1,000. Medical students who are residents of Berks, Lehigh, or Northhampton County are eligible.
To Apply: Applicants must be entering their first year of medical school. The completed application includes two reference letters and an essay indicating the reasons for becoming a physician and the contributions he/she expects to make in the field.
Deadline: The application deadline is in September. For more information, visit:

http://www.foundationpamedsoc.org/SFS/Scholarships/Allegheny.aspx

Northampton County Medical Society Alliance Scholarship

Description: The Northampton County Medical Society Alliance offers scholarships to medical students who reside in Northampton County and/or have a Bethlehem mailing address. The award amount is up to $1,000. Two students will be selected.

To Apply: Applicants must be enrolled in or accepted in an accredited medical school. Criteria for judging include academic achievement, community service involvement, and financial need.

Deadline: The application deadline is in March. For more information, visit:

http://www.ncmsa.org

Pennsylvania Geriatrics Society Western Division Award

Description: The Pennsylvania Geriatrics Society Western Division encourages medical students to submit abstracts. Winners will receive an honorarium of up to $1,500 to cover the costs of attending the American Geriatrics Society Annual Conference.

To Apply: Abstracts may be emailed to npopovich@acms.org, faxed to (412) 321 – 5323, or sent to:

Nadine Popovich
PA Geriatrics Society – Western Division
713 Ridge Avenue
Pittsburgh, PA 15212

Deadline: The application deadline is in March. For more information, contact Nadine Popovich as indicated above.

Ryu Family Foundation Scholarship (See Chapter 12)

Swiss Benevolent Society Scholarship (See Chapter 12)

Thomas M. Watson Memorial Scholarship

Description: The Thomas M. Watson Memorial Scholarship is offered by the Crawford Heritage Foundation. The award amount is $1,000. To be eligible, the medical school applicant must have been a resident of the central or western section of Crawford County, Pennsylvania for at least one year. Allopathic and osteopathic students may apply.

To Apply: For application information and instructions, visit the website below.

Deadline: For more information, visit:

http://www.crawfordheritage.org/scholarshipapp

Westmoreland County Medical Society Education Loan Program

Description: The Westmoreland County Medical Society offers loans to medical students attending accredited institutions. Applicants must be present or past residents of Westmoreland County.

To Apply: Medical students at all levels can apply for the loan. Criteria for judging include academic achievement, community service involvement, and financial need.

Deadline: The application deadline is in May. For more information, visit:

http://www.pamedsoc.org/

William Goldman Foundation Scholarship

Description: The William Goldman Foundation offers scholarships to medical students attending school in the Philadelphia area. Criteria for selection include scholastic achievement, financial need, and potential to make contributions to the Philadelphia community.

To Apply: For application information and instructions, contact the organization below.

Deadline: The application deadline is in March. For more information, contact William Goldman Scholarship Committee, 425 South 15th Street, Suite 1116, Philadelphia, PA 19102 or call (215) 568 – 0411.

Chapter 77

Medical Awards and Scholarships in Rhode Island

Medical students attending school in Rhode Island are eligible for a number of scholarships, awards, and grants. We recommend starting with your Office of Financial Aid and your school's website. Donors have provided funds, and you may be eligible for these school-specific internal awards and scholarships.

State medical associations often have information about scholarships and loans available for students from the state or attending school in the state:

Rhode Island Medical Society
235 Promenade St., Ste 500
Providence, RI 02908
(401) 331-3207
http://www.rimed.org/

Inquiries with your county medical society or association are recommended as well. We also encourage you to check with community foundations in the area in which you live to see if you are eligible for scholarships. Community Foundations in the State of Rhode Island include the Newport County Fund and Rhode Island Foundation.

Dr. Rudolph Jaworski Medical Scholarship

Description: The Rhode Island Polonia Scholarship Foundation provides this scholarship to a medical student of Polish-American descent. To be eligible, the applicant must be a resident of Rhode Island and a member of a Rhode Island Polish-American organization.
To Apply: Criteria for selection include academic record, character, financial need, and professional promise. For application information and instructions, visit the website below.
Deadline: The application deadline is in March. For more information, contact the organization at (401) 831 – 7177 or write to Rhode Island Polonia Scholarship Foundation, 866 Atwells Avenue, Providence RI 02909.

Paul and Mary Boghossian Memorial Trust

Description: Medical students who are of Armenian descent or a resident of Kent, Newport, or Washington counties in Rhode Island are eligible to apply for this scholarship.

To Apply: Criteria for selection include academic merit, financial need, and potential to make contributions. For application information and instructions, visit the website below.

Deadline: The application deadline is in April. For more information, contact the organization at (617) 434 – 0329 or write to Bank of America, Trustee, The Paul and Mary Boghossian Memorial Trust, Charitable Assets Division, PO Box 9477, Boston MA 02205, (617) 434-3223.

Ryu Family Foundation Scholarship (See Chapter 12)

Chapter 78

Medical Awards and Scholarships in South Carolina

Medical students from South Carolina and/or attending school in South Carolina are eligible for a number of scholarships, awards, and grants. We recommend starting with your Office of Financial Aid and your school's website. Donors have provided funds to each medical school, and you may be eligible for these school-specific internal awards and scholarships. Students may also benefit from reviewing scholarship and award opportunities posted on the websites of other South Carolina medical schools. South Carolina residents who are attending medical school in other states may also be eligible for scholarships posted on the financial aid websites of South Carolina medical schools. Below is a list of South Carolina medical schools along with their websites.

Financial Aid Websites of South Carolina Medical Schools	
Medical School	**Website**
University of South Carolina School of Medicine	http://financialaid.med.sc.edu/
Medical University of South Carolina	http://academicdepartments.musc.edu/esl/em/fin_aid/

State medical associations often have information about scholarships and loans available for students from the state or attending school in the state:

South Carolina Medical Assn.
P.O. Box 11188
Columbia, SC 29211
(803) 798-6207
https://www.scmedical.org/

Inquiries with your county medical society or association are recommended as well. We also encourage you to check with community foundations in the area in which you live to see if you are eligible for scholarships. Community Foundations in the State of South Carolina are listed on the next page.

Community Foundations in South Carolina

Central Carolina Community Foundation
Coastal Community Foundation of South Carolina
Eastern Carolina Community Foundation
Foothills Community Foundation
Community Foundation of Greenville
Greenwood County Community Foundation
Hilton Head Island Foundation
Spartanburg County Foundation
Waccamaw Community Foundation
Community Foundation of the Lowcountry

Dr. Grover White Scholarship (See Chapter 71)

South Carolina Medical Association Scholarships

Description: The South Carolina Medical Association Foundation offers a number of scholarships for medical students who are South Carolina residents. These scholarships include, but are not limited to, the following:

- Erick Crickman, MD Scholarship for a student from Darlington County with an interest in occupational medicine or family medicine
- Alice Ruth Folk Scholarship for a student from Spartanburg County
- M. Gordon Howle Scholarships for students from Greenville County
- Henry J. Stuckey Scholarship for a student from Bamberg County
- Spartanburg County Medical Society Scholarship for a student from Spartanburg County
- Cardiology Consultants of Spartanburg Scholarship for a student from Spartanburg, Laurens, Cherokee, or Union County
- Walter J. Roberts, Jr. MD Scholarship for a student who is a resident of South Carolina with financial need and GPA $\geq$ 3.0
- Florence County Medical Society Scholarship for a student from Florence County

To Apply: To be eligible, you must be attending medical school in South Carolina.
Deadline: The deadline is in March. For more information, contact Jan Price at (864) 327 - 9836

Chapter 79

Medical Awards and Scholarships in South Dakota

Medical students from South Dakota and/or attending school in South Dakota are eligible for a number of scholarships, awards, and grants. We recommend starting with your Office of Financial Aid and your school's website. Donors have provided funds, and you may be eligible for these school-specific internal awards and scholarships.

State medical associations often have information about scholarships and loans available for students from the state or attending school in the state:

South Dakota State Medical Association
P.O. Box 7406
Sioux Falls, SD 57117-7406
(605) 336-1965, ext. 3138
http://www.sdsma.org/

Inquiries with your county medical society or association are recommended as well. We also encourage you to check with community foundations in the area in which you live to see if you are eligible for scholarships. Community Foundations in the State of South Dakota are listed below.

Community Foundations in South Dakota

Black Hills Area Community Foundation
Milbank Community Foundation
Sioux Falls Area Community Foundation
South Dakota Community Foundation
Watertown Community Foundation

Amy Erickson Scholarship

Description: The Amy Erickson scholarship is given to medical students with an interest in complementary and alternative therapies. The award amount is $1,500.

To Apply: To be eligible, the applicant must be a third- or fourth-year medical student who is enrolled full-time. The applicant must submit an essay describing his interest in integrative medicine.

Deadline: The application deadline is in May. For more information, visit:

http://www.sfacf.org/ScholarshipDetails.aspx?CategoryID=7

Ashley Elizabeth Evans Medical School Scholarship

Description: The Ashley Elizabeth Evans Medical School Scholarship is given to graduates of Sioux Falls area high schools. The award amount is $2,500.

To Apply: To be eligible, the applicant must be admitted or enrolled in his first year of medical school at an accredited institution in the U.S. Criteria for judging include participation in school and community activities throughout high school and college. Academic excellence is also a consideration.

Deadline: The application deadline is in August. For more information, visit:

http://www.sfacf.org/ScholarshipDetails.aspx?CategoryID=7

Chapter 80

Medical Awards and Scholarships in Tennessee

Medical students from Tennessee and/or attending school in Tennessee are eligible for a number of scholarships, awards, and grants. We recommend starting with your Office of Financial Aid and your school's website. Donors have provided funds to each medical school, and you may be eligible for these school-specific internal awards and scholarships. Students may also benefit from reviewing scholarship and award opportunities posted on the websites of other Tennessee medical schools. Tennessee residents who are attending medical school in other states may also be eligible for scholarships posted on the financial aid websites of Tennessee medical schools. Below is a list of Tennessee medical schools along with their websites.

Financial Aid Websites of Tennessee Medical Schools	
Medical School	Website
Vanderbilt University School of Medicine	https://medschool.vanderbilt.edu/financial-services/medical-students
University of Tennessee College of Medicine	http://www.uthsc.edu/finaid/
East Tennessee State University James H. Quillen College of Medicine	http://www.etsu.edu/com/sa/finaid/
Meharry Medical College	http://www.mmc.edu/prospectivestudents/financial-aid/
Lincoln Memorial University Debusk College of Osteopathic Medicine	http://www.lmunet.edu/dcom/finaid/

State medical associations often have information about scholarships and loans available for students from the state or attending school in the state:

Tennessee Medical Association
P.O. Box 120909
Nashville, TN 37212-0909
(615) 385-2100
http://www.tnmed.org/

Inquiries with your county medical society or association are recommended as well. We also encourage you to check with community foundations in the area in which you live to see if you are eligible for scholarships. Community Foundations in the State of Tennessee are listed below.

Community Foundations in Tennessee

Community Foundation of Greater Chattanooga
Community Foundation of Cleveland and Bradley County
East Tennessee Foundation
Community Foundation of Greater Memphis
Community Foundation of Middle Tennessee
Community Foundation of Oblon County

Dr. Bill and Emily Jackson Medical Scholarship

Description: The Dr. Bill and Emily Jackson Medical Scholarship is given to a medical school student from certain counties in Tennessee. The award amount is up to $10,000.
To Apply: To be eligible, the applicant must have been a resident of Dickson, Hickman, or Humphreys Counties for at least one year before submission of the application. Criteria for judging include academic achievement and financial need.
Deadline: The deadline for the application is in May. For more information, visit:

http://www.goodlark.com/2014_01_30_new_goodlark_website_007.htm

Gordon W. and Agnes P. Cobb Scholarship

Description: The Cobb Scholarship provides support to students pursuing careers in medicine.
To Apply: To be eligible, the applicant must have graduated from a high school in Blount, Loudon, or Knox County. Financial need and strong work/volunteer history are considerations. Applicants from single parent families are given special consideration.
Deadline: For more information, visit:

http://www.easttennesseefoundation.org/receive/library_pages/gordon_w_and_agnes_p_cobb_scholarship.aspx

Linda P. Hare Scholarship

Description: Medical students from Meharry Medical College and Vanderbilt University School of Medicine may apply for this scholarship. The Community Foundation of Middle Tennessee administers this award.
To Apply: Criteria for judging include academic record. The applicant must submit a statement of their professional goals and commitment to addressing health equity. Preference is given to minority students.
Deadline: For more information, visit:

http://www.cfmt.org/request/scholarships/scholarships-specific-areas-study/

Tennessee Baptist Foundation Scholarship

Description: The Tennessee Baptist Foundation offers a scholarship to medical students.
To Apply: To be eligible, the applicant must have been a resident of Tennessee for at least one year prior to submission of the application. The applicant must also be a member of a church cooperating with the Tennessee Baptist Convention. Applicant must be enrolled full-time in an accredited medical school and maintain a GPA of at least 3.0. Criteria for judging include academic performance and involvement in church and Baptist Collegiate Ministries.
Deadline: For more information, visit:

http://www.tbfoundation.org/tbf.asp?cat=edu&subcat=qualischol

Chapter 81

Medical Awards and Scholarships in Texas

Medical students from Texas and/or attending school in Texas are eligible for a number of scholarships, awards, and grants. We recommend starting with your Office of Financial Aid and your school's website. Donors have provided funds to each medical school, and you may be eligible for these school-specific internal awards and scholarships. Students may also benefit from reviewing scholarship and award opportunities posted on the websites of other Texas medical schools. Texas residents who are attending medical school in other states may also be eligible for scholarships posted on the financial aid websites of Texas medical schools. Below is a list of Texas medical schools along with their websites.

Financial Aid Websites of Texas Medical Schools	
Medical School	Website
Baylor College of Medicine	https://www.bcm.edu/education/financial-aid
Texas A & M University College of Medicine	http://www.tamhsc.edu/education/finaid/index.html
Texas Tech University Paul L. Foster School of Medicine (El Paso)	http://elpaso.ttuhsc.edu/fostersom/studentaffairs/finaid.aspx
Texas Tech University (Lubbock)	http://www.ttuhsc.edu/financialaid/
Texas College of Osteopathic Medicine	http://web.unthsc.edu/departments/financialaid/
University of Texas Medical School at Houston	https://www.uth.edu/sfs/
University of Texas San Antonio	http://som.uthscsa.edu/FAME/tuition_fees.asp
University of Texas Southwestern	http://www.utsouthwestern.edu/about-us/administrative-offices/financial-aid/index.html
University of Texas Medical Branch	http://www.utmb.edu/enrollmentservices/financialaid.asp

State medical associations often have information about scholarships and loans available for students from the state or attending school in the state:

Texas Medical Association
401 West 15th St. Austin, TX
78701-1680
(512) 370-1300
http://www.texmed.org/

Inquiries with your county medical society or association are recommended as well. We also encourage you to check with community foundations in the area in which you live to see if you are eligible for scholarships. Community Foundations in the State of Texas are listed below.

Community Foundations in Texas	
Community Foundation of Abilene	Matagorda County Community
Amarillo Area Foundation	Foundation
Austin Community Foundation for the	McKenna Foundation
Capital Area	Montgomery County Community
Bandera Community Foundation	Foundation
Big Spring Area Community Foundation	New Braunfels Area Community
Community Foundation of Brazoria	Foundation
County	Community Foundation of North Texas
Brownsville Community Foundation	Permian Basin Area Foundation
Chautaqua Foundation	Rio Grande Valley Community
Coastal Bend Community Foundation	Foundation
Dallas Foundation	Greater Round Rock Community
Dallas Jewish Community Foundation	Foundation
Denison Community Foundation	San Angelo Area Foundation
East Texas Community Foundation	San Antonio Area Foundation
El Paso Community Foundation	Texas Area Fund Foundation
Foundation for Southeast Texas	Community Foundation of the Texas Hill
Community Foundation	Country
Chisholm Trail Communities Foundation	Texas Valley Communities Foundation
Heart of Texas Community Foundation	Communities Foundation of Texas
Greater Houston Community Foundation	Waco Foundation
Laredo Area Community Foundation	Wharton County Community Foundation
Levelland Area Endowment	Wichita Falls Area Community
Lubbock Area Foundation	Foundation

AMWA Southwest Chapter Student Scholarship

Description: The American Medical Writers Association offers this scholarship to encourage students who have an interest in medical writing to engage with the AMWA community. The winner will receive funds to cover the costs of attending the AMWA SW conference, including registration fee and lodging.
To Apply: To be eligible, applicants must be enrolled full-time in an accredited institution. The application includes letter of recommendation and essay

describing the student's reasons for wishing to attend the SW Regional AMWA conference.

Deadline: The deadline is in May. For more information, visit:

http://www.amwasouthwest.org/

Dr. Edgar Martin Harp Memorial Scholarship for Medical or Veterinary Students

Description: The Community Foundation of Abilene provides this scholarship to graduates of Nolan or Taylor County high schools.

To Apply: Applicants must be accepted to an accredited medical or veterinary school.

Deadline: For more information, visit:

http://cfabilene.org/available-college-scholarships

Harris County Medical Society Alliance Scholarship

Description: The Harris County Medical Society Alliance Scholarship is available to medical students at the Baylor College of Medicine and UT Houston Health Science Center. Applicants who reside in Harris County for one year or more prior to attending an accredited medical school out of Harris County may also apply.

To Apply: To be eligible, the applicant must be a U.S. citizen who is in his third or fourth year of medical school. The medical school determines the recipient. Contact your school for more information.

Deadline: For more information, visit:

https://www.tmaloanfunds.com/Content/Template.aspx?id=9#5

Montgomery County Medical Society Scholarship

Description: The Montgomery County Medical Society offers scholarships to medical students who are residents of Montgomery County, Texas.

To Apply: The application includes transcripts and letters of recommendation. A brief statement of your reasons for choosing the medical field as your profession is also required. For application information and instructions, visit the website below.

Deadline: For more information, visit:

http://www.montgomerycms.com/Template.aspx?id=126

North Texas Latin American Physicians Association Scholarship

Description: The North Texas Latin American Physicians Association offers scholarships to medical students in North Texas.
To Apply: To be eligible, the applicant must be:

- Enrolled (or will be) at UT Southwestern Medical School or University of North Texas Health Science Center OR
- College student from the North Texas Region who will be enrolled in a Texas medical school OR
- Current medical student from the North Texas Region enrolled in a Texas Medical School

The North Texas region includes the following counties: Collin, Dallas, Denton, Ellis, Franklin, Erath, Hood, Hunt, Grayson, Johnson, Kaufman, Navarro, Palo Pinto, Parker, Red River, Rockwall, Somervell, Tarrant, and Wise. The applicant (or parents/grandparents) must be descended from a Latin American country. For application information and instructions, visit the website below.
Deadline: The deadline is in May. For more information, visit:

http://www.ntlapa.com/about-us.html

Ridglea Lone Star Texas Vivian Eickoff Scholarship

Description: This scholarship supports students pursuing careers in health care and nursing. The award amount is up to $1,000.
To Apply: To be eligible, the applicant must be a citizen of the U.S. and Texas resident in the Greater Fort Worth Area.
Deadline: The deadline is in April. For more information, visit:

http://scholarships.site.swau.edu/ridglea-lone-star-texas-business-women-scholarship/

Smith County Medical Society Scholarship

Description: The Smith County Medical Society offers scholarships to medical students who are residents of Smith County, Texas.
To Apply: To be eligible, the applicant must be in the first, second, or third year of medical school. Financial need is a consideration. The application includes letters of recommendation.
Deadline: The deadline is in March. For more information, visit:

www.scmsalliance.com

Texas Academy of Family Practice Poster Competition

Description: The Texas Academy of Family Practice (TAFP) invites medical students, residents, and family physicians to submit their family medicine research for presentation at the TAFP Annual Session & Scientific Assembly in July.
To Apply: For more information, contact Samantha White at (512) 329-8666 Ext 16. Fax completed abstracts and applications to (512) 329-8237 or email them to Samantha at swhite@tafp.org.
Deadline: For more information, visit:

http://www.tafp.org/professional-development/assa/poster-competition

Texas Medical Association Fifty Year Club Scholarship

Description: The Texas Medical Association Fifty Year Club Scholarship is open to students at all Texas medical schools.
To Apply: To be eligible, the applicant must be a U.S. citizen who is in his second, third, or fourth year of medical school. The medical school determines the recipient. Contact your school for more information.
Deadline: For more information, visit:

https://www.tmaloanfunds.com/Content/Template.aspx?id=9

Texas Medical Association Minority Scholarship

Description: This scholarship is offered to minorities underrepresented in the physician workforce in the state of Texas. One scholarship is made available to each school annually. The amount of the award is $5,000.
To Apply: Applicants must be African American, Hispanic, or Native American. Only incoming medical school freshman are eligible. The application requires letter of medical school acceptance and essay. The essay should describe how the applicant would "improve the health of all Texans."
Deadline: For more information, visit:

https://www.tmaloanfunds.com/Content/Template.aspx?id=9

Texas Medical Liability Trust Scholarship

Description: The Texas Medical Liability Trust will award four $10,000 scholarships to students interested in finding creative and effective ways to enhance patient safety.
To Apply: According to the organization, "recipients will be chosen in a competition that weighs students' financial need along with their ability to evaluate the patient safety concerns in a closed claim study and communicate their recommendations in an essay."[1] To be eligible, the applicant must be entering their second, third, or fourth year at a Texas medical school. Only

current student members (or have a student application pending with) of the Texas Medical Association will be considered.
Deadline: The deadline is in June. For more information, visit:

http://www.tmlt.org/tmlt/about-tmlt/news-events/press-releases/tmlt-commits--40-000-in-scholarships-to-texas-medical-students.html

Travis County Medical Society Evans Swann Scholarship

Description: The Travis County Medical Society Foundation offers a scholarship to two medical students in Texas who graduated from a Travis County high school.
To Apply: Criteria for judging include character and ability. Financial need is a consideration. Applicants are asked to submit a personal essay addressing the role of the physician as a doctor, family member, and community member.
Deadline: The deadline is in May. For more information, visit:

http://www.tcms.com/member/documents/ScholarshipApplication.pdf

References

[1]Texas Medical Liability Trust. Available at: https://www.tmlt.org/tmlt/about-tmlt/news-events/press-releases/tmlt-commits--40-000-in-scholarships-to-texas-medical-students.html. Accessed July 2, 2014.

Chapter 82

Medical Awards and Scholarships in Utah

Medical students from Utah and/or attending school in Utah are eligible for a number of scholarships, awards, and grants. We recommend starting with your Office of Financial Aid and your school's website. Donors have provided funds, and you may be eligible for these school-specific internal awards and scholarships.

State medical associations often have information about scholarships and loans available for students from the state or attending school in the state:

Utah Medical Association
310 E. 4500 South, Ste. 500
Murray, UT 84107-4250
(801) 747-3500
http://www.utahmed.org/

Inquiries with your county medical society or association are recommended as well. We also encourage you to check with community foundations in the area in which you live to see if you are eligible for scholarships. Community Foundations in the State of Utah include the Park City Foundation and the Community Foundation of Utah.

Saccomanno Higher Education Foundation Scholarship (See Chapter 44)

Utah EMBA Alumni Service Scholarship

Description: The University of Utah Executive MBA Program offers this scholarship to students who have given back to their communities. Medical students are eligible. The award amount is $5,000. The scholarship program is administered by the Community Foundation of Utah.
To Apply: To be eligible, applicants must design and execute a service project. Only University of Utah students will be considered.
Deadline: For more information, visit:

http://utahcf.org/apply-for-a-grant/Apply-for-a-Scholarship/

Chapter 83

Medical Awards and Scholarships in Vermont

Medical students from Vermont and/or attending school in Vermont are eligible for a number of scholarships, awards, and grants. We recommend starting with your Office of Financial Aid and your school's website. Donors have provided funds, and you may be eligible for these school-specific internal awards and scholarships.

State medical associations often have information about scholarships and loans available for students from the state or attending school in the state:

Vermont Medical Society
P.O. Box 1457
Montpelier, VT 05601
(802) 223-7898
http://www.vtmd.org/

Inquiries with your county medical society or association are recommended as well. We also encourage you to check with community foundations in the area in which you live to see if you are eligible for scholarships. The Vermont Community Foundation is the major foundation in the state.

Kenneth and Bessie Ladeau Trust

Description: This is a scholarship fund for medical students. Preference is given to residents of New Hampshire and Vermont.
To Apply: To be eligible, applicants must have completed their first year of medical school. Criteria for judging include good academic standing and high moral character. The award amount is $300-500 per year.
Deadline: The deadline is in March. For more information, write to:

L. Raymond Massucco, Esq., Trustee
Kenneth & Bessie Ladeau Trust
c/o Massucco Law Offices, P.C.
90 Westminster Street
Bellows Falls , VT 05101
Tel: (802) 463-3303
Email: ray@massuccolaw.com

Ryu Family Foundation Scholarship (See Chapter 12)

Vermont Student Assistance Corporation

Description: This is a scholarship fund for medical students who are residents of Vermont.
To Apply: For application information and instructions, visit the website below.
Deadline: For more information, visit www.vsac.org or write to:

Scholarship Programs
Vermont Student Assistance Corporation
PO Box 2000
Champlain Mill
Winooski, VT 05404-2601
Email: info@vsac.org

Vermont Medical Society Education and Research Foundation Scholarship

Description: The Vermont Medical Society Education and Research Foundation Scholarship provide "an incentive for candidates to pursue a career in medicine and to provide motivation for graduates to practice in Vermont. All contributions to the foundation are tax deductible."[1]
To Apply: Visit the Society website for more information.
Deadline: For more information, visit:

http://www.vmsfoundation.org/scholarships

Profile of a Winner

Jen Makrides, a medical student at the University of Vermont College of Medicine, was a recent recipient of the Vermont Medical Society Education and Research Foundation Scholarship. As co-chair of the Vermont Human Trafficking Task Force's health subcommittee, Jen has been heavily involved in several research projects related to this important issue. She is also a writer, and her work has been published by Physicians for Human Rights, National Women's Law Center, and Human Strategies/Human Rights.[1]

References

[1]Vermont Medical Society Education and Research Foundation. Available at: http://www.vtmd.org/foundation-awards-scholarship-uvm-com-students. Accessed July 2, 2014.

Chapter 84

Medical Awards and Scholarships in Virginia

Medical students from Virginia and/or attending school in Virginia are eligible for a number of scholarships, awards, and grants. We recommend starting with your Office of Financial Aid and your school's website. Donors have provided funds to each medical school, and you may be eligible for these school-specific internal awards and scholarships. Students may also benefit from reviewing scholarship and award opportunities posted on the websites of other Virginia medical schools. Virginia residents who are attending medical school in other states may also be eligible for scholarships posted on the financial aid websites of Virginia medical schools. Below is a list of Virginia medical schools along with their websites.

Financial Aid Websites of Virginia Medical Schools	
Medical School	**Website**
University of Virginia School of Medicine	http://www.medicine.virginia.edu/education/medical-students/financial-aid/financial-aid
VCU School of Medicine	http://www.medschool.vcu.edu/studentaffairs/financial_aid/
Virginia Tech Carilion School of Medicine	http://www.vtc.vt.edu/education/admissions/tuition_fees.html
Edward Via College of Osteopathic Medicine	http://www.vcom.edu/financial/
Liberty University College of Osteopathic Medicine	https://www.liberty.edu/lucom/index.cfm?PID=27161

State medical associations often have information about scholarships and loans available for students from the state or attending school in the state:

Medical Society of Virginia
2924 Emerywood Pkwy.
Richmond, VA 23294
(800) 746-6768
http://www.msv.org/

Inquiries with your county medical society or association are recommended as well. We also encourage you to check with community foundations in the area in which you live to see if you are eligible for scholarships. Community Foundations in the State of Virginia are listed below.

Community Foundations in Virginia	
ACT for Alexandria Community Foundation of the Central Blue Ridge Charlottesville Area Community Foundation Community Foundation for Rockbridge Bath and Allegany Community Foundation of Northern Shenandoah Valley Foundation for Roanoke Valley Community Foundation of the Dan River Region Eastern Shore of Virginia Community Foundation Hampton Roads Community Foundation Community Foundation of Harrisonburg & Rockingham County Greater Lynchburg Community Trust Martinsville Area Community Foundation Community Foundation of the New River Valley	Northern Piedmont Community Foundation Community Foundation for Northern Virginia Peninsula Community Foundation of Virginia Piedmont Community Foundation Southeast Virginia Community Foundation Community Foundation of the Rappahannock River Region Community Foundation Serving Richmond & Central Virginia River Counties Community Foundation Rockbridge Area Community Foundation Shenandoah Community Foundation Suffolk Foundation Community Foundation Williamsburg Community Foundation Yorktown Community Foundation

ACAP – MAC Julian Cheng Hu Scholarship (See Chapter 58)

Chesapeake Medical Society Hubert W. Kuehn Scholarship

Description: The Chesapeake Medical Society offers the Hubert W. Kuehn Scholarship to medical students from Chesapeake, Virginia.
To Apply: For more information, contact the society. The award amount is $1,000.
Deadline: The deadline is in March. For more information, contact:

Ms. Leslie Phelps (Executive Director)
(757) 312 – 6192
leslie.phelps@chesapeakeregional.com

Hampton Roads Community Foundation

Description: Scholarships are available from the Hampton Roads Community Foundation:

- Florence L. Smith Medical (long-time Virginia residents attending medical school at Eastern Virginia Medical School, University of Virginia, or Virginia Commonwealth)
- Helen and Buzzy Schulwolf Fund for Smith Scholars (supplemental scholarship for recipient of the Smith Scholarship)
- Drs. Kirkland Ruffin & Willcox Ruffin Scholarship (students from Norfolk attending Eastern Virginia Medical School)
- Lewis K. Marin II, M.D. and Cheryl Rose Martin Scholarship (Virginia residents studying medicine at the University of Virginia)

To Apply: The application includes personal statement, two letters of recommendation, transcript, and financial need information.
Deadline: For more information, visit:

http://www.hamptonroadscf.org/scholarships/availableGraduateScholarships.html

Health Focus of Southwest Virginia Scholarship

Description: The Health Focus of Southwest Virginia offers these scholarships primarily to residents of Southwest Virginia. Award amounts vary from $250 to $3,500.
To Apply: Medical students from Southwest Virginia attending medical school in Virginia are given preference. The application includes transcripts, copy of tax return, personal summary, and proof of medical school admission or enrollment.
Deadline: The deadline is in May. For more information, visit:

http://healthfocusswva.org/scholarships/

Medical Society of Northern Virginia Scholarship

Description: The Medical Society of Northern Virginia offers scholarships to students attending medical school in Virginia. Candidates must be residents of Fairfax County or Loudon County. The award amount is $2,500.
To Apply: Only third-year medical students who are residents of Fairfax or Loudon County may apply. Candidates must be attending medical school in Virginia. The application includes CV, reference letters, and personal statement.
Deadline: The deadline is in April. For more information, visit:

http://www.msnva.org/foundation/

Mid-Tidewater Medical Society Scholarships

Description: The Mid-Tidewater Medical Society offers scholarships to students attending medical school in Virginia. Candidates must have connections to one of the following counties: Gloucester, Mathews, or Middlesex.

To Apply: The application includes the CV.

Deadline: The deadline is in October. For more information, email sarah.west@rivhs.com.

Roanoke Valley Academy of Medicine Alliance

Description: Multiple scholarships are available for students who attended high school in Roanoke Valley or who have lived and worked in the area for at least one year. Included in this area are Roanoke City and County, Salem, Botetourt County, Franklin County, and Craig County.

To Apply: For application information and instructions, contact the organization.

Deadline: The deadline is in May. For more information, contact:

Karen Davidson, Scholarship Committee
P.O. Box 8602
Roanoke, VA 24014
Email: rvam@rvam.org
(540) 345 - 8618

Chapter 85

Medical Awards and Scholarships in Washington

Medical students from Washington and/or attending school in Washington are eligible for a number of scholarships, awards, and grants. We recommend starting with your Office of Financial Aid and your school's website. Donors have provided funds to each medical school, and you may be eligible for these school-specific internal awards and scholarships. Students may also benefit from reviewing scholarship and award opportunities posted on the websites of other Washington medical schools. Washington residents who are attending medical school in other states may also be eligible for scholarships posted on the financial aid websites of Washington medical schools. Below is a list of Washington medical schools along with their websites.

Financial Aid Websites of Washington Medical Schools	
Medical School	Website
University of Washington	http://www.uwmedicine.org/education/md-program/admissions/financial-aid
College of Osteopathic Medicine of the Pacific-Northwest	http://www.pnwu.edu/students/financial-aid/

If you are a student from Washington attending medical school out of state, we encourage you to visit these websites to learn about scholarships that you may be eligible for.

State medical associations often have information about scholarships and loans available for students from the state or attending school in the state:

Washington State Medical Assn.
2033 6th Ave., Suite 1100
Seattle, WA 98121
(206) 441-9762
http://www.wsma.org/

Inquiries with your county medical society or association are recommended as well.

We also encourage you to check with community foundations in the area in which you live to see if you are eligible for scholarships. Community Foundations in the State of Washington are listed below.

Community Foundations in Washington	
Bainbridge Community Foundation Blue Mountain Community Foundation Columbia Basin Foundation Cowlitz Community Foundation Greater Everett Community Foundation Grays Harbor Community Foundation Inland Northwest Community Foundation Jefferson County Community Foundation Kent Community Foundation Kitsap Community Foundation Community Foundation of North Central Washington Orcas Island Community Foundation Preston Community Foundation Community Foundation of South Puget Sound	Renton Community Foundation San Juan Island Community Foundation Seattle Foundation Olympic View Community Foundation Skagit Community Foundation South Pacific County Community Foundation Community Foundation for Southwest Washington Stanwood-Camano Area Foundation Greater Tacoma Community Foundation Three Rivers Community Foundation Turtle Island Community Foundation Whatcom Community Foundation Yakima Valley Community Foundation

Arthur and Dorren Parrett Scholarship

Description: The US Bank National Association administers this scholarship. To be eligible, the applicant must be a resident of the state of Washington and have completed the first year of medical school. The award amount is $900 to $2,100.
To Apply: Criteria for selection include academic merit and financial need. For application information and instructions, contact the organization below.
Deadline: The application deadline is in July. For more information, contact:

US Bank National Assoc.
Trustee
Parrett Scholarship Foundation
PD-WA-T21P
1420 Fifth Avenue, Suite 2100
Seattle, WA 98101-4085

Jayne M. Perkins Memorial Scholarship (See Chapter 18)

Northwest Osteopathic Medical Association Scholarships (See Chapter 17)

Osteopathic Foundation of Central Washington Scholarship (See Chapter 17)

Washington Osteopathic Foundation Scholarship

Description: This scholarship program is available to osteopathic medical students who have completed two years of their training. The applicant must be a member of the Washington Osteopathic Medicine Association but does not have to attend medical school in Washington. The maximum loan is $5,000 per year.
To Apply: For application information and instructions, contact the organization below.
Deadline: For more information, contact:

Washington Osteopathic Foundation, Inc.
P.O. Box 16486
Seattle, WA 98116-6529
(206) 937-5358

Washington Student Achievement Council American Indian Endowed Scholarship

Description: The American Indian Endowed Scholarship provides scholarships to students who have ties to an American Indian tribe or community.
To Apply: Students can use scholarships at institutions in the state of Washington. Criteria for judging include academic merit and commitment to serve the American Indian community in Washington.
Deadline: For more information, visit:

http://www.wsac.wa.gov/american-indian-endowed-scholarship

Chapter 86

Medical Awards and Scholarships in West Virginia

Medical students from West Virginia and/or attending school in West Virginia are eligible for a number of scholarships, awards, and grants. We recommend starting with your Office of Financial Aid and your school's website. Donors have provided funds to each medical school, and you may be eligible for these school-specific internal awards and scholarships. Students may also benefit from reviewing scholarship and award opportunities posted on the websites of other West Virginia medical schools. "Students interested in pursuing careers in the health professions should not overlook the possibility of scholarship assistance in their own communities," writes the West Virginia University School of Medicine. "West Virginia has more than 100 community foundations, some of which offer scholarship support. These foundations may not have telephone listings because very few have paid staff. Check your local library for information on community foundations, or see if the reference desk has the West Virginia Foundation Directory, published by the Kanawha County Public Library."[1] Below is a list of West Virginia medical schools along with their websites.

Financial Aid Websites of West Virginia Medical Schools	
Medical School	**Website**
West Virginia University School of Medicine	http://financialaid.wvu.edu/home/hsc-office/aid-specific-to-certain-disciplines-of-study/medicine-m-d
Joan C. Edwards School of Medicine at Marshall University	http://jcesom.marshall.edu/students/financial-assistance/
West Virginia School of Osteopathic Medicine	http://www.wvsom.edu/OMS/financial-aid

State medical associations often have information about scholarships and loans available for students from the state or attending school in the state:

West Virginia State Medical Association
4307 MacCorkle Ave. SE
Charleston, WV 25304
(304) 925-0342
http://www.wvsma.com/

Inquiries with your county medical society or association are recommended as well. We also encourage you to check with community foundations in the area in which you live to see if you are eligible for scholarships. Community Foundations in the State of West Virginia are listed below.

Community Foundations in West Virginia	
Barbour County Community Foundation	Logan County Charitable and Educational
Beckley Area Foundation	Foundation
Boone County Community Foundation	Mason County Community Foundation
Doddridge County Community Foundation	Nicholas County Community Foundation
Eastern West Virginia Community Foundation	Community Foundation for the Ohio Valley
Hampshire County Community Foundation	Parkerburg Area Community Foundation
Hinton Area Foundation	Ritchie County Community Foundation
Jackson County Community Foundation	Lincoln County Community Foundation
Community Foundation of Jefferson County	Tucker County Community Foundation
Greater Kanawha Valley Foundation	Community Foundation of the Virginias
Little Kanawha Area Community Foundation	Your Community Foundation

Dr. A. Robert Marks Memorial Scholarship

Description: Medical students who have graduated from Harrison County High School or are residents of Harrison County may apply.
To Apply: For application information and instructions, contact the organization.
Deadline: For more information, contact:

Angela Urso
513 Heritage Road
Bridgeport, WV 26330
(304) 842 – 9557
aurso@bearcontracting.com

Family Medicine Foundation of West Virginia Educational Scholarship Program

Description: The Family Medicine Foundation of West Virginia offers these scholarships to medical students who are residents of West Virginia. Students must have plans to enter the field of family medicine in West Virginia. The award amount is $5,000, and four awards will be available. A service obligation following completion of training is required.
To Apply: Applicants must be residents of West Virginia, and entering the second, third, or fourth year of medical school. Only members of the West Virginia Chapter American Academy of Family Physicians are eligible. Two reference letters are required.
Deadline: The application is due in March. For more information, visit:

http://financialaid.wvu.edu/r/download/150670

Nicholas and Mary Trivillian Memorial Scholarship

Description: The Greater Kanawha Valley Foundation sponsors the Nicholas and Mary Trivillian Memorial Scholarship.
To Apply: Applicants must be residents of West Virginia enrolled full-time in medical school. Criteria for judging include minimum GPA, good moral character, and financial need.
Deadline: For more information, visit:

http://www.tgkvf.org

S. William & Martha R. Goff Educational Scholarship

Description: This is a scholarship administered by the Parkersburg Area Community Foundation.
To Apply: To be eligible, the medical school applicant must have attended high school in Wood County. Criteria for selection include merit and need.
Deadline: The deadline is in March. For more information, visit:

http://www.pacfwv.com/scholarships3.aspx#award

West Virginia Health Sciences Scholarship Program

Description: Medical students interested in practicing primary care and rural health in West Virginia may participate in the West Virginia Health Sciences Scholarship Program. Through this program, fifteen scholarships are awarded each year. The award amount is $20,000. Participants must sign a contract to complete a service obligation following training in an underserved area of West Virginia for a minimum of two years.
To Apply: Fourth-year students attending a West Virginia medical school are eligible to apply. Applicants must be entering a primary care internship or residency program (family medicine, internal medicine, pediatrics, combined medicine/pediatrics, obstetrics and gynecology, psychiatry). For application information and instructions, visit the website below.
Deadline: The application is due in October. For more information, visit:

https://secure.cfwv.com/Financial_Aid_Planning/Scholarships/Scholarships_and_Grants/WV_Health_Sciences_Scholarship_Program.aspx

References

[1]West Virginia University. Available at: http://financialaid.wvu.edu/home/hsc-office/aid-specific-to-certain-disciplines-of-study/medicine-m-d/md-specific-scholarships. Accessed July 2, 2014.

Chapter 87

Medical Awards and Scholarships in Wisconsin

Medical students from Wisconsin and/or attending school in Wisconsin are eligible for a number of scholarships, awards, and grants. We recommend starting with your Office of Financial Aid and your school's website. Donors have provided funds to each medical school, and you may be eligible for these school-specific internal awards and scholarships. Students may also benefit from reviewing scholarship and award opportunities posted on the websites of other Wisconsin medical schools. Wisconsin residents who are attending medical school in other states may also be eligible for scholarships posted on the financial aid websites of Wisconsin medical schools. Below is a list of Wisconsin medical schools along with their websites.

Financial Aid Websites of Wisconsin Medical Schools	
Medical School	**Website**
Medical College of Wisconsin	http://www.mcw.edu/medicalschool/financialaid.htm
University of Wisconsin School of Medicine and Public Health	http://finaid.wisc.edu/269.htm

State medical associations often have information about scholarships and loans available for students from the state or attending school in the state. Inquiries with your county medical society or association are recommended as well. We also encourage you to check with community foundations in the area in which you live to see if you are eligible for scholarships. Community Foundations in the State of Wisconsin are listed on the next page.

Amy Hunter – Wilson, M.D., Scholarship

Description: This scholarship award is open to American Indian students pursuing careers in medicine. Award amounts are $1,000 or more.
To Apply: Only U.S. citizens enrolled full-time in an accredited medical school who are members of a federally recognized American Indian tribe may apply. Preference will be given to Wisconsin residents who are attending school in Wisconsin. Criteria for judging include academic achievement, personal qualities and strengths, letters of recommendation, and financial need.

Deadline: The application deadline is in February. For more information, visit:

https://www.wisconsinmedicalsociety.org/_WMS/about_us/foundation/for_stu
dents/scholarships/2014/Victor%20A%20%20Baylon%20MD%20Scholarship
2014-2015.pdf

Community Foundations in Wisconsin	
Apostle Islands Area Community Foundation	Greater Green Bay Community Foundation
Ashland Foundation	Kenosha Community Foundation
Baldwin Area Community Foundation	La Crosse Community Foundation
Black River Falls Area Foundation	Lake Country Community Foundation
Chilton Area Community Foundation	Lakeshore Community Foundation
Clark County Community Foundation	Madison Community Foundation
Community Foundation of Central Wisconsin	Marshfield Area Community Foundation
Community Foundation of Chippewa County	Greater Milwaukee Foundation
Community Foundation of Dunn County	New Richmond Area Community Foundation
Community Foundation of Southern Wisconsin	Community Foundation of North Central Wisconsin
Grant County Community Foundation	Oshkosh Area Community Foundation
Community Foundation of Southern Wisconsin	Racine Community Foundation
Green County Community Foundation	Greater Sauk County Community Foundation
Community Foundation of Southern Wisconsin Rock	Shawano Area Community Foundation
Door County Community Foundation	Incourage Community Foundation
Eau Claire Community Foundation	Community Foundation of Southern Wisconsin
Fond du Lac Area Foundation	St. Croix Valley Foundation
Forest County Potawatomi Community Foundation	Stateline Community Foundation
Fort Atkinson Community Foundation	Watertown Area Community Foundation
Community Foundation of the Fox River Valley Region	Waukesha County Community Foundation
	Waupaca Area Community Foundation
	West Bend Community Foundation

Catherine Slota-Varma, MD Scholarship

Description: The Wisconsin Medical Society administers this award. Students attending medical school in Wisconsin may apply.

To Apply: Only full-time U.S. students in Wisconsin may apply. In the personal statement, applicants are asked to write about their desire to become a primary care physician. The personal statement should also include examples of leadership with organized medicine. Criteria for judging include academic achievement, personal qualities and strengths, letters of recommendation, and financial need.

Deadline: The application deadline is in February. For more information, visit: https://www.wisconsinmedicalsociety.org/_WMS/about_us/foundation/for_stu dents/scholarships/2014/Victor%20A%20%20Baylon%20MD%20Scholarship 2014-2015.pdf

Dr. J. Chris Kerr Memorial Scholarship

Description: The Mayo Clinic Health System – Northland offers this scholarship to students enrolled in medical school. Applicants must have graduated from high school in Barron County, Wisconsin.
To Apply: For application information, contact the organization below.
Deadline: The application deadline is in April. For more information, contact Sarah Salzgeber at (715) 537-3186 Ext. 7-1668.

Edmund J. and Estelle D. Walker and General Medical Education Scholarships

Description: The Wisconsin Medical Society administers this award through the Edmund J. and Estelle D. Walker Trust. Students attending medical school in Wisconsin may apply. Several awards are available each year.
To Apply: To be considered, applicants must have completed or be in the process of completing at least one year in medical school. Only full-time U.S. students in Wisconsin may apply. Preference will be given to those who are attending school in Wisconsin, and have a desire to practice in the state. Criteria for judging include academic achievement, personal qualities and strengths, letters of recommendation, and financial need.
Deadline: The application deadline is in February. For more information, visit:

https://www.wisconsinmedicalsociety.org/_WMS/about_us/foundation/for_stu dents/scholarships/2014/Victor%20A%20%20Baylon%20MD%20Scholarship 2014-2015.pdf

Goodman - Goodell Scholarship

Description: The Wisconsin Medical Society administers this award. Students attending medical school in Wisconsin may apply if they are from the Portage area.
To Apply: To be considered, applicants must currently be in their second year of medical school. Only full-time U.S. students in Wisconsin may apply. Preference will be given to those who are attending school in Wisconsin, and have a desire to practice family or pulmonary medicine. Criteria for judging include academic achievement, personal qualities and strengths, letters of recommendation, and financial need.
Deadline: The application deadline is in February. For more information, visit:

https://www.wisconsinmedicalsociety.org/_WMS/about_us/foundation/for_stu dents/scholarships/2014/Victor%20A%20%20Baylon%20MD%20Scholarship 2014-2015.pdf

John D. and Virginia Riesch Scholarship

Description: The Wisconsin Medical Society administers this award. Students attending UW School of Medicine and Public Health may apply.
To Apply: Only full-time U.S. students in Wisconsin may apply. In the personal statement, applicants are asked to show how they have demonstrated empathy, passion for learning, and desire to share their knowledge and educate others. Preference is given to those applicants who plan to practice in the state. Criteria for judging include academic achievement, personal qualities and strengths, letters of recommendation, and financial need.
Deadline: The application deadline is in February. For more information, visit:

https://www.wisconsinmedicalsociety.org/_WMS/about_us/foundation/for_stu dents/scholarships/2014/Victor%20A%20%20Baylon%20MD%20Scholarship 2014-2015.pdf

Robert Jason Gore Scholarship

Description: The Wisconsin Medical Society administers this award. Students attending medical school in Wisconsin may apply.
To Apply: To be considered, applicants must be full-time U.S. students in Wisconsin. In the personal statement, applicants should provide examples of how they have lived their lives with chivalry, honor, and loyalty. The statement should also indicate how applicants will use these qualities in patient care. Criteria for judging include academic achievement, personal qualities and strengths, letters of recommendation, and financial need.
Deadline: The application deadline is in February. For more information, visit:

https://www.wisconsinmedicalsociety.org/_WMS/about_us/foundation/for_stu dents/scholarships/2014/Victor%20A%20%20Baylon%20MD%20Scholarship 2014-2015.pdf

Rukmini and Joyce Vasudevan Scholarship

Description: The Wisconsin Medical Society administers this award. Students attending medical school in Wisconsin may apply.
To Apply: Only full-time U.S. students in Wisconsin may apply. This award is open to female medical students entering their third or fourth year of medical school. In the personal statement, applicants are asked to write about their compassion, caring, and courage, or hard work despite adversity in life. Criteria for judging include academic achievement, personal qualities and strengths, letters of recommendation, and financial need.
Deadline: The application deadline is in February. For more information, visit:

https://www.wisconsinmedicalsociety.org/_WMS/about_us/foundation/for_stu dents/scholarships/2014/Victor%20A%20%20Baylon%20MD%20Scholarship 2014-2015.pdf

Victor A. Baylon, M.D. Memorial Scholarship

Description: Medical students who are residents of Racine or Milwaukee counties in Wisconsin may apply for this award. Award amounts are $1,000 or more.
To Apply: Only U.S. citizens enrolled full time in an accredited medical school who are residents of Racine or Milwaukee County may apply. Exceptions will be made for nonresidents who graduated high school from these counties. Preference will be given to Wisconsin residents with an interest in pathology. Criteria for judging include academic achievement, personal qualities and strengths, letters of recommendation, and financial need.
Deadline: The application deadline is in February. For more information, visit:

https://www.wisconsinmedicalsociety.org/_WMS/about_us/foundation/for_stu
dents/scholarships/2014/Victor%20A%20%20%20Baylon%20MD%20Scholarship
2014-2015.pdf

Wisconsin Medical Society Presidential Scholar

Description: The Wisconsin Medical Society offers this award to recognize future medical leaders. The award amount is $3,000.
To Apply: Medical students who will be entering their fourth year are eligible to apply. Candidates should have demonstrated the attributes, skills and desire to become a medical leader in Wisconsin. Applicants must have been involved with the Wisconsin Medical Society or a County Medical Society. The application includes a letter of recommendation from a Wisconsin Medical Society member who has worked with the applicant in some capacity. A personal statement is also required.
Deadline: The application deadline is in February. For more information, visit:

https://www.wisconsinmedicalsociety.org/_WMS/about_us/foundation/for_stu
dents/scholarships/2014/Victor%20A%20%20%20Baylon%20MD%20Scholarship
2014-2015.pdf

Chapter 88

Medical Awards and Scholarships in Wyoming

Although the state of Wyoming does not have a medical school, the WWAMI program administered by the University of Washington School of Medicine reserves twenty seats annually for Wyoming residents. Students who are accepted into the program complete their first year at the University of Wyoming before continuing studies at the medical school. For these students, the search for scholarships should being with the Financial Aid Office at both institutions. Students may be eligible for internal awards. External awards may also be available through organizations and foundations throughout Wyoming.

State medical associations often have information about scholarships and loans available for students from the state. Inquiries with your county medical society or association are recommended as well. We also encourage you to check with community foundations in the area in which you live to see if you are eligible for scholarships. Community Foundations in the State of Wyoming are listed below.

Community Foundations in Wyoming

Casper Area Community Foundation
Dubois Area Community Foundation
Evanston Area Community Foundation
Community Foundation of Jackson Hole
Community Foundation for Park County
Rock Springs Area Community Foundation
Sheridan-Johnson Community Foundation
Wyoming Community Foundation

Success in Medical School: Insider Advice for the Preclinical Years

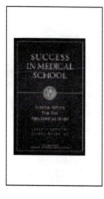

By Samir P. Desai, MD and Rajani Katta, MD

ISBN # 9781937978006

According to the AAMC, the United States will have a shortage of 90,000 physicians by 2020. In the mid-1990s, the AAMC urged medical schools to expand enrollment. Class sizes have increased, and new schools have opened their doors. Unfortunately, rising enrollment in medical schools has not led to a corresponding increase in the number of residency positions.

As a result, medical students are finding it increasingly difficult to match with the specialty and program of their choice. "Competition is tightening," said Mona Signer, Executive Director of the National Resident Matching Program. "The growth in applicants is more than the increase in positions."

Now more than ever, preclinical students need to be well informed so that they can maximize their chances of success. The decisions you make early in medical school can have a significant impact on your future specialty options.

To build a strong foundation for your future physician career, and to match into your chosen field, you must maximize your preclinical education. In *Success in Medical School*, you'll learn specific strategies for success during these important years of medical school.

"Overall, I recommend this book...The book has so much information about everything that there has to be a part of the book that will satisfy your interests."

- Medical School Success website

Medical School Interview: Winning Strategies from Admissions Faculty

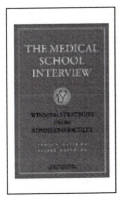

By Samir Desai, MD and Rajani Katta, MD

ISBN # 9781937978013

The medical school interview is the most important factor in the admissions process. Our detailed advice, based on evidence from research in the field and the perspectives of admissions faculty, will provide you with the insiders' perspective.

How can you best prepare for the MMI, group interview, panel interview, and behavioral interview? What qualities would make applicants less likely to be admitted? What personal qualities are most valued by admissions faculty? What can students do to achieve maximum success during the interview?

This book shows medical school applicants how to develop the optimal strategy for interview success.

"…this is an extremely thorough handbook, covering the questions applicants are likely to be asked and the appropriate and inappropriate answers…likely to be found indispensable by readers embarking on the arduous process of applying to medical school."

- Kirkus Reviews

Clinician's Guide to Laboratory Medicine: Pocket

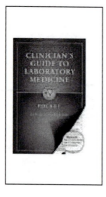

By Samir P. Desai, MD

ISBN # 9780972556187

In this book, you will find practical approaches to lab test interpretation. It includes differential diagnoses, step-by-step approaches, and algorithms, all designed to answer your lab test questions in a flash. See why so many consider it a "must-have" book.

"In our Medicine Clerkship, the Clinician's Guide to Laboratory Medicine has quickly become one of the two most popular paperback books. Our students have praised the algorithms, tables, and ease of pursuit of clinical problems through better understanding of the utilization of tests appropriate to the problem at hand."

- Greg Magarian, MD, Director, 3rd Year Internal Medicine Clerkship, Oregon Health & Science University

"It provides an excellent practical approach to abnormal labs."

- Northwestern University Feinberg School of Medicine Internal Medicine Clerkship website.

Success on the Wards: 250 Rules for Clerkship Success

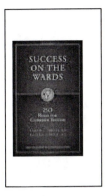

By Samir P. Desai, MD and Rajani Katta, MD

ISBN # 9780972556194

This is an absolute must-read for students entering clinical rotations.

The authors of *The Successful Match: 200 Rules to Succeed in the Residency Match* bring their same combination of practical recommendations and evidence-based advice to clerkships.

The book begins as a how-to guide with clerkship-specific templates, along with sample notes and guides, for every aspect of clerkships. The book reviews proven strategies for success in patient care, write-ups, rounds, and other vital areas.

Grades in required rotations are the most important academic criteria used to select residents, and this critical year can determine career choices. This book shows students what they can do now to position themselves for match success. An invaluable resource for medical students - no student should be without it.

"*Success on the Wards* is an essential tool for the rising medical student...This book offers insider information on how a medical student can excel on the wards…I strongly recommend this book. It should be a must-read for any motivated student doctor."

- AMSA *The New Physician* (Review from September 2012)

"*Success on the Wards* is easily the best book I have read on how to succeed in clerkship. It is comprehensive, thorough and jam-packed with valuable information. Dr. Desai and Dr. Katta provide an all encompassing look into what clerkship is really like."

- Review by Medaholic.com

The Successful Match: 200 Rules to Succeed in the Residency Match

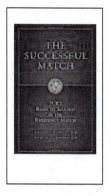

By Rajani Katta, MD and Samir P. Desai, MD

ISBN # 9780972556170

What does it take to match into the specialty and program of your choice?

The key to a successful match hinges on the development of the right strategy. This book will show you how to develop the optimal strategy for success.

Who actually chooses the residents? We review the data on the decision-makers. What do these decision-makers care about? We review the data on the criteria that matter most to them. How can you convince them that you would be the right resident for their program? We provide concrete, practical recommendations based on their criteria.

At every step of the process, our recommendations are meant to maximize the impact of your application. This book is an invaluable resource to help you gain that extra edge.

"Drs. Rajani Katta and Samir P. Desai provide the medical student reader with detailed preparation for the matching process. The rules and accompanying tips make the book user-friendly. The format is especially appealing to those pressed for time or looking for a single key element for a particular process."

- Review in the American Medical Student Association journal, *The New Physician*

The Resident's Guide to the Fellowship Match

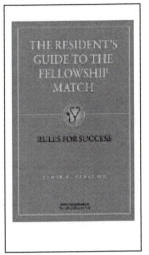

By Samir P. Desai, MD

ISBN # 9781937978020

What does it take to match into the subspecialty and fellowship program of your choice?

Our detailed advice, based on evidence from research in the field and the perspectives of fellowship program directors, will provide you with the insiders' perspective.

What are criteria most important to decision-makers? What can you do to have the best possible letters of recommendation written on your behalf? How can you develop a powerful and compelling personal statement? How can you overcome the obstacles of residency to publish research? What can you do to achieve maximum success during the interview?

This book shows fellowship applicants how to develop the optimal strategy for success - an invaluable resource to help applicants gain that extra edge.

The Successful Match website

Our website, TheSuccessfulMatch.com, provides medical school, residency and fellowship applicants with a better understanding of the admissions and selection process. You'll find:

- Match statistics for every specialty
- Conversations with program directors about the residency and fellowship selection process.
- Important information about the future of each specialty, including current challenges
- Resources to help you succeed in the preclinical years and clerkships

Consulting services

We also offer expert one-on-one consulting services to medical school, residency, and fellowship applicants. Whether you seek an overall strategy for match success, accurate assessment of your candidacy for a particular specialty or program, review of your curriculum vitae or personal statement, or thorough preparation for interviews, you can rest assured we have the knowledge, expertise, and insight to help you achieve your goals. If you are interested in our consultation services, please visit us at www.TheSuccessfulMatch.com. The website provides further details, including pricing and specific services.

MD2B Titles

The Medical School Interview: Winning Strategies from Admissions Faculty

Medical School Scholarships, Grants, & Awards: Insider Advice on How to Win Scholarships

Success in Medical School: Insider Advice for the Preclinical Years

Success on the Wards: 250 Rules for Clerkship Success

The Successful Match: 200 Rules to Succeed in the Residency Match

Resident's Guide to the Fellowship Match: Rules for Success

Clinician's Guide to Laboratory Medicine: Pocket

Available at www.MD2B.net

Bulk Sales

MD2B is able to provide discounts on any of our titles when purchased in bulk. The discount rate depends on the quantity ordered. For more information, please contact us at info@md2b.net or (713) 927-6830.